Bone remodeling and its disorders

Second edition

Bone remodeling and its disorders

Second edition

Gregory R Mundy MD

Heyser Professor of Bone and Mineral Metabolism and
Head, Division of Endocrinology and Metabolism

Program Director
Frederic C Bartter General Clinical Research Unit
The University of Texas Health Sciences Center
San Antonio
Texas, USA

Scientific Director
OsteoScreen Inc.
San Antonio
Texas, USA

The views expressed in this publication are those of the author and not necessarily those of Martin Dunitz Ltd.

© Martin Dunitz Ltd 1999

This edition first published in the United Kingdom in 1999 by

Martin Dunitz Ltd
The Livery House
7–9 Pratt Street
London
NW1 0AE

All rights reserved. No part of this publication may be reproduced, stored in a retrieval system, or transmitted, in any form or by any means, electronic, mechanical, photocopying, recording or otherwise, without the prior permission of the publisher or in accordance with the provisions of the Copyright Act 1988, or under the terms of any licence permitting limited copying issued by the Copyright Licensing Agency, 33–34 Alfred Place, London WC1E 7DP.

A CIP catalogue record for this book is available from the British Library.

ISBN 1-85317-429-7

Composition by Wearset, Boldon, Tyne and Wear
Printed and bound in Great Britain by
Biddles Ltd, Guildford and King's Lynn

CONTENTS

Preface to the Second Edition	vii	
1 Bone remodeling	1	
2 Cellular mechanisms of bone resorption	12	
3 Osteoblasts, bone formation and mineralization	30	
4 Factors regulating bone resorbing and bone forming cells	45	
5 Pharmacologic treatment for diseases of bone remodeling	83	
6 Hypercalcemia	107	
7 Metastatic bone disease	123	
8 Myeloma bone disease	147	
9 Primary hyperparathyroidism	162	
10 Paget's disease of bone	180	
11 Osteopetrosis	193	
12 Osteomalacia and rickets	200	
13 Osteoporosis	208	
14 Potential future treatments for osteoporosis	240	
Index	254	

PREFACE TO THE SECOND EDITION

Since the time of preparation for this book three years ago, there have been considerable advances in the field of bone and mineral metabolism, and I have attempted to incorporate them into this edition. These have included the identification and characterization of important genes involved in calcium homeostasis such as the calcium sensor and the PTH/PTH-rP receptors, as well as mutations in these genes that lead to disease states, the role of a number of important peptides and receptors in endochondral bone formation (for example, the FGF family of receptors and ligands and PTH-rP), improved understanding of the role of PTH-rP in bone metastasis, the registration and widespread use of powerful bisphosphonates in osteoporosis, osteolytic bone disease and Paget's disease, myeloma bone disease and metastatic bone disease, continued improvements in bone mineral density measurements and techniques for measuring rates of bone resorption and formation, reports of studies on drugs that mimic estrogen's efforts on bone but avoid some of the problems, the introduction of sestamibi imaging of the parathyroid glands and improved understanding of the molecular events and regulatory mechanisms involved in osteoblast and osteoclast differentiation. I have revised this edition to include all the new information of which I was aware at the time of writing. Inevitably, since there is a gap between this time and publication, and because this field is moving so fast, there will be omissions.

Nevertheless, this is an attempt to present one person's perspective of this field, which is growing rapidly in importance and interest. I am particularly grateful to all my longstanding colleagues in San Antonio, and particularly to those who advised me with the final chapters of this edition, namely Drs Theresa Guise, Brendan Boyce, Jan Bruder, David Roodman, Stephen Harris and Lynda Bonewald.

The front cover photomicrograph of metastatic human breast cancer cells was supplied by Dr Theresa Guise.

GR Mundy
January 1998

CHAPTER 1

Bone remodeling

Introduction

Abnormalities in bone remodeling occur in many of the more common diseases that affect humans. Age-related bone loss and its consequences are major public health problems in Western societies and affect more than 25% of the aging female population and 5–10% of the male population. Other common diseases associated with increased bone resorption include malignant disease, primary hyperparathyroidism and Paget's disease, which are also very common in the elderly population. Paget's disease affects 3% of people over the age of 40 in many Western societies, and primary hyperparathyroidism is now being recognized as an extremely common condition (prevalence estimated to be 1/1000 adults in the United States) since the advent of routine screening of serum samples for calcium concentrations.

Although these disorders are common and cause considerable suffering, in most cases little is known of mechanisms responsible for the dysfunctional bone remodeling that characterizes them. This is not unexpected, since at present we do not understand the mechanisms responsible for the control of normal bone remodeling, or how it is so highly coordinated and balanced. Under these circumstances, it is hardly surprising that we still do not understand the mechanisms responsible for the imbalance in bone remodeling which characterizes age-related bone loss, nor what is responsible for the aberrant rates of remodeling which occur in Paget's disease. However, new techniques for studying bone function at the cellular level (bone cell and organ culture), the availability of recombinant molecules and complementary DNA probes, the generation of gene deletions in animals, as well as new techniques for studying bone function at the clinical level (better measurement of bone mass and bone mineral density, and better markers for bone resorption and bone formation), should clarify the control mechanisms for the cellular events in normal bone remodeling. These new techniques and approaches seem certain to lead ultimately to new information and treatment measures to inhibit or prevent disorders of bone remodeling.

In this chapter, the natural history of the changes in bone which occur during life will be reviewed first from a whole body perspective, and then at the level of the morphologic changes that occur in different components of bone.

Natural history of the skeleton

Figure 1.1 is a diagrammatic representation illustrating how total body bone mass changes with age. Bone mass reaches a maximum about 10 years after linear growth stops, probably begins to decrease somewhere in the fourth decade, and declines to half its maximum value by the age of

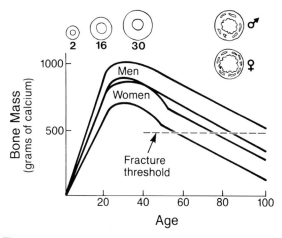

Figure 1.1

Changes in bone mass with age. Bone mass reaches a peak in young adult life, but then steadily declines in both men and women. In women there is a rapid phase of bone loss, which is associated with estrogen withdrawal and lasts for about 10 years after the menopause. The two critical determinants of bone mass are peak bone mass and rates of bone loss after mid-life. Since women have lower peak bone mass than men and lose bone rapidly because of estrogen withdrawal, bone mass in later life is less than it is in men.

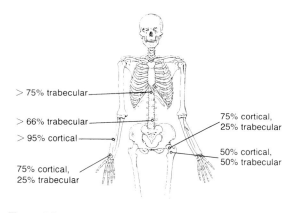

Figure 1.2

Proportions of cortical and cancellous (also called trabecular) bone in various parts of the skeleton. Note that the axial skeleton contains relatively more cancellous bone.

80. Peak bone mineral density (bone mass), which is reached in the 30s, is lower in women than it is in men, and lower in Caucasians than in African–Americans. Women of all ethnic groups show an additional accelerated phase of bone loss that occurs for about 10 years after the menopause. It has been estimated that a woman can expect to lose 35% of her cortical bone and 50% of her cancellous bone as she ages, and a man can expect to lose about two-thirds of these amounts (Smith et al 1975; Riggs et al 1981; Mazess 1982). About one-half of the loss in cancellous bone can be ascribed to the menopause, and about one-half to the aging process. It remains controversial as to when bone mineral density starts to decline, and whether there is a similar accelerated phase of bone loss in both cancellous and cortical bone after the menopause. Different techniques for measuring parameters of bone mass have given slightly different answers.

The bones of the adult skeleton consist of either cortical (or compact) bone and cancellous (or trabecular) bone. Current evidence indicates that cortical bone and cancellous bone do not change with age in exactly the same way, and so they probably should be considered as two separate functional entities. The proportions of cortical and cancellous bone differ at the different sites in the skeleton where osteoporotic fractures frequently occur (Figure 1.2). Cancellous bone is relatively prominent in the vertebral column, the most common site of fracture associated with osteoporosis, and the abnormality in the remodeling process that predisposes to this type of fracture is important to understand. In the lumbar spine, cancellous bone comprises more than 66% of the total bone. In the intertrochanteric area of the femur, bone is comprised of 50% cortical and 50% cancellous. In the neck of the femur, the bone is 75% cortical and 25% cancellous. In contrast, in the midradius more than 95% of the bone is cortical bone. The differences are most likely to reside in the different environments of the bone cells in cortical or cancellous bone. Bone remodeling cells on cancellous bone surfaces are in intimate contact with the cells of the marrow cavity, which produce a variety of potent osteotropic cytokines. It is likely that the cells in cortical bone, which are more distant from the influences of these cytokines, are influenced more by the systemic osteotropic hormones such as parathyroid hormone and 1,25-dihydroxyvitamin D_3. Osteoclasts and osteoblasts in cancellous bone may be controlled primarily by factors produced by adjacent bone marrow cells. Similar cells in Haversian systems of cortical bone are further removed from the myriad of osteotropic cytokines that are produced by marrow mononuclear cells.

Remodeling of cortical and cancellous bone

Cortical bone

Cortical bone is dense or compact bone. It comprises 85% of the total bone in the body, and is relatively most abundant in the long bone shafts of the appendicular skeleton. The volume of cortical bone is regulated by the formation of periosteal bone, by remodeling within Haversian systems and by endosteal bone resorption. Cortical bone is removed primarily by endosteal resorption and resorption within the Haversian canals. The latter leads to increased porosity of cortical bone. However, periosteal bone formation continues to increase the diameter of cortical bone throughout life. Cortical bone loss probably begins after the age of 40 (according to most studies) and there is an acceleration of cortical bone loss that occurs for 5–10 years after the menopause. This accelerated phase of cortical bone loss continues for 15 years and then gradually slows. There is irrefutable evidence that estrogen replacement therapy after the menopause may preserve cortical bone. In later life, women with osteoporosis lose cortical bone at similar rates to those of premenopausal women. Loss of cortical bone is the major predisposing factor for fractures that occur in the hip and around the wrist. Cortical bone is particularly prone to increased resorption in patients with primary hyperparathyroidism.

Cancellous bone

Although cancellous bone comprises only 15% of the skeleton, the changes that occur in this type of bone after the age of 30 determine whether the clinical features of osteoporosis will occur. Depending on the technique used, decline in cancellous bone mass begins in early adult life, occurring earlier than the decline in cortical bone mass (Riggs et al 1986). Other studies have disagreed with these findings, and suggested that the decline in cancellous bone mass begins later, after ovarian function ceases (Genant et al 1982). Riggs and Melton (1986) suggest that acceleration in cancellous bone loss occurring at the time of the menopause is not as prominent as the accelerated loss of cortical bone mass that occurs at this time.

Cancellous bone is the type of bone lost predominantly in patients with osteolytic bone disease due to malignancy. In this situation, the malignant cells lodge in the marrow cavity and produce local factors that stimulate adjacent osteoclasts on trabecular plates and on endosteal surfaces of cortical bone (Mundy et al 1974a,b). The loss of cancellous bone that occurs with aging is not due simply to a generalized thinning of the bone plates, but is rather due to complete perforation and fragmentation of trabeculae (Parfitt et al 1983; Kleerekoper et al 1985) (see also Chapter 13 on Osteoporosis). Since cancellous bone has a broad surface area, resorption may be modulated by focal osteoclastic resorption regulated by local hormonal factors produced by cells in the bone marrow microenvironment, including marrow cells as well as other types of bone cells.

The cellular events involved in the remodeling of bone

The process of bone remodeling is the key phenomenon in bone cell biology and understanding the mechanisms which control the remodeling process and its regulation will clarify not only local control of osteoclast and osteoblast function, but also the pathophysiology of age-related bone loss and osteoporosis (Figure 1.3). The adult skeleton is in a dynamic state, being continually broken down and reformed by the coordinated actions of osteoclasts and osteoblasts on trabecular surfaces and in Haversian systems. This turnover or remodeling of bone occurs in focal

Resorption Reversal Formation Resting

Figure 1.3

Bone remodeling. Sequence of events involved in normal bone remodeling. Bone remodeling is initiated by local events which lead to an increase in osteoclast activity. This is followed eventually by increased attraction and proliferation of osteoblast precursors, followed by the differentiation of these cells into mature osteoblasts, which lay down new bone and repair the resorption defects caused by the resorbing osteoclasts.

and discrete packets throughout the skeleton. The remodeling of each packet takes a finite period of time (estimated to be about 3–4 months). The remodeling which occurs in each packet (called a bone remodeling unit by Frost, who first described this sequence almost 30 years ago) (Frost 1964) is geographically and chronologically separated from other packets of remodeling. This suggests that activation of the sequence of cellular events responsible for remodeling is locally controlled, possibly by an autoregulatory mechanism, perhaps by autocrine or paracrine factors generated in the bone microenvironment. The sequence is always the same—osteoclastic bone resorption followed by osteoblastic bone formation to repair the defect. The new bone which is formed is called a bone structural unit (BSU) (Frost 1964).

Osteoclast activation is the initial step in the remodeling sequence. (A more detailed description of osteoclastic bone resorption is provided in Chapter 2). Osteoclasts are activated in specific focal sites by mechanisms which are still not understood. The activation of the osteoclast may occur because of interactions which take place between integral membrane proteins (integrins) on osteoclast cell membranes with proteins in bone matrix which contain RGD (arginine–glycine–asparagine) amino acid sequences (such as osteopontin). Miyauchi et al (1991) have demonstrated such a phenomenon in vitro. Osteoclast activation may also be due to stimulatory signals produced by local cells in the osteoclast microenvironment such as immune cells, but the potential trigger for activation of immune cells is unknown. The resorptive phase of the remodeling process has been estimated to last 10 days (Figures 1.4 and 1.5). This period is followed by repair of the defect by a team of osteoblasts which are attracted to the site of the resorption defect and then presumably proceed to make new bone. This part of the process takes approximately 3 months. The initial events in the formation phase are possibly unidirectional migration (chemotaxis) of osteoblast precursors to the site of the defect followed by enhanced cell proliferation. The complete sequence of cellular events which occur at the bone surface during the remodeling process has been described in detail by Baron et al (1984) from studies on the alveolar bone of the rat, and by Boyce et al (1989a,b) from the calvarial bone of the mouse. The cellular events which occur in these models are similar to those in adult human bone.

In the model described by Boyce et al (1989a), interleukin-1 was injected into the subcutaneous tissue overlying the calvarial bone of the normal mouse in small doses for 3 days. Quantitative histomorphometry was then performed on the calvarial bone at frequent intervals for the following 28 days. There is a phase of intense osteoclastic bone resorption that follows for several weeks, and lasts up to 21 days. Peak osteoclast number is observed at about 7 days, and following this the calvarial bone is almost entirely eroded through and through. Following this phase of bone resorption, the osteoclasts disappear and new bone formation begins. Re-evaluation of the sections from this experiment by Hughes and Boyce (Boyce et al 1989a) has shown that osteoclasts undergo apoptosis at the conclusion of the phase of bone resorption (Figure 1.6). The bone first formed is woven in nature and accumulates at the sites of resorption and is later replaced with lamellar bone. At 28 days, the bone that was previously removed by the action of the osteoclasts is completely replaced. (For diagram of these effects, see Figure 4.13.)

Interleukin-1 is clearly responsible for stimulating the initial phase of osteoclastic bone resorption. In part, this is prostaglandin-mediated

Figure 1.4

Diagram of early events involved in bone remodeling. (1) Resting osteoclast on a bone surface. (2) The mechanism by which osteoclasts are activated on remodeling surfaces still remains unclear, but may involve recognition by the osteoclasts of microdamage at mineralized bone surfaces. Osteoclast activity is modulated by cytokines. (3) As a consequence of activation, the osteoclasts become polarized and produce protons and lysosomal enzymes. (4) Bone resorption leads to the release of local growth regulatory factors for osteoblasts which are capable of stimulating all the subsequent events involved in bone formation.

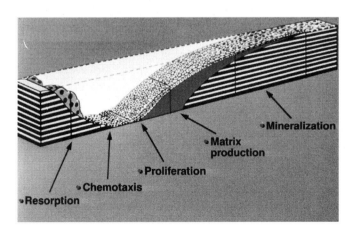

Figure 1.5

Diagram of the events involved in bone remodeling on a normal cancellous bone surface. Note that these cellular events are depicted chronologically. Bone resorption lasts for less than 2 weeks, but bone formation is prolonged over a period of several months. Note the cellular events involved in the bone formation process. (Redrawn from Eriksen (1986).)

Figure 1.6

Cells involved in the remodeling sequence demonstrated after local injection of interleukin-1 over the murine calvaria. Osteoclasts at the reversal site are undergoing apoptosis (Boyce et al 1989a).

(Boyce et al 1989a,b). However, the mechanisms which are responsible for stimulating osteoblasts to lay down new bone at the sites of the resorption defect are unclear. It appears that discontinuation of interleukin-1 is required as in the continued presence of interleukin-1, the phase of bone formation is impaired. A reasonable postulate is that local growth regulatory factors for osteoblasts are released as a result of the resorption process stimulated by interleukin-1, and they are subsequently responsible for the cellular events involved in the formation of new bone (see below).

All the diseases of bone are superimposed on this normal cellular remodeling sequence. In diseases such as primary hyperparathyroidism, hyperthyroidism and Paget's disease, in which osteoclasts are activated, there is a compensatory and (relatively) balanced increase in the formation of new bone. However, there are also a number of well-described conditions in which osteoblast activity does not completely repair the defect left by previous resorption by replacing all the bone removed. One example is myeloma, usually characterized by punched-out lytic bone lesions with little new bone formation (Snapper and Kahn 1971). In myeloma, there appears to be a specific defect in osteoblast maturation (Valentin-Opran et al 1982). There are probably increased numbers of osteoblasts around the edges of the lytic lesions, but the osteoblasts fail (in the great majority of patients) to synthesize more than thin osteoid seams. In solid tumors associated with malignancy, there is also a failure of bone formation to repair resorptive defects especially in patients dying from their malignancy (Stewart et al 1982). In elderly patients with osteoporosis, there is a decrease in mean wall thickness, presumably reflecting the inability of osteoblasts to repair adequately the resorptive defects made during normal osteoclastic resorption (Darby and Meunier 1981). It should also be stressed that progressive bone loss, beginning at about 35 years of age (depending on the bone), occurs in all humans and is indicative of a "physiological" imbalance between resorption and formation.

Although bone formation usually occurs on sites of previous osteoclastic resorption in normal adult humans, there are several special situations in which osteoblasts may lay down new bone on surfaces not previously resorbed. Two examples are osteoblastic metastases associated with tumors such as carcinoma of the prostate and breast, and during prolonged exposure to pharmacological doses of fluoride therapy. However, in most physiological and pathological circumstances, the coupling of bone formation to previous bone resorption occurs faithfully. The cellular and humoral mechanisms which are responsible for mediating the coupling process (or disrupting it, as in the diseases described above) are still not clear. Several theories have been proposed to account for coupling. Over 20 years ago, Rasmussen and Bordier (1974) suggested that the osteoclast, once it finishes the resorptive phase of the remodeling sequence, undergoes fission to form mononuclear cells which are the precursors of osteoblasts. However, it is now widely accepted that osteoclasts and osteoblasts have different origins. Osteoclasts arise from hematopoietic stem cells or at least stem cells in the marrow environment which have the capacity to circulate. Osteoblasts, in contrast, arise from stromal mesenchymal cells. Many workers have favored the notion that coupling is humorally mediated, that an osteoblast-stimulating factor (such as IGF-I, IGF-II or TGFβ) is released from bone matrix during the process of osteoclastic bone resorption and the stimulation of osteoblast activity leads to new bone formation (Howard et al 1981). A variation on this humoral concept is that the factor which stimulates resorption also acts directly (but slowly) on osteoblasts to cause their activation and subsequent new bone formation. There is an alternative to the humoral hypothesis to explain coupling. It is possible that since osteoblasts normally line bone surfaces, once the phase of osteoclastic resorption is over and osteoclasts disappear from the resorption site, osteoblasts and their precursors repopulate the resorption site and merely re-line the bone surface. They may thus repair the resorptive defect without the necessity for involvement of a humoral mediator that is specifically generated as a consequence of resorption. Manolagas and Jilka (1995) have proposed that coupling does not involve sequential signals released during the process of bone remodeling, but rather that factors that work through the GP-130 signal transduction mechanism are responsible for simultaneous stimulation of osteoclast and osteoblast lineages.

Obviously, understanding this sequence of cellular events may lead to clarification of the mechanism of decreased osteoblast activity that occurs in age-related bone loss, and possibly the pathophysiology of osteoporosis, as well as the specific defects in osteoblast function that occur in malignancies such as myeloma, breast cancer and prostate cancer. Based on observations that have been made possible in recent years of the effects of stimulatory factors such as transforming growth factor β(TGFβ) on bone in vivo (Marcelli et al 1990), a hypothesis for how coupling may be mediated will be proposed here, based on interpretation of the data available. Before this model is described, the events which are likely to be important in the formation phase of the remodeling sequence will be reviewed, together with the local osteotropic factors that may be responsible for mediating these events.

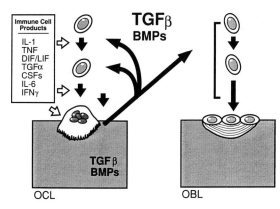

Figure 1.7

Potential role of TGFβ and related factors in the remodeling process. These growth factors are produced in active form as a consequence of bone resorption. They are then available locally to control subsequent events involved in bone formation.

Cellular events involved in the formation phase of the remodeling sequence

The specific cellular events following the phase of osteoclastic resorption are osteoclast apoptosis, followed by osteoblast chemotaxis, proliferation and differentiation, which in turn is followed by formation of mineralized bone and cessation of osteoblast activity. The initial event is likely to be osteoclast apoptosis, which can be enhanced by active TGFβ (Hughes et al 1996). This is followed by chemotactic attraction of osteoblasts or their precursors to the sites of the resorption defect. This attraction is also likely to be mediated by local factors produced during the resorption process. Resorbing bone has been shown to produce chemotactic factors for cells with osteoblast characteristics in vitro (Mundy et al 1982; Mundy and Poser 1983). One mediator which may be responsible for this effect is TGFβ (Figure 1.7), since active TGFβ is released by resorbing bone cultures (Pfeilschifter and Mundy 1987). Structural proteins such as collagen or the bone Gla protein could also be involved, since Type I collagen and bone Gla protein and their fragments cause the same effect (Mundy et al 1982; Mundy and Poser 1983). TGFβ, which is enriched in the bone matrix and released as a consequence of bone resorption, is also chemotactic for bone cells (Pfeilschifter et al 1990b). However, TGFβ is not the only potential chemo-attractant in bone. Platelet-derived growth factor (PDGF) is chemotactic for some mesenchymal cells, monocytes, neutrophils and smooth muscle cells (Grotendorst et al 1981; Deuel et al 1982; Seppa et al 1982; Senior et al 1983). Perhaps a combination of chemotactic factors is responsible for attraction of osteoblast precursors to resorption sites.

The next event involved in the formation phase of the coupling phenomenon is proliferation of osteoblast precursors. This is likely to be mediated by local osteoblast growth factors released during the resorption process. There are several leading candidates for these factors, which represent autocrine and paracrine factors. These include members of the TGFβ superfamily (TGFβs I and II). In addition, PDGF causes proliferation of cells with osteoblast characteristics. The insulin-like growth factors (IGFs) I and II and the heparin-binding fibroblast growth factors (FGFs) also cause osteoblast proliferation. All these factors are stored in the bone matrix.

The next sequential event during the formation phase is the differentiation of the osteoblast precursor into the mature cell. Several of the bone-derived growth factors can cause the appearance of markers of the differentiated osteoblast phenotype, including expression of alkaline phosphatase activity, Type I collagen and osteocalcin synthesis. Most prominent of these are IGF-I and bone morphogenetic protein 2 (BMP-2). Active TGFβ inhibits osteoblast differentiation in vitro, which suggests its role may be to "trigger" the process, after which it is removed or becomes inactivated, allowing the increased pool of precursors to undergo differentiation.

The final phase of the formation process must be cessation of osteoblast activity. The resorption lacunae are usually repaired either completely or almost completely. It is not known how this is achieved. One possibility is that factors produced during this process decrease osteoblast activity. Under the appropriate circumstances, one such factor could be TGFβ. Active TGFβ decreases differentiated function in osteoblasts, and as noted above is expressed by osteoblasts as they differentiate (Dallas et al 1994).

Osteoblastotropic factors which may be involved in the coupling process

Osteotropic factors which could be involved in the coupling phenomenon are TGFβ, BMPs, IGFs I and II, PDGF and FGFs. This area has also been recently reviewed by Canalis et al (1989b). These factors are likely to be released locally from bone as it resorbs, or by bone cells activated as a consequence of the resorption process. They may then act in a sequential manner to regulate all the cellular events required for the formation of bone.

The TGFβ superfamily may be particularly important in the coupling that links bone formation to prior bone resorption (Figure 1.8). Prolonged primary cultures of fetal rat calvarial osteoblasts show that the BMPs are expressed as these cells differentiate to form new bone in parallel with other differentiation markers such as osteocalcin and alkaline phosphatase. Transient exposure of these cells to TGFβ stimulates proliferation of the osteoblasts (continued exposure inhibits the formation of mineralized bone expression of differentiation markers). Addition of BMPs to culture leads to increased numbers of mineralized nodules. We suggest that the following events (Figures 1.5 and 1.7) occur during normal bone remodeling based on our in vitro observations (see also Chapters 4 and 14). Bone resorption

Figure 1.8

Potential role of the effects of TGFβ and related growth factors in the remodeling process. TGFβ is the most abundant factor in the bone matrix and is produced in large amounts in an active form when bone is resorbed. It may then trigger osteoblast chemotaxis and proliferation, leading to an autocrine/paracrine production of other growth regulatory factors for osteoblasts, including BMPs, FGFs and IGF-I and IGF-II. These factors may work as a cascade to complete the process of osteoblast differentiation and bone formation. (Redrawn from Eriksen (1986).)

leads to the release of active TGFβ, as has been shown previously (Pfeilschifter and Mundy 1987). TGFβ results in cessation of further osteoclastic bone resorption by causing osteoclasts to undergo apoptosis (Hughes et al 1996). Osteoblast precursors are recruited to the site of resorption. Exposure of osteoblast precursors to active TGFβ causes increased proliferation. However, this exposure to active TGFβ is transient, and as a consequence, the proliferating cells undergo differentiation and express bone morphogenetic proteins. This is also associated with expression of osteoblast differentiation markers such as alkaline phosphatase, Type I collagen and osteocalcin. The osteoid matrix becomes mineralized resulting in new bone. Thus, the bone resorption process results in a cascade of growth factors which are responsible for the subsequent events. Initially, one of the most abundant growth factors in the bone matrix, namely TGFβ, is released in an active form as a consequence of resorption. TGFβ then attracts osteoblast precursors to the site of the resorption defect and stimulates proliferation of osteoblast precursors (Gehron-Robey et al 1987; Pfeilschifter et al 1990b). The proliferating osteoblasts then begin to differentiate to form more mature osteoblasts and express differentiation markers such as alkaline phosphatase and osteocalcin, and also bone morphogenetic proteins. These bone morphogenetic proteins then are responsible for an autostimulatory effect on the osteoblasts and the formation of mineralized bone. Of course, it is unlikely that the TGFβ superfamily members are acting alone. Other growth factors such as the IGFs, the FGFs and the PDGFs are also likely to be having effects on osteoblast proliferation and differentiation. These factors are all bone growth stimulants. Recently, it has been shown that FGFs have comparable osteoblast stimulating effects on bone to those of TGFβ (Dunstan et al 1993).

The most convincing evidence that IGF-I may play a role as a coupling factor has been provided by the work of Canalis et al (1989a,b) on cultures of embryonic rat calvariae. This group showed that PTH stimulated expression of IGF-I by calvarial cultures. Thus, this mechanism has been suggested for the anabolic effect of PTH. In other words, PTH may stimulate bone cells to produce IGF-I upon transient exposure, and this production of IGF-I is responsible for subsequent bone formation. However, this is unlikely to be the only mechanism involved, and it remains unclear whether this is the mechanism responsible for the anabolic effect of IGF-I in vivo.

Hence, like hematopoiesis and differentiation of multipotent hematopoietic stem cells, bone formation may represent a complex multi-hierarchical organization of the cells in the osteoblast lineage. It is possible that the actions of these factors could be coordinated in a similar way to that suggested for the hematopoietic growth factors. These factors may work as a cascade, as suggested above for TGFβ and the BMPs, or they may act in concert together. Walker et al (1985) have suggested that the distinct colony stimulating factors (CSFs) for macrophages and granulocytes act on hematopoietic progenitor cells by causing direct effects on target cells, but also indirect effects by altering expression of receptors for other factors and therefore altering cell responsiveness to other factors. They have proposed that the capacity of each CSF to down-modulate other CSF receptors parallels the biological effects of the CSF. Such a hierarchical modulation of receptors and potential for alteration by one growth factor of the target cell's responses to other growth factors is also applicable to the osteoblast cell lineage. There is much evidence to suggest that there are synergistic as well as inhibitory interactions between the growth factors which act on osteoblasts. For example, TGFβ, PDGF, IGF-I and II, FGF-I and -II, and BMPs may all influence osteoblasts directly, but also may modulate osteoblast responsivity to each others' growth factor (Bowen-Pope et al 1983; Assoian et al 1984; Tucker et al 1984; Massague 1985; Massague et al 1985; Roberts et al 1985; Seyedin et al 1985). The potential interactions between these factors are extraordinarily complex, possibly even as complex as the interactions between the CSFs on hematopoiesis, but it will be essential to unravel them to understand the local control of bone formation. It is likely that the complicated interactions between these factors released locally in active form as a consequence of the resorption process are responsible for the carefully coordinated formation of new bone that occurs at these sites.

References

Assoian RK, Grotendorst GR, Miller DM et al (1984) Cellular transformation by coordinated action of three peptide growth factors from human platelets, *Nature* **309**: 804–6.

Baron R, Vignery A, Horowitz M (1984) Lymphocytes, macrophages and the regulation of bone remodeling. In: Peck WA, ed, *Bone and Mineral Research, Annual 2* (Elsevier: Amsterdam) 175–242.

Bowen-Pope DF, Dicorletto PE, Ross R (1983) Interactions between the receptors for platelet-derived growth factor and epidermal growth factor, *J Cell Biol* **96**: 679–83.

Boyce BF, Aufdemorte TB, Garrett IR et al (1989a) Effects of interleukin-1 on bone turnover in normal mice, *Endocrinology* **125**: 1142–50.

Boyce BF, Yates AJP, Mundy GR (1989b) Bolus injections of recombinant human interleukin-1 cause transient hypocalcemia in normal mice, *Endocrinology* **125**: 2780–3.

Canalis E, Centrella M, Burch W et al (1989a) Insulin-like growth factor I mediates selective anabolic effects of parathyroid hormone in bone cultures, *J Clin Invest* **83**: 60–5.

Canalis E, McCarthy T, Centrella M (1989b) Growth factors and the regulation of bone remodeling, *J Clin Invest* **81**: 277–81.

Dallas SL, Park-Snyder S, Miyazono K et al (1994) Characterization and autoregulation of latent TGFβ complexes in osteoblast-like cell lines: production of a latent complex lacking the latent TGFβ-binding protein (LTBP), *J Biol Chem* **269**: 6815–21.

Darby AJ, Meunier PJ (1981) Mean wall thickness and formation periods of trabecular bone packets in idiopathic osteoporosis, *Calcif Tissue Int* **33**: 199–204.

Deuel TF, Senior RM, Huang JS et al (1982) Chemotaxis of monocytes and neutrophils to platelet-derived growth factor, *J Clin Invest* **69**: 1046–9.

Dunstan C, Boyce B, Izbicka E et al (1993) Acidic and basic fibroblast growth factors promote bone growth in vivo comparable to that of TGFβ, *J Bone Miner Res* **8**: (Suppl 1): no 250.

Eriksen EF (1986) Normal and pathological remodeling of human trabecular bone: three dimensional reconstruction of the remodeling sequence in normals and in metabolic bone disease, *Endocrine Rev* **7**: 379–408.

Frost HM (1964) Dynamics of bone remodeling. In: *Bone biodynamics* (Little, Brown: Boston) 315.

Gehron-Robey PG, Young MF, Flanders KC et al (1987) Osteoblasts synthesize and respond to transforming growth factor type beta (TGFβ) in vitro, *J Cell Biol* **105**: 457–63.

Genant HK, Cann CE, Ettinger B et al (1982) Quantitative computed tomography of vertebral spongiosa: a sensitive method for detecting early bone loss after oophorectomy, *Ann Intern Med* **97**: 699–705.

Grotendorst GR, Seppa HEJ, Kleinman HK et al (1981) Attachment of smooth muscle cells to collagen and their migration toward platelet-derived growth factor, *Proc Natl Acad Sci U S A* **78**: 3669–72.

Howard GA, Bottemiller BL, Turner RT et al (1981) Parathyroid hormone stimulates bone formation and resorption in organ culture: evidence for a coupling mechanism, *Proc Natl Acad Sci U S A* **78**: 3204–8.

Hughes DE, Tiffee JC, Li HH et al (1996) Estrogen promotes apoptosis of murine osteoclasts mediated by TGFβ, *Nat Med* **7**: 1132–6.

Kleerekoper M, Villanueva AR, Stanciu J et al (1985) The role of three dimensional trabecular microstructure in the pathogenesis of vertebral compression fractures, *Calcif Tissue Int* **37**: 594–7.

Manolagas SC, Jilka RL (1995) Mechanisms of disease: bone marrow, cytokines, and bone remodeling—emerging insights into the pathophysiology of osteoporosis, *N Engl J Med* **332**: 305–11.

Marcelli C, Yates AJP, Mundy GR (1990) In vivo effects of human recombinant transforming growth factor beta on bone turnover in normal mice, *J Bone Miner Res* **5**: 1087–96.

Massague J (1985) Transforming growth factor β modulates the high affinity receptors of epidermal growth factor and transforming growth factor α, *J Cell Biol* **100**: 1508–14.

Massague J, Kelly B, Mottola C (1985) Stimulation by insulin-like growth factors is required for cellular transformation by Type β transforming growth factor, *J Biol Chem* **260**: 4551–4.

Mazess RB (1982) On aging bone loss, *Clin Orthop* **165**: 239–52.

Miyauchi A, Alvarez J, Greenfield EM et al (1991) Recognition of osteopontin and related peptides by an αvβ3 integrin stimulates immediate cell signals in osteoclasts, *J Biol Chem* **266**: 20 369–74.

Mundy GR, Poser JW (1983) Chemotactic activity of the gamma-carboxyglutamic acid containing protein in bone, *Calcif Tissue Int* **35**: 164–8.

Mundy GR, Luben RA, Raisz LG et al (1974a) Bone-resorbing activity in supernatants from lymphoid cell lines, *N Engl J Med* **290**: 867–71.

Mundy GR, Raisz LG, Cooper RA et al (1974b) Evidence for the secretion of an osteoclast stimulating factor in myeloma, *N Engl J Med* **291**: 1041–6.

Mundy GR, Rodan SB, Majeska RJ et al (1982) Unidirectional migration of osteosarcoma cells with osteoblast characteristics in response to products of bone resorption, *Calcif Tissue Int* **34**: 542–6.

Parfitt AM, Mathews CHE, Villanueva AR et al (1983) Relationships between surface, volume, and thickness of iliac trabecular bone in aging and in osteoporosis, *J Clin Invest* **72**: 1396–409.

Pfeilschifter J, Mundy GR (1987) TGFβ stimulates osteoblast activity and is released during the bone resorption process. In: Cohn DV, Martin TJ, Meunier PJ, eds, *Calcium regulation and bone metabolism: basic and clinical aspects* Vol 9 (Elsevier: Amsterdam) 450–4.

Pfeilschifter J, Bonewald L, Mundy GR (1990a) Characterization of the latent transforming growth factor β complex in bone, *J Bone Miner Res* **5**: 49–58.

Pfeilschifter J, Wolf O, Naumann A et al (1990b) Chemotactic response of osteoblast-like cells to transforming growth factor β, *J Bone Miner Res* **5**: 825–30.

Rasmussen H, Bordier P (1974) *The physiological and cellular basis of metabolic bone disease* (Williams and Wilkins: Baltimore).

Riggs BL, Melton LJ III (1986) Involutional osteoporosis, *N Engl J Med* **314**: 1676–86.

Riggs BL, Wahner HW, Dunn WL et al (1981) Differential changes in bone mineral density of the appendicular and axial skeleton with aging: relationship to spinal osteoporosis, *J Clin Invest* **67**: 328–35.

Riggs BL, Wahner HW, Melton LJ III et al (1986) Rates of bone loss in the axial and appendicular skeletons of women: evidence of substantial vertebral bone loss prior to menopause, *J Clin Invest* **77**: 1487–91.

Roberts AB, Anzano MA, Wakefield LM et al (1985) Type β transforming growth factor: a bifunctional regulator of cellular growth, *Proc Natl Acad Sci U S A* **82**: 119–23.

Senior RM, Griffin GL, Huang JS et al (1983) Chemotactic activity of platelet alpha granule proteins for fibroblasts, *J Cell Biol* **96**: 382–5.

Seppa H, Grotendorst G, Seppa S et al (1982) Platelet-derived growth factor is chemotactic for fibroblasts, *J Cell Biol* **92**: 584–8.

Seyedin SM, Thomas TC, Thompson AY et al (1985) Purification and characterization of two cartilage-inducing factors from bovine demineralized bone, *Proc Natl Acad Sci U S A* **82**: 2267–71.

Smith DM, Khairi MRA, Johnston CC Jr (1975) The loss of bone mineral with aging and its relationship to risk of fracture, *J Clin Invest* **56**: 311–18.

Snapper I, Kahn A (1971) *Myelomatosis* (Karger: Basel).

Stewart AF, Vignery A, Silvergate A et al (1982) Quantitative bone histomorphometry in humoral hypercalcemia of malignancy—uncoupling of bone cell activity, *J Clin Endocrinol Metab* **55**: 219–27.

Tucker RF, Shipley GD, Moses HL et al (1984) Growth inhibitor from BSC-1 cells closely related to platelet type B transforming growth factor, *Science* **226**: 705–7.

Valentin-Opran A, Charhon SA, Meunier PJ et al (1982) Quantitative histology of myeloma induced bone changes, *Br J Haematol* **52**: 601–10.

Walker F, Nicola NA, Metcalf D et al (1985) Hierarchical down-modulation of hemopoietic growth factor receptors, *Cell* **43**: 269–76.

CHAPTER 2

Cellular mechanisms of bone resorption

The major and possibly sole bone resorbing cell under normal conditions is the osteoclast, and this cell will be the main focus for this chapter. Other cells, however, have been linked to bone resorption. These include osteocytes, monocytes, tumor cells and osteoblasts. Osteocytic bone resorption, also called "osteocytic osteolysis", was first described over 30 years ago by histologists examining light microscopy sections. Osteocytic osteolysis was thought to be due to expansion of the lacunae in which osteocytes are embedded in bone. However, careful observations with scanning electron microscopy indicate that it is unlikely that osteocytes cause osteolysis (Jones et al 1985). Scanning electron microscopy shows that bone resorption by osteoclasts is characterized by easily discernible degradative changes in the structural proteins of the bone matrix, but these characteristic changes are not seen around osteocytes. Boyde and co-workers consider "osteocytic osteolysis" an artifact of observations made in bone that is rapidly turning over (fetal or woven bone) (Jones et al 1985). Other cells have also been linked to bone resorption. Monocytes and macrophages have been shown to degrade devitalized bone (Mundy et al 1977; Kahn et al 1978). These observations support the concept that monocytes and osteoclasts have a common precursor. Tumor cells also resorb devitalized bone in vitro by causing release of previously incorporated calcium (Eilon and Mundy 1978). There are no resorption pits associated with monocytes, macrophages or tumor cells when they lie against bone surfaces (Boyde et al 1986). Although this does not mean that they do not cause bone dissolution, it is unlikely that they play a major role. In vitro studies have suggested that osteoblasts act as helper cells in the process of osteoclastic resorption possibly by preparing the bone surface for later attack by osteoclastic enzymes, although there is still little direct evidence in vivo to support this interesting theory.

The morphology of the osteoclast

Osteoclasts are unique and highly specialized cells (Figure 2.1). They are found on endosteal bone surfaces, in Haversian systems and also occasionally on periosteal surfaces. They are not commonly seen on bone surfaces in normal individuals, but are seen frequently at sites undergoing rapid resorption such as the metaphyses of growing bones or adjacent to collections of metastatic tumor cells. They are large multinucleated cells, with up to 100 nuclei per cell in pathologic states (with even more nuclei in Paget's disease, but fewer in hematologic malignancies), although at sites of bone remodeling in normal subjects they have typically fewer than 10 nuclei per cell. The number of nuclei in osteoclasts is related to the species, with usually only a few in rodents, but more in other species such as cats.

CELLULAR MECHANISMS OF BONE RESORPTION

Figure 2.1
Osteoclasts in a resorption lacunae with a ruffled border. Note how the cell is polarized. Also note the intimate association with adjacent cells of the marrow cavity, including marrow mononuclear cells as well as bone cells on bone surfaces that produce factors that are powerful regulators of osteoclast formation and resorption.

The nuclei are centrally placed and usually contain one or two nucleoli. Osteoclasts have primary lysosomes, numerous and pleomorphic mitochondria and a specific area of the cell membrane which forms adjacent to the bone surface known as the ruffled border. This area of the cell membrane consists of folds and invaginations, which allow intimate contact with the bone surface. This is the site at which resorption of bone occurs and the resorption pit (also known as the Howship's lacuna or resorption bay) is formed (Figure 2.2). Some workers have likened the confined and circumscribed space between the ruffled border and the bone surface to a secondary lysosome (Baron et al 1983). The ruffled border is surrounded by a clear zone which appears free of organelles but in fact contains actin filaments and appears to anchor the ruffled border area to the bone surface undergoing resorption. This may be critical to the polarization of the osteoclast, which occurs when the cell is activated immediately prior to undergoing resorption.

Methods for studying osteoclast biology

Progress in understanding the cell biology and physiology of osteoclasts has been severely hampered by the absence of a useful osteoclast cell line. To circumvent this difficulty, a variety of model systems (Figure 2.3) have been developed for studying factors affecting osteoclast activity and formation and osteoclastic bone resorption.

Several investigators have developed techniques for isolating authentic osteoclasts from long bones. The most commonly used source has been the endosteal surface of chick long bones. Osdoby et al (1982) described the release of osteoclasts from embryonic chick tibiae. This method yields cell preparations that contain 50–75% osteoclasts, and the osteoclasts can be cultured for up to 10 days with retention of osteoclast morphology. The osteoclasts can be enriched by use of specific antibody-coated magnetic beads (Oursler et al 1991). A similar approach has been used by Zambonin Zallone et al (1982) in hypocalcemic chicks, by Boyde et al (1984) in embryonic chicks, by Chambers and Magnus (1982) in rats, by Chambers et al (1984) in

Figure 2.2
Isolated rat osteoclast attached to calcified matrix (sperm whale dentine). The activity of osteoclasts on calcified matrices can be examined by their capacity to form resorption pits, as depicted here by this rat osteoclast cultured on sperm whale dentine. (Kindly supplied by Professors Alan Boyde and Sheila Jones.) However, this technique is not without problems. It is not possible without special technology to measure the volume of resorption pits accurately. Moreover, some factors which stimulate osteoclastic bone resorption in vivo do not work well in this assay.

Figure 2.3
Current techniques used for studying osteoclast formation and action. Some techniques focus on specific aspects of the process such as osteoclast formation or activity of mature preformed cells. Organ culture and in vivo approaches examine the entire process of formation and resorption.

rabbits and by Roodman and Takahashi (unpublished observations, 1986) in baboon fetuses. Although this approach has been advocated as useful for acute studies, some investigators have questioned the viability of the cells. Zambonin Zallone et al (1982) isolated osteoclasts from medullary bone of laying hens rendered hypocalcemic by low-calcium diets in order to obtain higher yields. They claim that the osteoclasts remain viable for 3 weeks and preparations containing 90–95% osteoclasts can be obtained when the cells are cultured with cytosine arabinoside. However, it should be appreciated that these cells form only one resorption pit per 100 or more cells, and it is possible that many of them are sick or dying as the culture is prolonged. A substantial improvement in obtaining avian osteoclasts has recently been described by Alvarez et al (1991). They showed that mononuclear cells obtained after Ficoll–Hypaque separation of the marrow cells from hypocalcemic chickens or hens when cultured for 6 days formed essentially 100% multinucleated cells which stained positively with tartrate-resistant acid phosphatase and which formed resorption pits at the rate of approximately one pit/cell. (In our experience, the frequency of pit formation is much less.) Wesolowski et al (1995) have described an improvement in the preparation of greater numbers of highly enriched osteoclast precursors from murine bones. They take marrow mononuclear cells containing osteoclast precursors and enrich the osteoclast precursors by the use of echistatin, which binds osteoclasts through RGD sequences on the cell surface. Giant cell tumors of bone appear to be a particularly useful source of human osteoclast-like cells (Horton et al 1984). Antibodies to the vitronectin receptor can be used to separate giant cells from other cells found in these tumors, and with this approach the giant cells can be obtained in essentially homogeneous populations. They cause massive resorption in vitro. Since these cells have all the phenotypic characteristics of osteoclasts, and also function like osteoclasts, they are a very useful model for human cells with the osteoclast phenotype.

Methods such as these and others can be used to examine the morphologic changes of osteoclasts exposed to a variety of substances and osteoclastic bone resorption ultrastructurally, but can give essentially no information on the mechanisms responsible for regulation of osteoclast differentiation. In addition, because of the fragility of osteoclasts, obtaining reproducible and reliable cell preparations is extremely difficult.

Other methods have also been used to isolate osteoclasts and osteoclast-like cells from bone to overcome these problems. Dziak and Brand (1974), Wong and Cohn (1975), Peck et al (1977) and Braidman et al (1982) have employed sequential enzymatic digestion or selective digestion of rodent calvaria to obtain osteoclast-like cells. Although these cells have several osteoclast characteristics such as appropriate calcitonin responses and high acid phosphatase content, the majority are mononuclear and do not have the morphologic appearance of osteoclasts seen in situ.

Teitelbaum and co-workers have used rodent peritoneal macrophages (Kahn and Teitelbaum 1981; Teitelbaum et al 1981) as well as human monocytic cell lines (Bar-Shavit et al 1983) as model systems for osteoclasts. The murine macrophages release ^{45}Ca from dead bone fragments; release of ^{45}Ca is augmented when they become multinucleated (Fallon et al 1983). These authors (Bar-Shavit et al 1983) have also shown that HL-60 cells, a human promyelocytic leukemic cell line, can be induced to express the macrophage phenotype and release ^{45}Ca from devitalized bone matrix. Although this system has provided useful information on mechanisms of bone resorption, it has not been shown definitively that mature macrophages can form osteoclasts or that the mechanism by which macrophages cause ^{45}Ca release from bone is identical to bone resorption caused by osteoclasts. Recently, Yoneda et al (1991) have cultured HL-60 cells and produced a population of multinucleated cells that have the osteoclast phenotype. These cells were multinucleated, stained positively for tartrate-resistant acid phosphatase, had calcitonin receptors as assessed by autoradiography and responded to calcitonin, contained a vacuolar ATPase characteristic of the osteoclast proton pump, and formed resorption pits on sperm whale dentine. These data indicate that HL-60 cells share characteristics with cells in the osteoclast lineage, and particularly with osteoclast precursors. Since HL-60s have been likened to CFU-GM, this is further evidence of a common hematopoietic marrow precursor that osteoclasts share with the formed elements of the blood.

Baron and co-workers have studied osteoclast formation in vivo in alveolar bone (Tran Van et al 1982a,b). This system can also be used to study formation of osteoclasts from mononuclear precursors, as well as the fate of osteoclasts and the cells which line resorption bays after resorption is complete (reversal cells). Bone resorption may be induced in this model by extracting molars from adult rats. The absence of antagonist teeth leads to induction of remodeling along the periosteum of the mandible.

Bone organ culture systems (Stern and Raisz 1979) are very useful for studying factors controlling osteoclastic bone resorption. In the most commonly used models, pregnant rats or mice are injected with ^{45}Ca and the radius and ulna are dissected from the rat fetuses 24 hours later or the calvariae are harvested from neonatal mice. The explanted bones are then cultured for defined periods and various factors are added to the media and the percent of ^{45}Ca released from the bone relative to the total amount of ^{45}Ca in the bone fragments is determined. Light microscopic and ultrastructural studies can also be performed on the bone fragments. Although such systems cannot be used to determine if the effects on bone resorption result from direct or indirect effects on osteoclasts, since multiple cell populations are present, the same criticism can be made of currently available techniques for studying isolated cells, since none are perfectly homogeneous. Stern and Raisz (1979) have summarized the contribution of various organ culture systems to the field of bone resorption in an extensive review. The methods have been detailed in Mundy et al (1991).

Several laboratories have developed culture systems which support the formation of osteoclast-like cells. Burger et al (1982) developed a long-term culture system for murine marrow. Marrow cells are cultured with a source of colony-stimulating factor for 7 or 14 days in teflon bags, then resuspended in plasma clots which are wrapped around fetal bone rudiments. After 7 days the bones are examined for the presence of osteoclasts. No osteoclasts form unless bone marrow or fetal liver cells are cocultured with the bone rudiments. The system allows testing of various cell populations for the presence of osteoclast precursors and for factors which regulate osteoclastic bone resorption. This model has been expanded considerably by Lowik and co-workers, who have used it to assess effects of factors and drugs such as bisphosphonates on osteoclast precursor recruitment (Lowik et al 1986, 1989).

A different approach has been used by Testa et al (1981) who reported the formation of osteoclast-like cells in long-term feline marrow cultures. This culture system was very similar to that reported by Dexter and Testa (1976), in which marrow is cultured for several weeks and a stromal layer forms that supports long-term hematopoiesis. This long-term feline marrow culture system has been further characterized and modified (Ibbotson et al 1984). The multinucleated cells respond appropriately to osteotropic hormones, have several ultrastructural features of osteoclasts, contain tartrate-resistant acid phosphatase, and release ^{45}Ca from bone fragments. Heersche and co-workers (Pharoah and Heersche 1985) have also employed the feline marrow culture system to study the effects of 1,25-dihydroxyvitamin D_3 on the formation of osteoclast-like cells. These observations have been extended to murine (Takahashi et al 1988), baboon (Roodman et al 1985) and human (MacDonald et al 1987) marrow culture systems in which osteoclast-like multinucleated cells form in vitro. Such culture systems allow studies to determine if osteotropic factors stimulate proliferation of the precursors for osteoclasts, stimulate fusion of the precursors, or act on preformed multinucleated cells. These culture systems could potentially permit identification and purification of osteoclast precursors and determine the relative role that other cell types play in the activity and formation of osteoclasts. Further, the human marrow culture system may for the first time allow studies of osteoclast formation and activity in patients with metabolic bone disease. These culture systems are composed of mixed cell populations so that it is difficult to determine if a factor acts directly or indirectly on osteoclast precursors or on the multinucleated cells. The murine and human marrow culture models have been the most studied. The murine system is easier to use, since cells of the osteoclast phenotype can be identified after 6–7 days of culture. These cells contain calcitonin receptors, are multinucleated and form resorption pits on bone slices or on sperm whale dentine. The human marrow culture system must be carried out for longer periods using horse serum. Cells of the osteoclast phenotype are responsive to calcitonin and have calcitonin receptors as determined by autoradiography and by PCR (Kurihara et al 1990a,b; Takahashi et al 1993). The cells form fewer resorption pits than do the murine cultures. However, when marrow mononuclear cells from patients with Paget's disease are cultured in this system, the multinucleated cells have many of the morphologic characteristics of Pagetic osteoclasts, and contain viral sequences from the paramyxovirus family (Reddy et al 1992). Flanagan has described a technique which improves the capacity of human osteoclast-like cells to form pits (Sarma and Flanagan 1996).

Studying the biochemistry of the mammalian osteoclast has been markedly hindered by the lack of homogeneous populations of cells in sufficient quantities. There have been attempts to overcome this lack with cell lines which can be induced to form osteoclasts. Yoneda et al (1991) showed that multipotent HL-60 cells, which are capable of forming neutrophils or monocytes under appropriate stimulation, can form small numbers of osteoclasts when incubated with growth regulatory factors derived from tumor cells that enhance osteoclast formation. However, the numbers of mature osteoclasts formed are not sufficient to perform adequate studies. Similar such cell lines are those described by Gattei et al (1992) and Chambers et al (1993), but they suffer from this same problem. Recently, to overcome this problem, Roodman and colleagues (Hentunen et al 1996) have attempted a number of approaches in which they have introduced genes that immortalize cells in the osteoclast lineage with the use of the TRAP promoter which targets the cells in the osteoclast lineage. Initial attempts were made with SV40 large T antigen which induced osteoclast apoptosis, but cell lines could not be maintained (Boyce et al 1995). More recent attempts have been made using the Bcl-X_L gene which prevents programmed cell death in many cell types with large T antigen and may be more successful.

In recent years, some of the most important information in osteoclast biology has come from studies in osteopetrosis, the disease characterized by impaired osteoclast function. As the molecular defects responsible for this phenotype in different animal and human models have been identified, some of the critical mechanisms responsible for osteoclast formation and action have become apparent. These are discussed in more detail in the chapter on Osteopetrosis (Chapter 11).

Criteria for the definition of the osteoclast

This is one of the highly controversial topics in the bone field. Since osteoclasts are not readily obtainable, there are considerable variations from species to species in behavior of these cells, and each new model system for the study of cells with the osteoclast phenotype has been looked at with some skepticism by other workers in the field. Unfortunately, at this point in time, there is no single criterion which is pathognomonic for the osteoclast.

Some of the morphologic features of the osteoclast have been used as criteria for identification. These include multinuclearity, pleomorphic mitochondria and presence of the ruffled border adjacent to areas of resorbed bone. These criteria have received much attention in recent years as investigators have attempted to isolate osteoclasts in vitro and distinguish them from other cells. The major distinction is from the macrophage polykaryon, which is a related cell with a similar lineage. Some of the features of the osteoclast that aid in the distinction from macrophage polykaryons include the capacity to resorb bone, capacity to form a ruffled border, contraction of the cytoplasm on exposure to calcitonin, crossreactivity with osteoclast-specific monoclonal antibodies (although it has not been convincingly shown that any current antibodies are absolutely specific for the osteoclast), appropriate responses to calciotropic hormones, and absence of the Fc receptor. The 23C6 antibody to the vitronectin receptor has been widely used as a marker for the osteoclasts (Horton and Davies 1989). This has turned out to be a useful marker not only for identifying osteoclasts but also for use in purifying these cells. Unfortunately, the 23C6 marker is not unique to the osteoclast, although its expression on the osteoclast seems to be much greater than it is in other multinucleated giant cells. Much has been made of the presence of calcitonin receptors for identifying osteoclasts, but as is the case for 23C6 antibodies, other cells in the marrow microenvironment may have calcitonin receptors, particularly cells in the monocyte–macrophage family. Moreover, in some species, osteoclasts themselves appear not to have calcitonin receptors. The presence of tartrate-resistant acid phosphatase is a helpful marker, but not useful for distinguishing human osteoclasts from macrophage polykaryons. Responsivity to osteotropic hormones also has been used as a criterion for identification of osteoclasts. Osteoclast stimulating agents including parathyroid hormone, interleukin-1, tumor necrosis factor, transforming growth factor α and 1,25-dihydroxyvitamin D_3 activate osteoclasts. Inhibitors of osteoclast activity include calcitonin, gamma interferon and transforming growth factor β. However, the effects of some of these factors are not specific for osteoclasts. For example, 1,25-dihydroxyvitamin D_3 promotes not only the fusion of osteoclasts but also enhances the fusion of macrophages to form polykaryons (Roodman et al 1985). Moreover, some of these factors are species-specific. For example, calcitonin does not necessarily cause contraction of embryonic avian osteoclasts (Nicholson et al 1987).

Origin and cell lineage

The multinucleated osteoclast is the primary bone resorbing cell. For years, the origin of the osteoclast has been the subject of dispute, although now most workers agree that it is derived from a multipotent precursor it shares with cells of the monocyte–macrophage lineage in the bone marrow (Figures 2.4 and 2.5). A variety of studies have shown that the osteoclast is blood-borne, in contrast to osteoblasts. Walker (1972, 1973) showed that parabiotic linkage of an osteopetrotic mouse with a normal litter-mate caused a marrow cavity to form due to the formation of osteoclasts. Studies using quail-chick chimeras (Kahn and Simmons 1975), in which quail-bone rudiments are grafted onto chick allantoic membrane, have disclosed that the osteoclasts formed are predominantly of host origin. This system takes advantage of the distinctive nuclear morphology of quail and chick cells and permits identification of host and donor cells. Jotereau and LeDouarin (1978) have confirmed that osteoclasts in quail-chick chimeras are not bone-derived.

Transplantation of hemopoietic tissue into lethally irradiated osteopetrotic recipients suggests that osteoclast precursors must be present in hemopoietic tissues. Walker (1975) showed that transplantation of spleen or marrow cells into osteopetrotic mice resulted in removal of excessive bone present in these animals. Marks (1976) showed that in the ia osteopetrotic rat, transplantation of spleen cells could cure the disease. Infusion of the mononuclear cell fraction from the spleen (Marks 1978) was responsible for formation of osteoclasts with ruffled borders, something not seen in untreated ia rats. These studies revealed that transplantation of cells derived from

Figure 2.4

Model for osteoclast formation, showing the life cycle of the osteoclast and the sites at which hormones and cytokines regulate osteoclast numbers.

hemopoietic tissue could cure osteopetrosis, and suggest that the critical cells which are transplanted are osteoclast precursors. However, the results do not exclude the possibility that the transplanted cells act instead by producing a factor that permits normal differentiation of osteopetrotic osteoclasts. Results with transplantation of cells which contained markers showed that osteopetrosis was in fact cured by formation of donor-derived osteoclasts. For example, Coccia et al (1980) and Sorell et al (1981) transplanted marrow from HLA-matched male siblings into female patients who had osteopetrosis, and showed by Y-body analysis that the osteoclasts formed in the patients were donor in origin. Studies in osteopetrotic rodents using fetal liver cells (Marks 1978) and mononuclear cells from thymus (Marks and Schneider 1978), as well as a cell suspension containing hemopoietic stem cells (Loutit and Nisbit 1982), also indicate that osteopetrosis can be cured by transplantation of hemopoietic cells. These studies all support the concept that the osteoclast precursor is a mononuclear cell derived from hemopoietic tissue.

Osteoclasts form by fusion of mononuclear precursors. This was shown in studies by Kahn and Simmons (1975) using quail-chick chimeras, who found that some osteoclasts that formed contained nuclei with both quail and chick characteristics. Young (1962) showed in experiments using [^{3}H]thymidine that osteoclasts formed by fusion of mononuclear precursors rather than mitotic division. Using autoradiography, it has been shown that osteoclast-like cells grown in long-term marrow cultures are formed by fusion (Ibbotson et al 1984; MacDonald et al 1986). More recent studies have shown that the cell attachment molecule E-cadherin is involved in the process, since E-cadherin is expressed by osteoclasts as they fuse and either peptide antagonists or neutralizing antibodies to E-cadherin, both of

- common fate at reversal sites
- precipitated by resorption inhibitors, TGFβ
- change in pattern of gene expression

Figure 2.5

Morphologic characteristics of apoptotic osteoclasts. The features are condensation of nuclear chromatin, darker staining of the cytoplasm, loss of ruffled border and withdrawal of the cells from the bone surface.

which interfere with the cell attachment function of E-cadherin, block osteoclast formation (Mbalaviele et al 1995).

Taken together, these data derived from diverse experimental systems all support the notion that the multinucleated osteoclast is formed by fusion of mononuclear cells which are hemopoietic rather than bone-derived in origin.

The leading candidate for the mononuclear precursor for the osteoclast appears to be a stem cell of the monocyte–macrophage family. The classic experiments of Fischman and Hay (1962) demonstrated in regenerating newt limb that osteoclasts were formed by the fusion of labeled leukocytes which were probably monocytes histologically. Tinkler et al (1981) infused [^{3}H]thymidine-labeled peripheral blood murine monocytes into syngeneic recipients treated with 1,25-dihydroxyvitamin D_3, and observed that the osteoclasts that formed contained labeled nuclei. Similarly, Zambonin Zallone et al (1984) found that some peripheral blood monocytes can fuse with purified osteoclasts in vitro. Burger et al (1982) reported that the osteoclast precursors in mouse marrow cells were immature monocytes by morphologic criteria. Similar nonadherent cells were identified as potential human osteoclast precursors in an entirely different system (Ibbotson et al 1984; Kurihara et al 1990a,b).

We propose the following model of osteoclast development based on the above data (Figure 2.4). We suggest that the osteoclast arises from a progenitor cell similar to that for other members of the monocyte–macrophage family. In this model, the colony stimulating factors (CSFs) stimulate the proliferation and differentiation of the granulocyte–macrophage committed progenitor cells (CFU-GM). These CSFs probably include CSF-1 and GM-CSF, and possibly other cytokines such as interleukin-6 and interleukin-3. This model is consistent with the observations of Burger et al (1982) that incubation of marrow with colony stimulating activity responsible for the proliferation of monocyte–macrophage progenitors increases the number of osteoclast progenitors, and our finding (MacDonald et al 1986) that recombinant human CSF-1 increased formation of osteoclast-like cells in long-term marrow cultures. CFU-GM stimulated by CSF-1 form promonocytes, which are immature nonadherent progenitors of mononuclear phagocytes and osteoclasts. Also consistent are the studies in op/op osteopetrotic mice, which do not have competent osteoclasts. In this disease, biologically active CSF-1 is not produced and osteoclasts do not form (Felix et al 1990a,b; Wiktor-Jedrzejczak et al 1990; Yoshida et al 1990; Kodama et al 1991). Both Burger et al (1982) and Ibbotson et al (1984) have identified the precursor for these cells as a nonadherent immature monocyte. The promonocyte can presumably proliferate and differentiate along the macrophage pathway and eventually form a tissue macrophage or can differentiate along the osteoclast pathway, depending on the factors to which it is exposed.

The first osteoclast precursors, the early preosteoclasts, can still proliferate and circulate in the peripheral blood. These cells are a specialized subpopulation of peripheral blood monocytes but are morphologically indistinguishable from other monocytes by light microscopy. In this regard, Zambonin Zallone et al (1984) have shown that some peripheral blood monocytes fuse with osteoclasts. The concentration of early pre-osteoclasts may be increased in states of primary hyperparathyroidism (MacDonald et al 1987), Paget's disease (Demulder et al 1991) or other conditions in which bone resorption or turnover is increased. The early pre-osteoclast contains nonspecific esterase but not tartrate-resistant acid phosphatase according to the observations of Baron et al (1986). Based on in vitro data with long-term marrow cultures (Roodman et al 1985; Takahashi et al 1986; MacDonald et al 1987), PTH, 1,25-dihydroxyvitamin D_3 and other factors such as transforming growth factor alpha (TGFα) and epidermal growth factor (EGF) stimulate the formation of these cells, while calcitonin inhibits their formation. The early pre-osteoclast gives rise to a late pre-osteoclast, a step which is regulated by 1,25-dihydroxyvitamin D_3, PTH or possibly other osteotropic factors. The late pre-osteoclast has decreased or absent proliferative potential and has lost some of its monocytic surface antigens.

Once the late pre-osteoclast "homes" to bone, it expresses osteoclast-specific antigens (Horton et al 1985; Oursler et al 1985) and fuses with other cells to form a multinucleated osteoclast. The late pre-osteoclast may have ultrastructural features of osteoclasts as reported for mononuclear osteoclasts (Ries and Gong 1982), and expresses a calcitonin receptor. This cell also has the capacity to bind through integrins to RGD sequences in bone matrix proteins (Miyauchi et al 1991). In this model, mature multinucleated osteoclasts would not express the majority of the monocytic surface antigens, would strongly express osteoclast-specific antigens, and develop all the ultrastructural features of mature osteoclasts. This model is proposed as a continuum rather than as distinct stages of differentiation. Vaananen and colleagues (Salo et al 1996) have shown that the cell membrane of the osteoclast is divided into several domains using enveloped viral glycoproteins and lectins as markers. During active resorption, when the osteoclast is polarized, the basolateral domain is distinct from the ruffled border and sealing zone.

Osteoclast apoptosis

Recently, it has been observed that osteoclasts undergo morphologic apoptosis at the conclusion of the resorbing phase of the bone remodeling process (Hughes et al 1995). The morphologic characteristics of osteoclast apoptosis are condensation of the nuclear chromatin, darker staining of the osteoclast cytoplasm, loss of ruffled border and detachment from the mineralized bone matrix, and cessation of bone resorption. Observations by Hughes and Boyce (Boyce et al 1989a) suggest that osteoclast apoptosis is a common occurrence at reversal sites (see Chapter 1) and may be precipitated by resorption inhibitors such as estrogen and bisphosphonates, and also by TGFβ (Hughes et al 1996). Regulation of the process of osteoclast apoptosis may be potentially important during bone resorption, since this represents a step by which bone resorption could be controlled.

Molecular mechanisms of bone resorption (Figure 2.6)

Osteoclasts resorb bone by the production of proteolytic enzymes and hydrogen ions in the localized environment under the ruffled border of the cell. Hydrogen ions are generated in the cell by the enzyme carbonic anhydrase Type II. They are then pumped across the ruffled border by a proton pump, apparently related but not identical to the proton pump in the intercalated cells of the kidney (Blair et al 1989). Lysosomal enzymes are also released by the osteoclast, and the hydrogen ions produced by the proton pump provide an optimal environment for these proteolytic enzymes to degrade the bone matrix.

The production of protons under the ruffled border of the osteoclast is required for normal bone resorption. This probably occurs because the osteoclast needs to release mineral from the bone matrix, and provide an optimal environment for the maximal proteolytic activity of lysosomal enzymes as well as activation of growth factors such as TGFβ and the insulin-like growth factors. A molecular mechanism for the translocation of protons from the osteoclast cytosol to the area

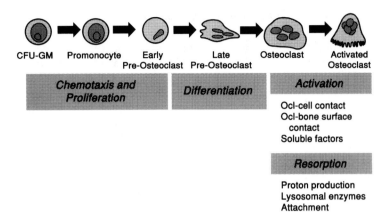

Figure 2.6

Events involved in osteoclastic bone resorption. To resorb bone, osteoclasts are required to form from pluripotent precursors. Bone resorption is mediated in large part by mature multinucleated cells, which use specific molecular mechanisms to accomplish this process. These mechanisms include, but are not limited to, proton production and secretion across the ruffled border, polarization of the cell, attachment of the cell to the mineralized bone matrix, production of lysosomal enzymes and expression of the proto-oncogenes c-src and c-fos.

under the ruffled border has recently been identified by several workers. This molecular mechanism may be a variation of the complex vacuolar ATPase found in the intercalated cells of the kidney (Blair et al 1989), although there has been some controversy on this point (Chatterjee et al 1992). Although this ATPase may not be typical of the renal ATPase, this is a complex enzyme and pharmacologic inhibition may depend on the specific subunit composition of the enzyme.

There are a number of ion exchangers, pumps and channels in the basolateral membrane of the osteoclast which are required for the extrusion of protons across the ruffled border of the cell (apical surface). These are required to maintain the electrochemical balance of the osteoclast. These ion exchangers, pumps and channels include an Na^+/H^+ antiporter, an Na^+/K^+ ATPase, a HCO_3^-/Cl^- exchanger, a Ca^{++} ATPase, and a K^+ channel.

There has been considerable controversy over the capacity of osteoclasts to produce collagen-degrading enzymes. For many years it has been thought that the osteoblast was the major source of collagenase activity in the microenvironment of the resorbing osteoclast (Sakamoto et al 1984), and that osteoclasts caused matrix degradation by the production of lysosomal cysteine proteinases, which caused collagen degradation at low pH (Vaes et al 1968; Eilon and Raisz 1978). Using immunolocalization studies, Delaisse et al (1993) have demonstrated the presence of intracellular collagenase (matrix metalloproteinase-1) as well as collagenase in the extracellular sub-osteoclastic resorbing compartment, using anti-mouse antibodies. These more recent studies on matrix metalloproteinases have suggested that the osteoclast itself may be a rich source of collagen-digesting enzymes, which certainly makes sense for a cell responsible for resorbing the bone matrix, which consists of more than 90% Type I collagen. Other enzymes are likely to be important in bone resorption. Cathepsin K has been recently identified in osteoclasts (Drake et al 1996). It has significant primary sequence homology to members of the papain cysteine protease superfamily, including cathepsins S, L and B. Cathepsin K is a potential target for inhibitors of bone destruction (Bossard et al 1996).

The osteoclast is a motile cell. It resorbs bone to form a lacuna and then moves across the bone surface to resorb a separate area of bone. The tracks of its path can often be followed (Jones et al 1985). Periods of locomotion are not associated with resorption. When the cell stops moving, it usually starts resorbing bone.

Disruption of any of the critical molecular mechanisms responsible for bone resorption causes osteopetrosis. For example, it has recently been shown that there is an unusual form of inherited osteopetrosis in children in which there is a deficiency of the carbonic anhydrase Type II isoenzyme (Sly et al 1985). The osteoclasts in this disease are incompetent, bone is not resorbed and the bone marrow cavity is not formed. Children with this disease also have renal tubular acidosis, due to a similar enzyme defect in renal tubular cells leading to impairment of hydrogen ion secretion. In another well studied model of osteopetrosis that occurs in mice, the op/op variant, it has recently been found that osteopetrosis is due to a defect in osteoclast formation caused by an abnormality in the coding region for CSF-1. As a consequence of this genetic abnormality, defective CSF-1 is produced by stromal cells in the osteoclast microenvironment, and osteoclast formation is impaired. The disease can be cured by treatment with exogenous CSF-1 (Felix et al 1990a,b; Kodama et al 1991).

Osteopetrosis has been a very informative disease for studying molecular mechanisms responsible for osteoclast formation and action. Not only has the study of this disease led to observations that carbonic anhydrase Type II and CSF-1 are required for normal osteoclast function, but recently it has been shown that the expression of the proto-oncogenes src and fos is also necessary for osteoclasts to function (Soriano et al 1991; Johnson et al 1992; Wang et al 1992). This has been demonstrated by targeted disruption of the normal proto-oncogenes for src and fos in embryonic stem cells followed by homologous recombination and observations in mutant mice which fail to express these oncogenes. In both cases, osteopetrosis occurs. In the case of src, the defect is not in osteoclast formation but in osteoclast action (Boyce et al 1992a). Src is a nonreceptor tyrosine kinase bound to the cytoplasmic plasma membrane which may be involved in polarization and activation of the osteoclasts. There are approximately 40 or 50 proteins inside cells which are phosphorylated on tyrosine residues by src, and the essential substrate in the osteoclast or in any other cell remains unknown. Two possibilities have recently been suggested. A cytoskeletal protein associated with actin which is phosphorylated by src is localized to the ruffled border in active osteoclasts and may be important (Boyce et al 1992b). Boyce has favored the notion that cortactin, a cytoskeletal protein expressed in the ruffled border of the osteoclast, may be an essential src substrate. Tanaka et al (1995, 1996) have suggested that another cytoskeletal protein, c-cbl, is an important 120 kilodalton substrate for src in osteoclastic resorption, and showed by immunofluorescence studies and confocal microscopy that c-cbl and c-src may co-localize. It is possible that a number of important cytoskeletal proteins are responsible for the effects of src during the bone resorption process. Similarly, it has been shown that PI3 kinase, an enzyme involved in phosphoinositol metabolism, which is activated by interactions between osteopontin and the $\alpha_v\beta_3$ integrin receptor on osteoclasts, co-precipitates with src in osteoclast lysates (Hruska et al 1992). A model integrating the role of c-src into the mechanisms by which osteoclasts resorb bone is shown in Figure 2.7. The role of c-src in osteoclast function is also reviewed in Chapter 11.

The early response gene c-fos is essential for normal osteoclast formation. Gene knockout experiments have shown in mice that null-mutations for c-fos introduced into the germ line lead to mice with absent osteoclast formation and severe osteopetrosis (Johnson et al 1992; Grigoriadis et al 1994). Since the defect is in the osteoclast lineage, this type of osteopetrosis is

Figure 2.7

Proposed model for osteoclastic bone resorption. In this model, the factors which influence osteoclastic bone resorption (systemic hormones such as parathyroid hormone and 1,25-dihydroxyvitamin D_3 and local factors such as the osteotropic cytokines) increase the formation of osteoclasts from pluripotent precursors. The actual resorption process by mature multinucleated cells requires attachment to the bone surface. This may result in activation of the osteoclast by stimulation of the nonreceptor tyrosine kinase $pp60^{c-src}$.

different from either op/op osteopetrosis (where the defect in accessory cells is critical) or from c-src deficiency (where osteoclasts form but have impaired functional capacity). Surprisingly, overexpression of c-fos leads to osteogenic sarcomas and related mesenchymal tumors (Ruther et al 1987). In this case, the defect seems to be specific for the osteoblast lineage. The relationship between defects caused by overexpression of c-fos and lack of expression of c-fos remains unclear.

Adhesion molecules on osteoclast cytoplasmic membranes are clearly important for normal osteoclast function and particularly for bone resorption. These integral membrane proteins (integrins) have been shown recently to bind to molecules present in the bone matrix such as osteopontin through specific RGD (Arg–Gly–Asp) amino acid sequences, an event which leads to osteoclast activation, accumulation of intracellular calcium and activation of the phosphoinositol pathway (Miyauchi et al 1991). Several other RGD containing matrix proteins have been identified, including Type I collagen and bone sialoprotein II, which could act as integrin-binding proteins in bone (Teti et al 1991). A major integrin on the osteoclast surface is the $\alpha_v\beta_3$ dimer, which appears to be closely related to the vitronectin receptor (Davies et al 1989). The importance of this process in bone resorption has recently been demonstrated by Sato et al (1990) who have found that synthetic peptide antagonists to RGD sequences inhibit osteoclastic bone resorption in vitro. Recently, it has been shown that echistatin, which inhibits binding to RGD sequences in vivo, also blocks bone resorption in vivo (Fisher et al 1993). Surprisingly, the $\alpha_v\beta_3$ integrin is expressed predominantly at the basolateral membrane, suggesting that other integrins may be important at the apical (ruffled border) membrane (Baron et al 1993).

Several other processes may be involved in the complex mechanism of osteoclastic bone resorption. Some workers have suggested that the surface of the bone is prepared for the osteoclast by the actions of collagenase released by bone lining cells or osteoblasts (Chambers 1985). The osteoclasts then produce acid and lysosomal enzymes which complete the process. Since osteoblasts have the capacity to produce enzymes which could activate latent collagenase such as plasminogen activator, such a mechanism is possible. However, Boyde has claimed that studies with scanning electron microscopy show that osteoclasts do not necessarily require osteoblast preparation of the bone surface for resorption to occur, and isolated osteoclasts can resorb bone surfaces without the support of any other cells.

It appears that oxygen-derived free radicals are also involved in the resorption of bone by osteoclasts (Garrett et al 1990). Many degradative processes by phagocytic cells are associated with free radical production, and bone resorption seems another. The use of radical generating systems in vivo and in vitro show that enzymes which deplete tissues of radicals such as superoxide dismutase block osteoclastic bone resorption stimulated by parathyroid hormone or interleukin-1. Staining reactions with nitroblue tetrazolium show that radical generation occurs within osteoclasts. Radicals could be involved in the degradation of bone under the ruffled border. However, the demonstration that radical generation is associated with new osteoclast formation in vivo suggests that radicals also have a cellular effect on the formation of osteoclasts (Garrett et al 1990). There is some debate over the relative importance of specific reactive oxygen species (Suda et al 1993; Fraser et al 1996). However, Steinbeck et al (1994) have clearly shown expression of NADPH-oxidase in osteoclasts, as well as the capacity of osteoclasts to produce superoxide actively.

Nitric oxide has recently been shown to be a potential intermediate in the mode of action of some cytokines on bone resorption (MacIntyre et al 1991; Lowik et al 1994; Brandi et al 1995; Ralston et al 1995; Evans and Ralston 1996). Nitric oxide synthase inhibitors block bone resorption which is stimulated by IL-1 or TNF, suggesting that nitric oxide is in part responsible for the effects of these cytokines. However, larger concentrations of nitric oxide inhibit bone resorption, and this may be relevant to the inhibitory effects of gamma interferon on osteoclastic bone resorption stimulated by cytokines.

Regulation of osteoclast activity

Osteoclasts lie on bone surfaces in a bed of elliptical or fusiform spindle-shaped cells called lining

THE BONE RESORBING UNIT

Calvarial Surface Isolated Cells

Figure 2.8

Osteoclasts on a bone surface. When bone resorption is stimulated, lining cells covering the bone surface retract, allowing osteoclasts access to the mineralized surface. They are then able to resorb bone. The left panel in this figure shows bone cells on the calvarial surface of the rat exposed to parathyroid extract. An osteoclast is occupying the space vacated by the retracted lining cells. (Kindly supplied by Professors Alan Boyde and Sheila Jones.)

Figure 2.9

Local factors which have been associated with osteoclastic bone resorption. These were formerly known as osteoclast activating factors (OAFs). Some of these factors activate osteoclastic bone resorption and some inhibit it. Their major effects on bone resorption are probably not on the mature cell but rather on precursors as indicated above. Other mediators not included in this Figure, but which are likely to be important, are leukotrienes and leukemia inhibitory factor (stimulatory) and osteoprotegerin and interleukin-4 (inhibitory).

Figure 2.10

Fetal rat long bone organ cultures showing effects of osteoclast activating factor (OAF). When peripheral blood leukocytes are stimulated with phytohemagglutinin or an antigen to which they have previously been exposed, they produce a bone resorbing activity that stimulates osteoclastic resorption. The right-hand panel shows an intense increase in osteoclast number and activity, with degradation of mineralized bone matrix. Note how the control bone is less cellular but contains more mineralized matrix.

cells, which are probably members of the osteoblast lineage. When exposed to a bone resorbing agent, the first response is that these lining cells retract and the osteoclasts insinuate themselves into the retracted area, a ruffled border forms and bone is resorbed at the exposed surface (Jones et al 1985). The molecular mechanisms by which these complicated processes are controlled are unknown. Why lining cells retract at specific sites and how the osteoclast is activated is still not clear (Figure 2.8). Although some have suggested that the osteoclast is activated by a soluble signal released from the lining cell (Rodan and Martin 1981; McSheehy and Chambers 1986), it is possible the major mechanism for activation of the mature cell may be by interactions between integrins on osteoclast cell membranes with extracellular bone constituents such as osteopontin (Miyauchi et al 1991).

Many hormones and local factors have not been shown to stimulate osteoclast activity directly (Figures 2.9 and 2.10). Their mechanisms of action differ. Osteoclastic resorption may be stimulated by factors which enhance proliferation of osteoclast progenitors, which cause differentiation of committed precursors into mature cells or activation of the mature multinucleated cell to resorb bone (Mundy and Roodman 1987). Similarly, osteoclasts could be inhibited by agents which block proliferation of precursors, which inhibit differentiation or fusion, or which inactivate the mature multinucleated resorbing cell. Current evidence indicates that most factors which stimulate or inhibit osteoclasts act on at least two of these steps. The factors that regulate osteoclastic bone resorption are considered in Chapter 4.

References

Alvarez JI, Teitelbaum SL, Blair HC et al (1991) Generation of avian cells resembling osteoclasts from mononuclear phagocytes, *Endocrinology* **128**: 2324–35.

Baron R, Chakraborty M, Chatterjee D (1993) The biology of the osteoclast. In: Mundy GR, Martin TJ, eds, *Physiology and pharmacology of bone. Handbook of experimental pharmacology* (Springer-Verlag: Berlin) 111–47.

Baron R, Vignery A, Horowitz M (1983) Lymphocytes, macrophages and the regulation of bone remodeling. In: Peck WA, ed, *Bone and Mineral Research, Annual 2* (Elsevier: Amsterdam) 175–242.

Baron R, Neff L, Van PT et al (1986) Kinetic and cytochemical identification of osteoclast precursors and their differentiation into multinucleated osteoclasts, *Am J Pathol* **121**: 363–78.

Bar-Shavit Z, Teitelbaum SL, Reitsma P et al (1983) Induction of monocytic differentiation and bone resorption by 1,25-dihydroxyvitamin D_3, *Proc Natl Acad Sci USA* **80**: 5907–11.

Blair HC, Teitelbaum SL, Ghiselli R et al (1989) Osteoclastic bone resorption by a polarized vacuolar proton pump, *Science* **245**: 855–7.

Bossard MJ, Tomaszek TA, Thompson SK et al (1996) Proteolytic activity of human osteoclast cathepsin K–expression, purification, activation, and substrate identification, *J Biol Chem* **271**: 12 517–24.

Boyce BF, Yoneda T, Lowe C et al (1992a) Requirement of pp60[c-src] expression of osteoclasts to form ruffled borders and resorb bone, *J Clin Invest* **90**: 1622–7.

Boyce BF, Chen H, Bouton A et al (1992b) A src tyrosine phosphoprotein substrate (P80/85) is localized to the ruffled border of osteoclasts, *J Bone Miner Res* **7** (Suppl 1): no 50.

Boyce BF, Wright K, Reddy SV et al (1995) Targeting simian virus 40T antigen to the osteoclast in transgenic mice causes osteoclast tumors and transformation and apoptosis of osteoclasts, *Endocrinology* **136**: 5751–9.

Boyde A, Ali NN, Jones SJ (1984) Resorption of dentine by isolated osteoclasts in vitro, *Br Dent J* **156**: 216–20.

Boyde A, Maconnachie E, Reid SA et al (1986) Scanning electron microscopy in bone pathology: review of methods. Potential and application, *Scanning Electron Microsc* **4**: 1537–54.

Braidman IP, Hales M, Anderson DC (1982) Comparison of binding of 1,25-dihydroxycholecalciferol and 25-hydroxycholecalciferol intact tissue and cytosol preparations from bone and other tissues in the fetal rat, *J Endocrinol* **92**: 147–55.

Brandi ML, Hukkanen M, Umeda T et al (1995) Bidirectional regulation of osteoclast function by nitric oxide synthase isoforms, *Proc Natl Acad Sci USA* **92**: 2954–8.

Burger EH, Vander Meer JWM, Gevel JS et al (1982) In vitro formation of osteoclasts from long-term cultures, bone marrow and splenic transplants, *J Exp Med* **192**: 651–63.

Chambers TJ (1985) The pathobiology of the osteoclast, *J Clin Pathol* **38**: 241–52.

Chambers TJ, Magnus CJ (1982) Calcitonin alters the behavior of isolated osteoclasts, *J Pathol* **136**: 27–40.

Chambers TJ, Thomson BM, Fuller K (1984) Resorption of bone by isolated rabbit osteoclasts, *J Cell Sci* **66**: 383–99.

Chambers TJ, Owens JM, Hattersley G et al (1993) Generation of osteoclast-inductive andosteoclastogenic cell lines from the H-2K (b) tsA58 transgenic mouse, *Proc Natl Acad Sci USA* **90**: 5578–82.

Chatterjee D, Chakraborty M, Leit M et al (1992) Sensitivity to vanadate and isoforms of subunits A and B distinguish the osteoclast proton pump from other vacuolar H^+ ATPases, *Proc Natl Acad Sci USA* **89**: 6257–61.

Coccia PF, Krivit W, Cervenka J et al (1980) Successful bone marrow transplantation for infantile malignant osteopetrosis, *N Engl J Med* **302**: 701–8.

Davies J, Warwick J, Totty N et al (1989) The osteoclast functional antigen, implicated in the regulation of bone resorption, is biochemically related to the vitronectin receptor, *J Cell Biol* **109**: 1817–26.

Delaisse JM, Eeckhout Y, Neff L et al (1993) (Pro)collagenase (matrix metalloproteinase-1) is present in rodent osteoclasts and in the underlying bone-resorbing compartment, *J Cell Sci* **106**: 1071–82.

Demulder A, Singer F, Roodman GD (1991) Granulocyte macrophage progenitors (CFU-GM) are abnormal in Paget's disease, *J Bone Miner Res* **6**: 433a.

Dexter TM, Testa NG (1976) Differentiation and proliferation of haemopoietic cells in culture. In: Prescott DM, ed, *Methods in cell biology*, Vol 14 (Academic Press: New York) 387–405.

Drake FH, Dodds RA, James IE et al (1996) Cathepsin K, but not cathepsins B, L, or S, is abundantly expressed in human osteoclasts, *J Biol Chem* **271**: 12 511–6.

Dziak R, Brand JS (1974) Calcium transport in isolated bone cells. I. Bone cell isolation procedures, *J Cell Physiol* **84**: 75–84.

Eilon G, Mundy GR (1978) Direct resorption of bone by human breast cancer cells in vitro, *Nature* **276**: 726–8.

Eilon G, Raisz LG (1978) Comparison of the effects of stimulators and inhibitors of resorption on the release of lysosomal enzymes and radioactive calcium from fetal bone in organ culture, *Endocrinology* **103**: 1969–75.

Evans DE, Ralston SH (1996) Nitric oxide and bone, *J Bone Miner Res* **11**: 300–5.

Fallon MD, Teitelbaum SL, Kahn AJ (1983) Multinucleation enhances macrophage-mediated bone resorption, *Lab Invest* **49**: 159–64.

Felix R, Cecchini MG, Fleisch H (1990a) Macrophage colony stimulating factor restores in vivo bone resorption in the op/op osteopetrotic mouse, *Endocrinology* **127**: 2592–4.

Felix R, Cecchini MG, Hofstetter W et al (1990b) Impairment of macrophage colony-stimulating factor production and lack of resident bone marrow macrophages in the osteopetrotic op/op mouse, *J Bone Miner Res* **5**: 781–9.

Fischman DA, Hay ED (1962) Origin of osteoclasts from mononuclear leukocytes in regenerating newt limbs, *Anatomical Res* **143**: 329–38.

Fisher JE, Caulfield MP, Sato M et al (1993) Inhibition of osteoclastic bone resorption in vivo by echistatin, an arginyl–glycyl–aspartyl (RGD)-containing protein, *Endocrinology* **132**: 1411–13.

Fraser JHE, Helfrich MH, Wallace HM (1996) Hydrogen peroxide, but not superoxide, stimulates bone resorption in mouse calvariae, *Bone* **19**: 223–6.

Garrett IR, Boyce BF, Oreffo ROC et al (1990) Oxygen-derived free radicals stimulate osteoclastic bone resorption in rodent bone in vitro and in vivo, *J Clin Invest* **85**: 632–9.

Gattei V, Bernabei PA, Pinto A et al (1992) Phorbol ester induced osteoclast-like differentiation of a novel human leukemic cell line (FLG 29.1), *J Cell Biology* **116**: 437.

Grigoriadis AE, Wang ZQ, Cecchini MG et al (1994) c-Fos: a key regulator of osteoclast-macrophage lineage determination and bone remodeling, *Science* **266**: 443–8.

Hentunen JJ, Windle SV, Reddy RD et al (1996) Targeting BCL-XL to the osteoclast in transgenic mice enhances osteoclast forming capacity, *J Bone Miner Res* **11** (Suppl 1): no 13.

Horton MA, Davies J (1989) Perspectives—adhesion receptors in bone, *J Bone Miner Res* **4**: 803–8.

Horton MA, Rimmer ET, Lewis D et al (1984) Cell surface characterization of the human osteoclast: phenotypic relationship to other bone marrow-derived cell types, *J Pathol* **144**: 281–94.

Horton MA, Lewis D, McNulty K et al (1985) Human fetal osteoclasts fail to express macrophage antigens, *Br J Exp Pathol* **66**: 103–8.

Hruska KA, Rolnick F, Huskey M (1992) Occupancy of the osteoclast $\alpha_v\beta_3$ integrin by osteopontin stimulates a novel src associated phosphatidylinositol 3 kinase (PI_3 kinase) resulting in phosphatidylinositol trisphosphate (PIP_3) formation, *J Bone Miner Res* **7** (Suppl 1): no 55.

Hughes DE, Wright KR, Uy HL et al (1995) Bisphosphonates promote apoptosis in murine osteoclasts in vitro and in vivo, *J Bone Miner Res* **10**: 1478–87.

Hughes DE, Tiffee JC, Li HH et al (1996) Estrogen promotes apoptosis of murine osteoclasts mediated by TGFβ, *Nat Med* **7**: 1132–6.

Ibbotson KJ, Roodman GD, McManus LM et al (1984) Identification and characterization of osteoclast-like cells and their progenitors in cultures of feline marrow mononuclear cells, *J Cell Biol* **94**: 471–80.

Johnson RS, Spiegelman BM, Papaloannou V (1992) Pleiotropic effects of a null mutation in the c-fos proto-oncogene, *Cell* **71**: 577–86.

Jones SJ, Boyde A, Ali NN et al (1985) A review of bone cell substratum interactions, *Scanning* **7**: 5–24.

Jotereau FV, LeDouarin NM (1978) The developmental relationship between osteocyte and osteoclasts: a study using quail-chick nuclear marker in endochondral ossification, *Develop Biol* **63**: 255–65.

Kahn AJ, Simmons DJ (1975) Investigation of the cell lineage in bone using a chimera of chick and quail embryonic tissue, *Nature* **258**: 325–7.

Kahn AJ, Teitelbaum SL (1981) Endotoxin inhibition of macrophage mediated bone resorption, *Calcif Tissue Int* **33**: 269–75.

Kahn AJ, Stewart CC, Teitelbaum SL (1978) Contact-mediated bone resorption by human monocytes in vitro, *Science* **199**: 988–90.

Kodama H, Yamasaki A, Nose M et al (1991) Congenital osteoclast deficiency in osteopetrotic (op/op) mice is cured by injections of macrophage colony-stimulating factor, *J Exp Med* **173**: 269–72.

Kurihara N, Gluck S, Roodman GD (1990a) Sequential expression of phenotype markers for osteoclasts during differentiation of precursors for multinucleated cells formed in long-term human marrow cultures, *Endocrinology* **127**: 3215–21.

Kurihara N, Chenu C, Civin CI et al (1990b) Identification of committed mononuclear precursors for osteoclast-like cells formed in long-term marrow cultures, *Endocrinology* **126**: 2733–41.

Loutit JF, Nisbit NW (1982) The origin of osteoclasts, *Immunobiology* **161**: 193–203.

Lowik CWGM, Nibbering PH, Vanderuit M (1994) Inducible production of nitric oxide in osteoblast-like cells and in fetal mouse bone explants is associated with suppression of osteoclastic bone resorption, *J Clin Invest* **93**: 1465–72.

Lowik CW, Boonekamp PM, Van de Pluym G et al (1986) Bisphosphonates can reduce osteoclastic bone resorption by two different mechanisms, *Adv Exp Med Biol* **208**: 275–81.

Lowik CWGM, Van Der Pluijm G, Bloys H et al (1989) Parathyroid hormone (PTH) and PTH-like protein (Plp) stimulate interleukin-6 production by osteogenic cells—a possible role of interleukin-6 in osteoclastogenesis, *Biochem Biophys Res Commun* **162**: 1546–52.

MacDonald BR, Mundy GR, Clark S et al (1986) Effects of human recombinant CSF-GM and highly purified CSF-1 on the formation of multinucleated cells with osteoclast characteristics in long-term bone marrow cultures, *J Bone Miner Res* **1**: 227–33.

MacDonald BR, Takahashi N, McManus LM et al (1987) Formation of multinucleated cells with osteoclastic characteristics in long-term human bone marrow cultures, *Endocrinology* **120**: 2326–33.

MacIntyre I, Zaidi M, Alam ASMT et al (1991) Osteoclastic inhibition—an action of nitric oxide not mediated by cyclic GMP, *Proc Natl Acad Sci USA* **88**: 2936–40.

Marks SC Jr (1976) Osteopetrosis in the ia rat cured by spleen cells from a normal littermate, *Am J Anat* **146**: 331–8.

Marks SC Jr (1978) Studies of the cellular cure for osteopetrosis by transplanted cells. Specificity of the cell type in ia rats, *Am J Anat* **151**: 131–7.

Marks SC Jr, Schneider GB (1978) Evidence for a relationship between lymphoid cells and osteoclasts: bone resorption restored in ia (osteopetrotic) rats by lymphocytes, monocytes and macrophages from a normal littermate, *Am J Anat* **152**: 331–41.

Mbalaviele G, Chen H, Boyce BF et al (1995) The role of cadherin in the generation of multinucleated osteoclasts from mononuclear precursors in murine marrow, *J Clin Invest* **95**: 2757–65.

McSheehy PMJ, Chambers TJ (1986) Osteoblastic cells mediate osteoclastic responsiveness to parathyroid hormone, *Endocrinology* **118**: 824–8.

Miyauchi A, Alvarez J, Greenfield EM et al (1991) Recognition of osteopontin and related peptides by an $\alpha_v \beta_3$ integrin stimulates immediate cell signals in osteoclasts, *J Biol Chem* **266**: 20 369–74.

Mundy GR, Roodman GD (1987) Osteoclast ontogeny and function. In: Peck W, ed, *Bone and Mineral Research, Annual 5* (Elsevier: Amsterdam) 209–80.

Mundy GR, Altman AJ, Gondek M et al (1977) Direct resorption of bone by human monocytes, *Science* **196**: 1109–11.

Mundy GR, Roodman GD, Bonewald LF et al (1991) Assays for bone resorption and bone formation. In: Barnes D, Mather JP, Sato GH, eds, *Methods in Enzymology*, Vol 198. Peptide growth factors, Part C, Section VII: Techniques for study of growth factor activity (Academic Press: New York) 502–10.

Nicholson GC, Moseley JM, Sexton PM et al (1987) Chicken osteoclasts do not possess calcitonin receptors, *J Bone Miner Res* **2**: 53–9.

Osdoby P, Martini MC, Caplan AI (1982) Isolated osteoclasts and their presumed progenitor cells, the monocyte, in culture, *J Exp Zoology* **224**: 331–4.

Oursler MJ, Bell LV, Clevinger B et al (1985) Identification of osteoclast specific monoclonal antibodies, *J Cell Biol* **100**: 1592–1600.

Oursler MJ, Collin-Osdoby P, Anderson F et al (1991) Isolation of avian osteoclasts—improved techniques to preferentially purify viable cells, *J Bone Miner Res* **6**: 375–85.

Peck WA, Burke JK, Wilkins J et al (1977) Evidence for preferential effects of parathyroid hormone, calcitonin and adenosine in bone and periosteum, *Endocrinology* **100**: 1357–61.

Pharoah MJ, Heersche JNM (1985) 1,25-Dihydroxyvitamin D_3 causes an increase in the number of osteoclast-like cells in cat bone marrow cultures, *Calcif Tissue Int* **37**: 276–81.

Ralston SH, Ho LP, Helfrich MH et al (1995) Nitric oxide: a cytokine-induced regulator of bone resorption, *J Bone Miner Res* **10**: 1040–9.

Reddy KB, Mangold GL, Tandon AK et al (1992) Inhibition of breast cancer cell growth *in vitro* by a tyrosine kinase inhibitor, *Cancer Res* **52**: 3636–41.

Ries WL, Gong JK (1982) A comparative study of osteoclasts: in situ versus smear specimens, *Anatomical Record* **203**: 221–32.

Rodan GA, Martin TJ (1981) Role of osteoblasts in hormonal control of bone resorption—a hypothesis, *Calcif Tissue Int* **33**: 349–51.

Roodman GD, Ibbotson KJ, MacDonald BR et al (1985) $1,25(OH)_2$ Vitamin D_3 causes formation of multinucleated cells with osteoclast characteristics in cultures of primate marrow, *Proc Natl Acad Sci USA* **82**: 8213–17.

Ruther U, Garber C, Komitowski D et al (1987) Deregulated c-fos expression interferes with normal bone development in transgenic mice, *Nature* **325**: 412–16.

Sakamoto S, Sakamoto M (1984) Isolation and characterization of collagenase synthesized by mouse bone cells in culture, *Biomed Res* **5**: 39.

Salo J, Metsikko K, Palokangas H et al (1996) Bone-resorbing osteoclasts reveal a dynamic division of basal plasma membrane into two different domains, *J Cell Sci* **109**: 301–7.

Sarma U, Flanagan AM (1996) Macrophage colony-stimulating factor induces substantial osteoclast generation and bone resorption in human bone marrow cultures, *Blood* **88**: 2531–40.

Sato Y, Tsuboi R, Lyons R et al (1990) Characterization of the activation of latent TGFβ by co-cultures of endothelial cells and pericytes or smooth muscle cells—a self regulating system, *J Cell Biol* **111**: 757–63.

Sly WS, Whyte MP, Sundaram V et al (1985) Carbonic anhydrase II deficiency in 12 families with the autosomal recessive syndrome of osteopetrosis with renal tubular acidosis and cerebral calcification, *N Engl J Med* **313**: 139–45.

Sorell M, Kapoor N, Kirkpatrick D et al (1981) Marrow transplantation for juvenile osteopetrosis, *Am J Med* **70**: 1280–7.

Soriano P, Montgomery C, Geske R et al (1991) Targeted disruption of the c-src proto-oncogene leads to osteopetrosis in mice, *Cell* **64**: 693–702.

Steinbeck MJ, Appel WH, Verhoeven AJ et al (1994) NADPH-oxidase expression and in situ production of superoxide by osteoclasts actively resorbing bone, *J Cell Biol* **126**: 765–72.

Stern PA, Raisz LG (1979) Organ culture of bone. In: Simmons DJ, Kunin AS, eds, *Skeletal research and experimental approaches* (Academic Press: New York) 21–59.

Suda N, Morita I, Kuroda T (1993) Participation of oxidative stress in the process of osteoclast differentiation, *Biochem Biophys Acta* **1157**: 318–23.

Takahashi N, MacDonald BR, Hon J et al (1986) Recombinant human transforming growth factor alpha stimulates the formation of osteoclast-like cells in long term human marrow cultures, *J Clin Invest* **78**: 894–8.

Takahashi N, Yamana H, Yoshiki S et al (1988) Osteoclast-like cell formation and its regulation by osteotropic hormones in mouse bone marrow cultures, *Endocrinology* **122**: 1373–82.

Takahashi S, Goldring S, Roodman GD (1993) Detection of calcitonin receptor (CTR) mRNA at multiple stages in the osteoclast (OCL) lineage by the polymerase chain reaction (PCR), *J Bone Miner Res* **8** (Suppl 1): no 381.

Tanaka S, Neff L, Baron R et al (1995) Tyrosine phosphorylation and translocation of the c-Cbl protein after activation of tyrosine kinase signaling pathways, *J Biol Chem* **270**: 14 347–51.

Tanaka S, Amling M, Neff L et al (1996) c-Cbl is downstream of c-Src in a signalling pathway necessary for bone resorption, *Nature* **383**: 528–31.

Teitelbaum SL, Malone JD, Kahn AJ (1981) Glucocorticoid enhancement of bone resorption by rat peritoneal macrophages in vitro, *Endocrinology* **108**: 795–9.

Testa NG, Allen TD, Lajtha LG et al (1981) Generation of osteoclasts in vitro, *J Cell Sci* **44**: 127–37.

Teti A, Rizzoli R, Zallone AZ (1991) Parathyroid hormone binding to cultured avian osteoclasts, *Biochem Biophys Res Commun* **174**: 1217–22.

Tinkler SMB, Williams DM, Johnson NW (1981) Osteoclast formation in response to intraperitoneal injection of 1, alpha hydroxycholecalciferol in mice, *J Anat* **133**: 91–7.

Tran Van P, Vignery A, Baron R (1982a) Cellular kinetics of the bone remodeling in the rat, *Anatomical Record* **202**: 445–56.

Tran Van P, Vignery A, Baron R (1982b) An electron-microscopic study of the bone remodeling sequence in the rat, *Cell Tissue Res* **225**: 283–92.

Vaes E (1968) The action of parathyroid hormone on the excretion and synthesis of lysosomal enzymes and on the extracellular release of acid by bone cells, *J Cell Biol* **39**: 676–97.

Walker DG (1972) Congenital osteopetrosis in mice cured by parabiotic union with normal siblings, *Endocrinology* **91**: 916–20.

Walker DG (1973) Osteopetrosis cured by temporary parabiosis, *Science* **180**: 875.

Walker DG (1975) Control of bone resorption by hematopoietic tissue. The induction and reversal of congenital osteopetrosis in mice through the use of bone marrow mononuclear phagocytes, *J Exp Med* **142**: 651–63.

Wang ZQ, Ovitt C, Grigoriadis AE et al (1992) Bone and haematopoietic defects in mice lacking c-fos, *Nature* **360**: 741–5.

Wesolowski G, Duong LT, Lakkakorpi PT et al (1995) Isolation and characterization of highly enriched, prefusion mouse osteoclastic cells, *Exp Cell Res* **219**: 679–86.

Wiktor-Jedrzejczak W, Bartocci A, Ferrante AWJ et al (1990) Total absence of colony-stimulating factor 1 in the macrophage-deficient osteopetrotic (op/op) mouse, *Proc Natl Acad Sci USA* **87**: 4828–32.

Wong GL, Cohn DV (1975) Target cells in bone for parathyroid hormone and calcitonin are different: enrichment for each cell type by sequential digestion of mouse calvaria and adhesion to polymeric surfaces, *Proc Natl Acad Sci USA* **72**: 3167–71.

Yoneda T, Alsina MM, Garcia JL et al (1991) Differentiation of HL-60 cells into cells with the osteoclast phenotype, *Endocrinology* **129**: 683–9.

Yoshida H, Hayashi S, Kunisada T et al (1990) The murine mutation osteopetrosis is in the coding region of the macrophage colony stimulating factor gene, *Nature* **345**: 442–4.

Young RW (1962) Cell proliferation and specialization during endochondral osteogenesis in young rats, *J Cell Biol* **141**: 357.

Zambonin Zallone A, Teti A, Primavera MV (1982) Isolated osteoclasts in primary culture: first observations on structure and survival in cultured media, *Anat Embryol* **165**: 405–13.

Zambonin Zallone A, Teti A, Primavera MV (1984) Monocytes from circulating blood fuse in vitro with purified osteoclasts in primary culture, *J Cell Sci* **66**: 335–42.

CHAPTER 3

Osteoblasts, bone formation and mineralization

Bone formation is an extremely complex process which is not well understood. This is hardly surprising when the multiple requirements of the process are considered. For example, not only is bone a unique mineralized connective tissue that provides the structural support for the body, it is also a storehouse for essential ions. The skeleton is a repository for 99% of the body's calcium, 80% of the phosphate, and a major proportion of the body's stores of magnesium, sodium and carbonate. The skeleton is a source of these ions during times of systemic deficiency, so that during calcium deficiency, bone resorption maintains the serum calcium at the expense of the skeleton. The skeleton also provides a defense mechanism against systemic acidosis and assists renal and respiratory systems in maintaining acid–base balance. During bone resorption, additional phosphate and carbonate are released to help buffer systemic acidosis. The cellular events involved in bone formation restore packets of this complex tissue which has been lost during resorption. The bone formation process varies in different parts of the skeleton—endochondral bone formation in the long bones is characterized by an intermediate cartilage phase, whereas intramembranous bone growth occurs without an intermediate phase in the flat bones. A variation of the latter is the appositional bone formation that occurs at sites of previous resorption on endosteal surfaces and within Haversian systems. The formation of bone is not surprisingly more difficult to study than bone resorption, a relatively simpler process, and the in vitro systems for studying bone resorption are much better developed.

Cells in the osteoblast lineage

Osteoblasts

Osteoblasts represent a heterogeneous family of cells (Figure 3.1), which are derived from the stromal cell system (Owen 1985). This family includes mature osteoblasts, which synthesize the proteins of the bone matrix, osteocytes, which are buried within bone and communicate with each other via the canalicular system, and the bone lining cells, which cover bone surfaces. Since the function of each of these different cells of the osteoblast lineage is different, they will be considered separately. Cells in the osteoblast lineage have a common stromal cell precursor shared with adipocytes, reticular cells, fibroblasts and chondrocytes (Owen 1985). The factors involved in controlling differentiation of cells in the osteoblast lineage have not yet been fully identified, although a number of growth regulatory factors that influence osteoblast proliferation and differentiation have recently been implicated.

Mature osteoblasts are cuboidal cells that have a single eccentric nucleus and a well developed endoplasmic reticulum and Golgi apparatus. They have the capacity to synthesize the proteins of the

OSTEOBLASTS, BONE FORMATION AND MINERALIZATION

Figure 3.1

Cells involved in bone formation as demonstrated by local injection of transforming growth factor β into subcutaneous tissue over the calvarium of a normal mouse. TGFβ (0.1 µg) was given by subcutaneous injection for 3 days, and the bone was sectioned 2 days later. Note the marked increase in cellular activity, involving all cells linked to the bone formation process, including proliferating cells as well as differentiating cells. Also note woven bone adjacent to the normal bone periosteal surface. (Reproduced from Marcelli et al (1990).)

bone matrix such as Type I collagen and the bone Gla protein (osteocalcin). They also contain the membrane-bound ectoenzyme alkaline phosphatase, which probably plays an essential role in bone mineralization and which is frequently used by bone cell biologists as a marker for cells with the osteoblast phenotype, as well as by clinicians as a serum marker of osteoblast activity.

Of some interest are the cell attachment molecules utilized by osteoblasts. It appears from in vitro studies that cell clustering and possibly attachment are important in bone nodule formation and subsequent bone mineralization (Bellows et al 1986), and it has long been thought that heterotypic interactions between osteoblast lineage cells and osteoclast lineage cells are important in bone resorption. Recently, members of the cadherin family of molecules have been implicated in these interactions. An OB-cadherin has recently been cloned from osteoblasts and appears specific for these cells (Okazaki et al 1994). We have found a role for E-cadherin in osteoclast formation (Mbalaviele et al 1995), and more recently a possible role for cadherin-6 (also called cadherin-K) and its isoforms in osteoblast–osteoclast heterotypic interactions (Mbalaviele et al 1996). Of course, these are not the only cell attachment molecules likely to be involved in mediating direct cell–cell contact in the bone microenvironment.

Functions

- Osteoblasts are responsible for the production of the proteins of the bone matrix, including Type I collagen and osteocalcin, which are often used as markers, and others such as osteopontin, bone sialoproteins and osteonectin.

- Osteoblasts secrete the growth factors which are stored in the bone matrix, such as transforming growth factor β, bone morphogenetic proteins, platelet-derived growth factor and the insulin-like growth factors (Hauschka et al 1986).

- Osteoblasts mineralize newly formed bone matrix. This may be mediated in part by subcellular particles known as matrix vesicles, which are generated from the osteoblast cytoplasm (Bonucci 1971). Matrix vesicles are enriched in alkaline phosphatase. Osteoblasts also produce other bone matrix constituents that may be important in the mineralization process such as phospholipids and proteoglycans (see below).

- Osteoblasts may be required for normal bone resorption to occur. Experimental data suggest that osteoblasts or their progeny (bone lining cells) may act as accessory cells for osteoclastic resorption (Rodan and Martin 1981; McSheehy and Chambers 1986). Interactions may occur either between these cells by cell–cell contact with osteoclasts or osteoclast precursors, by the production of soluble mediators that are required for osteoclasts to resorb bone, or by preparing the bone surface for osteoclastic resorption by the production of proteolytic enzymes.

Osteocytes

Osteocytes are buried within the mineralized matrix of bone. They are the most abundant of the bone cells. There are ten times as many osteocytes as osteoblasts (Parfitt 1977). They are derived from osteoblasts which have successfully synthesized bone matrix and then become incorporated within that matrix. Osteocytes communicate with each other and with cells on the bone surface via their dendritic processes encased in canaliculi. Their normal function is unknown. One function that has long been ascribed to them is the capacity to resorb bone by enlarging osteocyte lacunae, but more recent evidence suggests that this "osteocytic osteolysis" may represent fixation artefact (Boyde 1980). Osteocytes have been shown to express transforming growth factor β (TGFβ) and possibly other growth factors. Whether this observation has physiological significance requires further study. It has been suggested that weight-bearing loads may influence behavior of bone remodeling cells on bone surfaces by effects on osteocytes buried within bone, which subsequently release mediators such as TGFβ into the canalicular system. Bone lining cells, which are probably osteocytes present on the bone surface, have been implicated as accessory cells in the bone resorption process (see above).

Recently, attempts have been made to culture isolated populations of osteocytes in order to understand better their cell biology (Nijweide and Mulder 1986; Kato et al 1996). Kato et al (1997) have established a cell line from primary osteocyte cultures in which the cells were derived from transgenic mice where the transgene was the large T antigen linked to the osteocalcin promoter. These cells may make it possible to study the mechanisms by which load-bearing alters bone remodeling, and the means by which osteocytes communicate with cells on bone surfaces.

There is a specific bone fluid that circulates through the canalicular system and bathes the bone surface. It is separated from the extracellular fluid by a bone "membrane" which probably consists of bone lining cells. These lining cells function to keep calcium in the extracellular fluid, where it is supersaturated with respect to bone (Parfitt 1987). Their overall function may be to "buffer" short-term fluctuations in extracellular fluid calcium concentrations. It is unknown whether this process of exclusion of calcium from the bone fluid by the bone lining cells is hormone-regulated, although this seems highly likely.

Experimental models used to study the osteoblast phenotype and bone formation

For over 25 years, bone cell biologists have been studying the functions of isolated cells with the osteoblast phenotype in culture. The first attempts were made with rodent bone cells derived from the calvariae of fetal rat pups (Peck et al 1964). During the following 10 years, attempts were made to separate cells from explanted rodent calvariae into the osteoblast and osteoclast subpopulations by using sequential enzyme digestion (Wong and Cohn, 1974; Luben et al 1976). Early in the digestion process, cells with "osteoclast" characteristics are released. The cells released later after enzyme digestion are more osteoblastic, at least as assessed by their hormonal responsiveness. As an alternative to freshly dispersed bone cells, some workers began to characterize osteosarcoma cell lines for their osteoblastic characteristics (Martin et al 1976; Majeska et al 1978, 1980). However, cultured osteosarcoma cells do not behave in the same manner in vitro as do freshly dispersed primary osteoblasts, and even differ significantly from each other in behavior (Mundy et al 1993). This has raised the possibility that these transformed cells are either "frozen" at a specific stage in differentiation, or their proliferation and differentiation programs overlap so that they do not represent any normal cell in the osteoblast lineage. It seems more likely that the latter explanation is probably correct.

Aubin and colleagues have used normal fetal rat calvarial cells in prolonged culture that have been subcloned to reveal different characteristics and studied differentiation of these cells in response to different types of hormones (Grigoriadis et al 1988). Other investigators have also tried to establish permanent cell lines from rodent calvarial cultures, and have been most notably successful with murine cultures. One cell line, MC3T3-E1, has now been widely studied as a nontransformed osteoblast-like cell derived from normal calvarial cells (Kodama et al 1982). Other workers have used stromal cells, loosely defined cells of the stromal system which may have the capacity to support osteoclast activation or osteoclast formation. In the case of murine ST2 and PA6 cells, cell–cell contact may be involved in osteoclast activation (Udagawa et al 1989). In the case of C433 cells, a stromal cell line derived from a giant cell tumor of bone, it has been shown that the cells produce 5-lipoxygenase metabolites that may be important both for osteoclast and giant cell activation (Gallwitz et al 1993).

Although cell lines are convenient to use and readily renewable, they are not reliable for determining lineage. The variations in responsivity from one cell line to the next led workers to develop a method for prolonged primary culture of isolated fetal rat calvarial osteoblasts with β-glycerophosphate to enhance mineralization and ascorbic acid to support matrix formation (Bellows et al 1986). The bone cells formed clusters over several weeks, which in turn became surrounded by nodules of woven bone. Owen et al (1990) have used the same model of freshly isolated rodent calvarial cells to compare protein production and gene expression during differentiation with different types of osteosarcoma cells (Figure 3.2). They have suggested the osteosarcoma cells give limited information in this regard compared with freshly isolated rodent cells. Using cultures of fetal rat calvarial cells for 3 weeks or more, a developmental cascade of gene expression can be followed. Initially, there is expression of histone proteins during the proliferative phase, followed later by genes associated with bone matrix formation such as Type I collagen, then later by genes associated with mineralization such as Type I collagen, alkaline phosphatase and osteocalcin. Harris et al (1994) have also used cultures of primary fetal rat calvarial osteoblasts to show that growth factors such as the BMPs, TGFβ and FGF–II are expressed by osteoblasts as they differentiate.

One of the major problems with studying bone cells in culture is their heterogeneity as well as their inaccessibility and the inconvenience of handling freshly dispersed cells. To overcome this problem, we have established a number of cell lines using promoters which are specifically utilized at different stages in the osteoblast lineage linked to SV40 large T-antigen, which immortalizes cells (Ghosh-Choudhury et al 1994, 1996). We have found that several of these cell lines behave identically to fetal rat calvarial osteoblasts in culture. These cell lines have been cloned and can be used now as surrogates for fetal rat calvarial cells. These have many advantages over many of the osteosarcoma cell lines, which are trans-

Figure 3.2

Technique for studying capacity of fetal rat calvarial osteoblasts to form mineralized bone nodules in prolonged primary culture (Bellows et al 1986, Owen et al 1990). Note how as the cells differentiate there is a sequential expression of genes involved in bone cell differentiation. (These data were kindly supplied by Drs Gary Stein and Jane Lian.)

formed cells and do not neatly fit into the behavior of normal freshly isolated osteoblasts and their precursors. These cells respond appropriately to growth regulatory factors, including BMPs, TGFβ and the FGFs, in a similar manner to rat calvarial osteoblasts.

Attempts have also been made to study human bone cells in vitro (Beresford et al 1984). These have also been isolated by enzyme digestion from cancellous bone surfaces. Various manipulations of cell isolation have been performed to enrich for the osteoblast phenotype. However, difficulties have been encountered because of variability in cell populations and unreliable hormone responses, presumably due to variable cellular compositions from isolation to isolation.

Organ culture methods have been made to study bone forming cells. Raisz and co-workers used organ cultures of fetal rat calvariae and studied collagenase-digestible protein synthesis as a parameter of bone collagen synthesis and bone formation (Dietrich et al 1976). This particular system has been responsible for much information about the effects of hormones and factors on bone collagen synthesis (Canalis et al 1989), although the effects observed in this system in response to factors such as 1,25-dihydroxyvitamin D_3, cortisol and transforming growth factor β are hard to reconcile with known effects of these factors in vivo. Nevertheless, they are similar to those observed in prolonged cultures of fetal rat calvarial cells, which form mineralized nodules.

Structural composition of bone

There are two major types of bone. Cortical or compact bone is present mainly in the long bone shafts. Cancellous bone occurs predominantly in the vertebrae, proximal ends of the long bones and ribs. Cortical bone makes up approximately 75% of the total skeleton and cancellous bone 20%. The approximate proportions of cortical and cancellous components of different parts of the skeleton are shown in Chapter 1.

Bone collagen

There are at least 13 genetically distinct types of collagen molecules which have been identified in mammalian connective tissues (Gordon et al 1987; Mayne and Burgeson 1987; Tikka et al 1988; Eyre et al 1990). Bone consists predominantly of Type I collagen, which belongs to the fibril-forming Class I collagens (types I, II, III, V and XI) which are the products of at least eight separate genes. These collagens are similar in size, comprising a single uninterrupted triple helix of three alpha chains, each about 1015 amino acids in length.

Type I collagen, which comprises about 90% of the bone matrix, is a complex molecule that consists of a heterotrimer of two pro-α1(I) and one pro-α2(I) polypeptide chains. These peptide chains are structurally very similar but genetically distinct. The genes for the pro-α1(I) and pro-α2(I) chains are located on different chromosomes. The Type I collagen molecule is highly coiled because every third amino acid residue in the helical domain is glycine, which does not have a bulky side chain and allows these coils to occur.

Type I procollagen is characterized by the repeating triplet (Gly–X–Y), and where glycine is frequently followed by a proline. The steps involved in collagen synthesis are extremely complicated, and there are multiple potential sites for regulation, both during and subsequent to translation. The post-translational modifications of Type I collagen that are specific for bone include hydroxylation of some proline and lysine residues, and glycosylation of hydroxylysyl residues to form galactosyl–hydroxylysyl residues (in contrast to skin, where glucosyl–galactosyl–hydroxylysyl residues are formed). Other post-translational modifications include assembly of the two pro-α1(I) chains and the single pro-α2(I) chain into a triple helix, and translocation of the product through the Golgi complex to a secretory pathway. Bone Type I collagen is very insoluble due to the intra- and intermolecular crosslinks. This crosslinking occurs within the extracellular space. Collagen molecules are cleaved in the extracellular space at both the N-terminal and C-terminal by specific N-terminal and C-terminal peptidases. Crosslinking of the molecules occurs and the collagens become packed in a one-quarter stagger array. Electron microscopy of collagen fibrils shows that bone Type I collagen molecules are organized in a characteristic staggered arrangement with gaps between the end of one molecule and the beginning of the next, the so-called "hole zones" where mineralization occurs. Specific interactions occur between collagen and other extracellular macromolecules, such as fibronectin, osteonectin, and the proteoglycans. Once the alignment of the collagen molecule and related macromolecules occurs, the mineralization process can presumably take place.

Osteogenesis imperfecta is a hereditable disorder of Type I collagen. It is due to a variety of point mutations in either the pro-α1(I) or pro-α2(I) chains, the two distinctive polypeptide chains that comprise the precursor of Type I collagen known as Type I procollagen. Over 100 different procollagen mutations have been identified in unrelated probands with osteogenesis imperfecta. In a few cases, the mutations cause decreased synthesis of pro-α1(I) or pro-α2(I) chains, although in most cases the disease is associated with the synthesis of structurally abnormal collagen chains that lead to abnormalities in collagen function. For example, mutations that produce subtle changes in the conformation of the procollagen molecule can interfere with fibril assembly markedly, and the patients present with the clinical picture of osteoporosis (Spotila et al 1991). N-terminal mutations are associated with the mildest disease. Definitive proof that these abnormalities in collagen are responsible for the disease phenotype has been shown in transgenic mice expressing these mutations (Stacey et al 1988).

A number of animal models have been developed that indicate the relationship between abnormal expression of Type I collagen genes and osteoporosis. The Mov 13 mouse contains the Moloney leukemia virus inserted into the first intron of the pro-α1(I) gene for collagen, leading to impaired production of Type I collagen. Homozygous mice have lethal osteogenesis imperfecta, but heterozygous mice develop milder osteopenic skeletal disease (Stacey et al 1988; Bonadio et al 1990). In another transgenic model of osteogenesis imperfecta, a pro-α1(I) minigene containing an internal deletion of exon 45 also leads to impaired production of pro-α1(I) collagen. Some of the resultant transgenic mice have the clinical phenotype of osteoporosis. In a third model of osteoporosis, the OIM mouse, there is a naturally occurring mutation in pro-α2(I) gene that impairs synthesis of normal procollagen heterotrimer. Heterozygotes with this disorder also have the clinical phenotype of osteoporosis (Chipman et al 1993).

The relationship between abnormalities and expression of Type I collagen and osteoporosis is intriguing, but is not well understood at the pathophysiologic level. Why mutations in the Type I collagen gene or impaired procollagen synthesis should cause bone fragility with a propensity to fractures and the characteristic histologic picture of osteoporosis is not clear.

Noncollagenous proteins in bone

In recent years, a series of noncollagen proteins have been isolated in bone, with potentially important biological activities.

Bone Gla protein (osteocalcin) and related proteins

Bone Gla protein, also called osteocalcin, is a highly conserved 6000 dalton protein that contains three γ-carboxyglutamic acid residues that allow it to bind calcium. It composes about 20% of the noncollagen proteins in human bone. The γ-carboxylation of osteocalcin is caused by post-translational modifications of the protein and is dependent on vitamin K. Bone Gla protein is probably made exclusively by osteoblasts, but it is not released constitutively. It is produced by cells with the characteristics of osteoblasts when they are incubated with 1,25-dihydroxyvitamin D_3. Osteocytes produce even more osteocalcin than osteoblasts (Mikuni-Takagaki et al 1996). Although the function of the bone Gla protein is entirely unknown, it has been postulated that the bone Gla protein could retard mineralization (Price et al 1982). Bone Gla protein can also act as a chemoattractant for osteoclast progenitors, attracting them towards bone surfaces (Malone et al 1982). However, rats treated with the anticoagulant warfarin, an antagonist of vitamin K activity, have essentially no osteocalcin in their skeletons but have no detectable bone abnormalities (Price et al 1982). Like alkaline phosphatase, the bone Gla protein is currently being used as a marker of osteoblast activity in clinical states, although there are some discrepancies between the circulating levels of these two proteins in disorders of increased bone turnover.

Recently, Ducy et al (1996) have shown that when a null mutation is introduced into the germ line of mice, the resultant mice that are osteocalcin deficient have a peculiar abnormality in bone formation resulting in increased cortical bone thickness. This suggests that osteocalcin has a negative or inhibitory effect on osteoblast differentiation. Much work needs to be done to clarify the precise role of osteocalcin in osteoblast function, but for the first time there seems to be a reasonable start for studying the physiological effects of osteocalcin on bone formation.

The serum bone Gla protein can be measured by radioimmunoassay (Price et al 1980) and serves as a marker of increased bone turnover, and in particular as a parameter of enhanced osteoblast activity. It is widely believed that expression of osteocalcin is a unique characteristic of osteoblasts (Delmas 1993), although as noted above osteocytes also express osteocalcin. Recently developed sandwich assays using monoclonal antibodies have improved the sensitivity and specificity of osteocalcin assays. Since circulating concentrations of osteocalcin do not correlate perfectly with measurements of serum alkaline phosphatase, it seems likely that these two osteoblast products are probably produced by cells at different stages in the osteoblast lineage. The clinical usefulness of measurements of bone Gla protein remain to be determined.

There is a second γ-carboxylated (Gla protein) in bone known as the matrix Gla protein. Its function in bone is entirely unknown (Otawara and Price 1986; Price 1987). It is approximately 9 kilodaltons in size, is found in cartilage in bone, and has some structural homology to bone Gla protein. It is presumably a naturally occurring inhibitor of extracellular calcification in blood vessels, since knockout mice die within 4 weeks of birth with massive calcification of elastic arteries leading to rupture (McKee et al 1996).

Osteonectin

Osteonectin is a 32-kilodalton acidic glycoprotein that was also purified from the bone matrix (Termine et al 1981). It is the most abundant non-collagen protein in bone. Although it is synthesized by osteoblasts, it is also synthesized by skin fibroblasts, tendon cells and odontoblasts. Its function is unknown, although it is phosphorylated, glycosylated, highly crosslinked and binds avidly to collagen and to mineral surfaces. It binds strongly to Type I collagen and hydroxyapatite, and promotes or initiates crystal growth in vitro. Osteonectin is found in teeth and in bone, but not in tendon.

Other macromolecules

Other macromolecules found in bone have recently been studied, including a number of proteoglycans whose physiological functions are unknown. These proteoglycans are composed of a central protein core to which glycosoaminoglycans (namely chondroitin sulfate or heparan sulfate) are attached (Fisher and Termine 1985). Proteoglycan-II (also called decorin) has a core protein of about 45 kilodaltons and is different from similar proteoglycans found in cartilage and tendon. It contains a single chondroitin sulfate and occurs in a periodic manner within collagen fibrils, thus "decorating" collagen fibrils. Decorin appears to regulate collagen fibril formation.

Proteoglycan-I (biglycan), like decorin, also has a central core protein of 45 kilodaltons, but it contains two chondroitin sulfates rather than one, and is thus distinct from decorin. A bone sialoprotein of 60 kilodaltons has also recently been identified. Bone also contains α-2 HS glycoprotein, which is about 80 kilodaltons in size. It is synthesized in the liver but trapped within bone, where it binds to hydroxyapatite.

Cell attachment proteins

The bone matrix contains a number of different cell attachment proteins which have the common RGD (arginine–glycine–aspartic acid) amino acid sequence which is responsible for mediating attachment of these proteins to integrins (integral membrane proteins) on cell surfaces (Baron 1993). These cell attachment proteins include fibronectin, osteopontin, thrombospondin and several other bone sialoproteins, including one protein called bone sialoprotein and a second called BAG (bone acidic glycoprotein). Osteopontin has attracted particular interest, because recently it has been shown to bind the $\alpha_v\beta_3$ integrin receptor on osteoclasts by its RGD sequence (Tanaka et al 1991). This binding of osteopontin to the osteoclast integrin receptor leads to activation of the phospholipase C pathway in osteoclasts and increases in intracellular calcium. This process may involve the src tyrosine kinase which may be responsible for phosphorylating tyrosine residues on specific components of this pathway. Osteopontin also contains calcium binding sites. It is synthesized by both osteoclasts and osteoblasts. Osteopontin is a highly phosphorylated phosphoprotein which exists in multiple forms, due both to alternate splicing as well as post-translational variations in degrees of phosphorylation (Nemir et al 1989). Fibronectin is a ubiquitous cell attachment protein (Weiss and Reddi 1980) which is made locally by bone cells, but could also be synthesized elsewhere and brought in by the vasculature. It is not known if fibronectin has a special function in bone. Thrombospondin also contains calcium binding sites in addition to the RGD sequence. It is a trimer of approximately 450 000 molecular weight. It mediates cell attachment, but its particular function in bone remains unknown. Bone sialoprotein (BSP) (Herring 1972; Fisher et al

1983) and the other bone sialoprotein, BAG, have functions that are still not clear. However, recent studies in knockout mice show that marrow spaces are smaller in mice that do not express BSP (Aubin et al 1996). These observations are still preliminary, but the results seem more likely to indicate an increase in bone formation rather than an abnormality in osteoclast function. It is possible that all these cell attachment proteins in bone can maintain osteoclasts or other bone cells in particular locations by the interaction between the specific integrin receptors on these cells and the relevant bone attachment proteins. As shown in the case of osteopontin and osteoclasts, this attachment process may lead to cell activation.

Regulatory growth factors in bone

Recently, it has become apparent that there are a number of biologically active proteins in bone that have the potential to regulate bone cell activity. Most of these proteins are growth regulatory factors, including transforming growth factor β-I, transforming growth factor β-II, the bone morphogenetic proteins, platelet-derived growth factor, fibroblast growth factors, and insulin-like growth factors I (IGF-I) and II (IGF-II) (Hauschka et al 1986). The bone morphogenetic proteins are bone-derived peptides that are members of the extended transforming growth factor β (TGFβ) family, and which share approximately 30% amino acid homology with TGFβ. More than a dozen have been identified. These proteins are synthesized by bone cells locally, unlike α-2 HS glycoprotein, which is synthesized elsewhere and trapped within bone. The presence of BMPs in the bone microenvironment and their potent effects on bone cells may be very important for understanding the regulation of normal bone remodeling. They will be discussed in more detail under hormonal control of bone remodeling.

Cbfa-1 transcription factor

One of the most interesting findings recently reported has been the identification of a transcription factor for cis-acting elements in the osteocalcin promoter which appears to be osteoblast-specific. This transcription factor, called Cbfa-1, was cloned from nuclear extracts of osteoblasts and appears to be specifically expressed in osteoblasts (Ducy et al 1997). Null mutant mice have shown complete absence of bone at birth, but the presence of cartilage (Komori et al 1997; Otto et al 1997). A counterpart has been described in humans called cleidoocranial dysplasia (Mundlos et al 1997). This transcription factor is apparently responsible for causing differentiation of pre-osteoblasts to osteoblasts, and its direct role in regulation of expression of other osteoblast related genes is a current focus for attention which may represent one of the more important findings in osteoblast biology in recent years.

Different types of bone formation

The cellular mechanisms responsible for bone formation are different in different parts of the skeleton. The two major types are intramembranous and endochondral. A major difference between the two types is whether bone is formed de novo (intramembranous) or is preceded by a cartilage phase (endochondral).

Intramembranous bone formation

Intramembranous bone formation occurs in the periosteal column of long bones and the flat bones of the skull and face. The mechanism responsible for the flat bones of the calvarium and the face is presumably the mechanism that determines the width of the long bones. Intramembranous bone formation begins with the condensation of an island of mesenchymal cells that gradually differentiate into osteoblasts. The osteoblasts produce an extracellular matrix that enlarges and gradually mineralizes. As these bone-forming cells become buried in the matrix, they cease synthesizing bone and become osteocytes (see above). This process occurs independently of prior cartilage formation.

Endochondral bone formation

Endochondral bone formation is an entirely different process from intramembranous bone formation. Here, bone formation occurs on an anlage of cartilage. The cartilage is formed by chondroblasts and the cartilage anlage is eventually penetrated by blood vessels and gradually resorbed by multinucleated cells. A collar of bone gradually develops around this anlage to form the midshaft of the bone (diaphysis). At each end of the cartilage anlage, specialized areas contain hypertrophic chondrocytes that become the epiphyseal plates (growth plates). This is the area responsible for the continued elongation of the long bones during growth. Following resorption of the cartilage by the multinucleated cells, bone is laid down on the cartilaginous trabecular structure and is then remodeled by the action of osteoclasts and osteoblasts. A similar process probably occurs during fracture repair. This process of endochondral bone formation is disturbed by vitamin D deficiency. The resultant bone disease is called rickets. In this bone disease, the growth plate expands and mineralization of the bone matrix fails to occur.

Considerable insights have been gained in recent years into some of the regulatory mechanisms involved in endochondral bone formation. A key step is the transition from prehypertrophic cartilage cells to hypertrophic cartilage cells which occurs at the cartilage–bone transition zone. This step appears to be regulated by PTH-rP. In null mutant mice in which PTH-rP is deleted, there is enhanced cartilage cell differentiation (Karaplis et al 1994). The null mutant mice show the early appearance of hypertrophic chondrocytes, together with shortened columns of proliferating chondrocytes at the growth plate and premature appearance of mineralized osteoid tissue adjacent to the hypertrophic chondrocytes. PTH-rP clearly regulates this final step in chondrocyte differentiation negatively. When PTH-rP is added to limb explants of day 16.5 normal mouse embryos, there is suppression of differentiation of hypertrophic chondrocytes. PTH-rP inhibits cartilage cell differentiation in null mutant mice in which the PTH-rP gene is deleted. However, PTH-rP has no effect when added to limb explants from PTH/PTH-rP receptor knockout mice. A member of the hedgehog family of secreted proteins, Indian hedgehog, appears to be involved. Indian hedgehog is expressed by prehypertrophic chondrocytes and seems also to regulate the final step of cartilage cell differentiation negatively. Vortkamp et al (1996) have suggested that Indian hedgehog mediates its effects on cartilage cell differentiation indirectly by enhancing production of PTH-rP in perichondrial cells. The role of BMPs in this process, and how they fit into this series of sequential signals, remains unclear. BMP-6 is found in high concentrations in hypertrophic cartilage cells and BMP-2 can accelerate differentiation of growing chondrocytes to mature matrix producing chondrocytes.

Prehypertrophic cartilage cells appear to have a distinct phenotype. They synthesize Indian hedgehog protein and Type X collagen. They are also responsive to 1,25-dihydroxyvitamin D_3, and thyroid hormones as well as PTH-rP. The cartilage cells at the growth plate, hypertrophic and prehypertrophic, secrete angiogenic factors which in turn attract endothelial cell outgrowths, which are required for the process of endochondral bone formation.

One of the age-old questions in endochondral bone formation is the fate of the cartilage cell in general, and in particular whether there is a direct transformation of chondrocytes to osteoblasts. The evidence for transformation appears fairly convincing in avian species, although not definitive as yet in mammals. Several in vitro studies have demonstrated that chondrocytes associated with calcifying cartilage matrix can acquire properties of osteoblasts (Canceddda et al 1992; Lian et al 1993). Recently, Scammell and Roach (1996) have shown evidence for direct bone formation by former chondrocytes by histologic examination of rapid fracture callus. However, this is a very difficult issue to prove. Some cartilage cells clearly undergo apoptosis, and others are likely to differentiate to cells in the osteoblast lineage. At earlier stages these cells clearly have multiple potentials in the stromal cell system, although whether the fully differentiated hypertrophic or prehypertrophic cartilage cell itself can differentiate to the osteoblast remains unclear.

There is also circumstantial evidence that hypertrophic chondrocytes can differentiate into osteoblasts based on transmission electron microscopy (Holtrop 1966, 1972), as well as immunofluorescence studies which show expression of both Types I and X collagen in fetal human epiphyseal chondrocytes (Kirsch et al 1992). New bone formation has been observed at the sites where chondrocytes derived from growth cartilage were implanted in the abdominal cavity of rats (Shimomura et al 1975). Transition of chondrocytes to osteoblasts was observed in co-cultures of cartilage fragments with the chorioallantoic membranes of chick embryos (Kahn and Simmonds 1977; Thesingh et al 1991) and also in cultures of the mandibular condyle (Strauss et al 1990). In culture, chondrocytes from chick embryo tibia and the ventral part of chick embryo vertebrae express osteoblast-like markers, such as osteocalcin, Type I collagen, osteonectin and osteopontin (Cancedda et al 1992; Lian et al 1993). Roach et al (1995) have recently demonstrated that chondrocytes in vivo, which are located within one lacunae, undergo asymmetric cell division, where one cell dies by apoptosis while the other divides again and differentiates into a bone forming cell. More recently, it has been shown that chondrocytes within the cartilage struts of rabbit fracture callus may alter their phenotype to become bone forming cells, which then directly replace the central cartilage core with bone (Scammell and Roche 1996).

Appositional growth

Endochondral bone formation ceases when the epiphyses close following puberty because of exposure to sex hormones. However, bone growth continues by appositional bone formation, a process that is probably analogous to intramembranous bone formation. This type of growth occurs in the periosteum, increasing the diameter of the long bone shafts. Appositional bone formation can also occur on cancellous bone surfaces in certain pathologic situations, which include osteoblastic metastases, fluoride treatment and electrical stimulation.

Remodeling

In adults, bone is removed in discrete packets by osteoclasts and then replaced by osteoblasts, a process known as bone remodeling and discussed in more detail in Chapter 1. It seems likely that the hormonal factors responsible for bone remodeling in Haversian systems and on endosteal bone surfaces could be similar or identical to the factors that regulate intramembranous and endochondral bone formation.

Mineralization

One of the unique and important aspects of the bone formation process is the biological mineralization of the bone proteins to form a mineralized matrix. Following the production of osteoid tissue (nonmineralized bone-matrix) by osteoblasts, the osteoid tissue is mineralized in an orderly and controlled manner by the dispersion of mineral within this matrix. The chemistry and processes initiating and controlling mineralization of bone are unclear. Bone many mineralize by several processes, i.e., collagen fibrils deposition or matrix vesicles. One thing that is clear is that calcium and phosphate are required and calcium is a suitable surface for crystal nucleation. Collagen may not only act as a nucleator but also as an organizer of crystal formation. It is distributed initially within the hole zones of collagen, the gaps between the ends of two collagen molecules, in a way that does not cause disruption to the spatial orientation of the collagen fibril. Although it is evident that the physicochemical process of mineralization must be carefully and tightly regulated, the precise nature of this regulation is still not understood.

Posner has reviewed the nature of bone mineral and the process of mineralization (Posner 1987), which has been an area of controversy for over 30 years. Long-standing data suggest that mineral is initially deposited as amorphous calcium phosphate, the initial solid phase formed at neutral pH. This phase is randomly and poorly ordered and amorphous when viewed by X-ray diffraction, which means that it generates no coherent X-ray diffraction pattern. Following deposition of amorphous calcium phosphate, a series of solid-phase transformation steps occur that lead to poorly crystalline hydroxyapatite as the final stable solid phase. The initiation of mineralization is probably caused by heterogeneous nucleation, the active binding of calcium, phosphate, and calcium-phosphate complexes at the nucleation site in the matrix, rather than by simple precipitation that would result in a random organization of the crystals. In mature bone, it is possible that poorly crystalline calcium carbonate-containing hydroxyapatite is deposited rather than an amorphous calcium phosphate or hydroxyapatite.

Factors potentially important in mineralization

Mineralization of bone is clearly influenced by the proteins present in the bone matrix, some of which act as inhibitors and some as enhancers of the mineralization process.

Collagen

There are several ways in which collagen is uniquely equipped to be mineralized. Collagen provides an oriented support for newly formed mineral crystals. There are structural and chemical differences in Type I bone collagen compared with other Type I collagens from skin, fascia or tendon, which are due to post-translational changes in the molecule. These changes may allow the ready diffusion of relatively large hydrated ions, such as calcium-phosphate ion complexes, into the fibril where they can participate in nucleation and growth of crystals. There are sites on the collagen molecule that have the capacity to initiate precipitation of crystals, such as free side chain groups of the positively charged amino acids lysine and hydroxylysine.

The specific longitudinal and lateral staggering of the collagen molecules in the fibril results in holes and pores in which nucleation, crystal growth, secondary nucleation, and multiplication of the solid phase can occur. This unique packing arrangement of fibrils allows more available space for mineral than is present in other soft-tissue collagens that do not mineralize. As a result of enzymatic post-translational phosphoryl transfer from adenosine triphosphate (and possibly other high-energy phosphate bonds), a sufficient number of organically bound collagen–phosphate groups and phosphate groups of other proteins are strategically placed within the collagen fibrils. These may then facilitate the formation of a solid phase from a solution. Thus, collagen may provide an oriented support for newly formed mineral crystals, allow for orderly mineralization by the structural arrangement of the fibrils, and regulate mineral size. However, collagen itself does not have the capacity to initiate mineralization.

Phosphoproteins

Bone sialoproteins and proteoglycans are minor constituents of the bone matrix. Phosphoproteins in the bone matrix may bind calcium to promote crystal deposition and growth and thereby act as nucleators. Crystal growth could then depend on the conformational change in these proteins after calcium binding. The initiation of mineralization is coincident with depolymerization of proteoglycan molecules. Proteoglycans may inhibit calcification by a number of mechanisms that include shielding the collagen fibrils and thereby diminishing the rate of diffusion, by chemical interactions with certain side-chain groups of collagen, by sequestering calcium ions or calcium-phosphate ion complexes and excluding phosphate ions, or by occupying critical spaces or volumes within the fibril. Different phosphoproteins probably have varying degrees of importance in regulating the mineralization process.

Pyrophosphate

Pyrophosphate is a naturally occurring inhibitor of calcification. Pyrophosphate has a short half-life in the circulation due to its rapid enzymatic degradation by pyrophosphatases. Pyrophosphate is widely expressed in the body fluids and increases the stability of the solution phase of calcium-phosphate. The bisphosphonates are stable pyrophosphate analogs that also inhibit calcification in large doses.

Bone Gla protein (osteocalcin)

The bone Gla protein (osteocalcin), a highly conserved and abundant protein found in the bone matrix, contains γ-carboxyglutamic acid residues that bind to calcium. Its role in physiological bone formation is undergoing reappraisal. Depletion of this protein from newly formed bone by treatment of animals with anticoagulants such as warfarin results in no impairment of mineralization (Price et al 1982; Price 1987). It has been suggested recently that bone Gla protein could act as an inhibitor rather than a promoter of the mineralization process. Recent studies in osteocalcin knockout mice showing an increase in cortical bone width necessitate re-evaluation of all these earlier studies (Ducy et al 1996). These latter results suggest that it functions as a physiological inhibitor of bone formation.

Lipids and proteolipids

Within bone there are acidic phospholipids that form complexes with calcium-phosphate and could thereby influence the mineralization process. These acidic phospholipids have the capacity to bind to calcium.

Alkaline phosphatase

Alkaline phosphatase is an ecto-enzyme produced by osteoblasts that is a useful marker of osteoblast activity and is likely to be involved in the mineralization process from circumstantial in vitro data. In support of this, patients with the disease hypophosphatasia, which is characterized by reduced circulating alkaline phosphatase activity, have impaired bone mineralization. Bone alkaline phosphatase is present in high concentrations in matrix vesicles, but its precise role in mineralization is still not clear. Alkaline phosphatase may be involved in the degradation of inorganic pyrophosphate, thus providing a sufficient local concentration of phosphate or inorganic pyrophosphate for mineralization to proceed.

Cellular components involved in the mineralization process

A nucleation site is required for calcium-phosphate crystal formation for initiation of mineralization. The initial site of mineral deposition in some tumors such as calcifying cartilage appears to be the matrix vesicle. Matrix vesicles are extracellular organelles, derived from both chondroblasts and osteoblasts, which appear to form nucleation sites for precipitation of hydroxyapatite crystals. These matrix vesicles have been observed in growth-plate cartilage as well as in maturing bone (Anderson 1969). They are likely to be more important in calcifying cartilage and rapidly forming woven bone rather than in lamellar bone, since unlike the former they are rarely seen in lamellar bone. Extrusion of the vesicle and its contents occurs at the cell surface into the osteoid next to the mineralizing bone. They are highly enriched in alkaline phosphatase, ATP, proteases, peptidase, proteolipids and phospholipase A_2. They presumably function by concentrating calcium and phosphate, removing inhibitors of mineralization, and by creating a favorable environment for the mineralization process. For review see Sela et al (1992).

Mitochondria have also been implicated in the mineralization process (Anderson 1983). Mitochondria are highly enriched in calcium and phosphate, and they may release calcium-phosphate ion complexes during mineral deposition. Moreover, mitochondria in cells derived from tissues that are calcified contain more calcium-phosphate than mitochondria from noncalcifying tissues. However, their precise role in mineralization is unknown.

Hormonal control of mineralization

Although mineralization is highly influenced by the structural molecules present in the bone matrix, it is also apparent that mineralization is under hormonal control. One clear requirement for the normal mineralization of bone is the availability of active vitamin D metabolites. Impaired mineralization (diseases known as rickets in children or osteomalacia in adults) can be caused by deficiencies in vitamin D or by abnormalities in vitamin D metabolism. Whether vitamin D regulates mineralization by a direct effect or whether its effects are indirect and due to an adequate supply of calcium and phosphate provided at the mineralization site by the actions of vitamin D metabolites remains unclear.

Impairment of normal mineralization may be caused by vitamin D deficiency, by aluminum intoxication, by fluoride intoxication, and by a deficiency of phosphate. The precise mechanisms by which aluminum and fluoride cause impaired mineralization are still not clear.

Proposed scheme of mineralization

Although there are many events in the mineralization process that are not understood, the following is a possible scheme for cartilage calcification. Chondroblasts at the growth plate secrete collagen and other bone matrix proteins. Collagen may provide the major structural background for the deposition of mineral that can be laid down in an orderly manner, and the acidic phosphoproteins and proteolipids may regulate crystal size and rate of deposition. Matrix vesicles are budded off from chondroblasts or osteoblasts, possibly under control of vitamin D metabolites. These matrix vesicles are highly enriched in enzymes such as alkaline phosphatase and ATPases which are necessary to initiate mineralization on the structural protein support. Once crystal growth is initiated, its size and shape is then regulated in an orderly manner by the macromolecules in the matrix in which it is laid down.

References

Anderson HC (1969) Vesicles associated with calcification in the matrix of epiphyseal cartilage, *J Cell Biol* **41**: 59–72.

Anderson HC (1983) Calcific diseases—a concept, *Arch Pathol Lab Med* **107**: 341–8.

Aubin JE, Gupta AK, Zirngbl R et al (1996) Knockout mice lacking bone sialprotein expression have bone abnormalities, *J Bone Miner Res* **11** (Suppl 1): no 30.

Baron R (1993) The biology of the osteoclast. In: Mundy GR, Martin TJ, eds, *Physiology and pharmacology of bone. Handbook of experimental pharmacology* (Springer-Verlag: Berlin) 111–47.

Bellows CG, Aubin JE, Heersche JN et al (1986) Mineralized bone nodules formed in vitro from enzymatically released rat calvaria cell populations, *Calcif Tissue Int* **38**: 143–54.

Beresford JN, Gallagher JA, Poser JW et al (1984) Production of osteocalcin by human bone cells in vitro. Effects of 1,25(OH)$_2$D$_3$, 24,25(OH)$_2$D$_3$, parathyroid hormone, and glucocorticoids, *Metab Bone Dis Relat Res* **5**: 229–34.

Bonadio J, Saunders TL, Tsai E et al (1990) Transgenic mouse model of the mild dominant form of osteogenesis imperfecta, *Proc Natl Acad Sci USA* **87**: 7145–59.

Bonucci E (1971) The locus of initial calcification in cartilage and bone, *Clin Orthop* **78**: 108–39.

Boyde A (1980) Electron microscopy of the mineralizing front. In: Jee WS, Parfitt AM, eds, *Bone histomorphometry. Third International Workshop* (Société Nouvelle de Publications Médicales et Dentaires: Paris) 69–78.

Canalis E, McCarthy T, Centrella M (1989) The role of growth factors in skeletal remodeling, *Endocrinol Metab Clin N Am* **18**: 903–18.

Cancedda FD, Gentili C, Manduca P et al (1992) Hypertrophic chondrocytes undergo further differentiation in culture, *J Cell Biol* **117**: 427–35.

Chipman SD, Sweet HO, McBride DJ et al (1993) Defective proalpha2(I) collagen synthesis in a recessive mutation in mice—a model of human osteogenesis imperfecta, *Proc Natl Acad Sci USA* **90**: 7701–5.

Delmas P (1993) Biochemical markers of bone formation. In: Mundy GR, Martin TJ, eds, *Physiology and pharmacology of bone. Handbook of experimental pharmacology* (Springer-Verlag: Berlin) 673–724.

Dietrich JW, Canalis EM, Maina DM et al (1976) Hormonal control of bone collagen synthesis in vitro: effects of parathyroid hormone and calcitonin, *Endocrinology* **98**: 943–9.

Ducy P, Desbois C, Boyce BF et al (1996) Increased bone formation in osteocalcin-deficient mice, *Nature* **382**: 448–52.

Ducy P, Zhang R, Geoffroy V et al (1997) Osf 2/Cbfa 1: A transcriptional activator of osteoblast differentiation, *Cell* **89**: 747–54.

Eyre DR, Wu JJ, Nizibizi C (1990) The collagens of bone and cartilage: molecular diversity and supramolecular assembly. In: Cohn DV, Glorieux FH, Martin TJ, eds, *Calcium regulation and bone metabolism* (Elsevier: Amsterdam) 188–94.

Fisher LW, Termine JD (1985) Purification of the non-collagenous proteins from bone: technical pitfalls and how to avoid them. In: Ornoy A, Harell A, Sela J, eds, *Current advances in skeletogenesis* (Elsevier: Amsterdam) 467.

Fisher LW, Whitson SW, Avioli LV et al (1983) Matrix sialoprotein of developing bone, *J Biol Chem* **258**: 12 723–7.

Gallwitz WE, Mundy GR, Lee CH et al (1993) 5-Lipoxygenase metabolites of arachidonic acid stimulate isolated osteoclasts to resorb calcified matrix, *J Biol Chem* **368**: 10 087–94.

Ghosh-Choudhury N, Windle JJ, Koop BA (1996) Immortalized murine osteoblasts derived from BMP 2-T-antigen expressing transgenic mice, *Endocrinology* **137**: 331–9.

Ghosh-Choudhury N, Harris MA, Feng JQ et al (1994) Expression of the BMP 2 gene during bone cell differentiation, *Crit Rev Eukaryot Gene Expr* **4**: 345–55.

Gordon MK, Gerecke DR, Olsen BR (1987) Type XXI collagen: distinct extracellular matrix component discovered by cDNA cloning, *Proc Natl Acad Sci USA* **84**: 6040–4.

Grigoriadis AE, Heersche JNM, Aubin JE (1988) Differentiation of muscle, fat, cartilage and bone from progenitor cells present in a bone-derived clonal cell population, *J Cell Biol* **106**: 2139–51.

Harris SE, Bonewald LF, Harris MA et al (1994) Effects of TGFβ on bone nodule formation and expression of bone morphogenetic protein-2, osteocalcin, osteopontin, alkaline phosphatase and Type I collagen mRNA in prolonged cultures of fetal rat calvarial osteoblasts, *J Bone Miner Res* **9**: 855–63.

Hauschka PV, Mavrakos AE, Iafrati MD et al (1986) Growth factors in bone matrix, isolation of multiple types by affinity chromatography on heparin-sepharose, *J Biol Chem* **261**: 12 665–74.

Herring GM (1972) The organic matrix in bone. In: Bourne GH, ed, *The biochemistry and physiology of bone* (Academic Press: New York) 127.

Holtrop ME (1966) The origin of bone cells in endochondral ossification. In: Fleisch H, ed, *Calcified tissues* (Springer-Verlag: Berlin-Heidelberg-New York) 32-6.

Holtrop ME (1972) The ultrastructure of the epiphyseal plate. II. The hypertrophic chondrocytes, *Calcif Tissue Res* **9**: 140.

Kahn AJ, Simmonds DJ (1977) Chondrocyte-to-osteocyte transformation in grafts of perichondrium-free epiphyseal cartilage, *Clin Orthop* **129**: 299–304.

Karaplis AC, Luz A, Glowacki J et al (1994) Lethal skeletal dysplasia from targeted disruption of the parathyroid hormone-related peptide gene, *Genes Dev* **8**: 277–89.

Kato Y, Qiao M, Windle J et al (1996) Establishment of a murine osteocyte-like cell line, *J Bone Miner Res* **11** (Suppl 1): T356.

Kato Y, Windle JJ, Koop BA et al (1997) Establishment of an osteocyte-like cell line MLO-Y4, *J Bone Miner Res*, in press.

Kirsch T, Swoboda B, von der Mark K (1992) Ascorbate independent differentiation of human chondrocytes in vitro: simultaneous expression of Types I and X collagen and matrix mineralization, *Differentiation* **52**: 89–100.

Kodama HA, Amagai Y, Koyama H et al (1982) Hormonal responsiveness of a preadipose cell line derived from newborn mouse calvaria, *J Cell Physiol* **112**: 83–8.

Komori T, Yagi H, Nomura S et al (1997) Targeted disruption of Cbfa 1 results in a complete lack of bone formation owing to maturational arrest of osteoblasts, *Cell* **89**: 755–64.

Lian JB, McKee MD, Todd AM et al (1993) Induction of bone-related proteins, osteocalcin and osteopontin, and their matrix ultrastructural localization with development of chondrocytes hypertrophy in vitro, *J Cell Biochem* **52**: 206–19.

Luben RA, Wong GL, Cohn DV (1976) Biochemical characterization with parathormone and calcitonin of isolated bone cells: provisional identification of osteoclasts and osteoblasts, *Endocrinology* **99**: 526–34.

Majeska RJ, Rodan SB, Rodan GA (1978) Maintenance of parathyroid hormone response in clonal rat osteosarcoma lines, *Exp Cell Res* **111**: 465–8.

Majeska RJ, Rodan SB, Rodan GA (1980) Parathyroid hormone-responsive clonal cell lines from rat osteosarcoma, *Endocrinology* **107**: 1494–503.

Malone JD, Teitelbaum SL, Hauschka PV et al (1982) Presumed osteoclast precursors (monocytes) recognize two or more regions of osteocalcin, *Calcif Tissue Int* **84**: 511.

Marcelli C, Yates AJP, Mundy GR (1990) In vivo effects of human recombinant transforming growth factor beta on bone turnover in normal mice, *J Bone Miner Res* **5**: 1087–96.

Martin TJ, Ingleton PM, Underwood JC et al (1976) Parathyroid hormone-responsive adenylate cyclase in induced transplantable osteogenic rat sarcoma, *Nature* **260**: 436–8.

Mayne R, Burgeson RE (1987) *Structure and function of collagen types* (Academic Press: Orlando).

Mbalaviele G, Chen H, Boyce BF et al (1995) The role of cadherin in the generation of multinucleated osteoclasts from mononuclear precursors in murine marrow, *J Clin Invest* **95**: 2757–65.

Mbalaviele G, Nishimura R, Reddy R et al (1996) Characterization of the molecular mechanisms of heterotypic osteoclast–osteoblast interactions during bone resorption—role of a novel cadherin-6 isoform, *J Bone Miner Res* **11** (Suppl 1): no 70.

McKee MD, Nanci A, Ducy P et al (1996) Extracellular matrix calcification in elastic and muscular arteries in matrix gla protein-deficient mice, *J Bone Miner Res* **11** (Suppl 1): no M593.

McSheehy PMJ, Chambers TJ (1986) Osteoblastic cells mediate osteoclastic responsiveness to parathyroid hormone, *Endocrinology* **118**: 824–8.

Mikuni-Takagaki Y, Suzuku Y, Kawase T et al (1996) Distinct responses of different populations of bone cells to mechanical stress, *Endocrinology* **137**: 2028–35.

Mundlos S, Otto F, Mundlos C et al (1997) Mutations involving the transcription factor Cbfa 1 cause cleidocranial dysplasia, *Cell* **89**: 773–80.

Mundy GR, Harris SE, Sabatini M et al (1993) The use of osteosarcoma cells to characterize factors which regulate bone cell function. In: Novak JF, McMaster JH, eds, *Frontiers of osteosarcoma research* (Hogrefe & Huber Publishers: Seattle, WA) 449–56.

Nemir M, DeVouge MW, Mukherjee BB (1989) Normal rat kidney cells secrete both phosphorylated and non-phosphorylated forms of osteopontin showing different physiological properties, *J Biol Chem* **264**: 18 202–8.

Nijweide PJ, Mulder RJP (1986) Identification of osteocytes in osteoblast-like cell cultures using a monoclonal antibody specifically directed against osteocytes, *Histochemistry* **84**: 342–7.

Okazaki M, Takeshita S, Kawai S et al (1994) Molecular cloning and characterization of OB-cadherin, a new member of cadherin family expressed in osteoblasts, *J Biol Chem* **269**: 12 092–8.

Otawara Y, Price PA (1986) Developmental appearance of matrix Gla protein during calcification in the rat, *J Biol Chem* **261**: 10 828–32.

Otto F, Thornell AP, Crompton T et al (1997) Cbfa 1, a candidate gene for cleidocranial dysplasia syndrome is essential for osteoblast differentiation and bone development, *Cell* **89**: 765–72.

Owen M (1985) Lineage of osteogenic cells and their relationship to the stromal system. In: Peck WA, ed, *Bone and Mineral Research, Annual 3* (Elsevier: Amsterdam) 1–26.

Owen TA, Holthuis J, Shalhoub V et al (1990) Evidence for a functional relationship between proliferation and initiation of osteoblast phenotype development. In: Cohn DV, Glorieux FH, Martin TJ, eds, *Calcium regulation and bone metabolism* (Elsevier: Amsterdam) 371–6.

Parfitt AM (1977) The cellular basis of bone turnover and bone loss, *Clin Orthop* **127**: 236–47.

Parfitt AM (1987) Bone plasma calcium homeostasis, *Bone* **8** (Suppl): S1–S8.

Peck WA, Birge SJ, Fedak SA (1964) Bone cells: biochemical and biological studies after enzymatic isolation, *Science* **146**: 1476–7.

Posner AS (1987) Bone mineral and the mineralization process. In: Peck WA, ed, *Bone and Mineral Research, Annual 5* (Elsevier: Amsterdam) 65–116.

Price PA (1987) Vitamin K-dependent bone proteins. In: Cohn DV, Martin TJ, Meunier PJ, eds, *Calcium regulation and bone metabolism: basic and clinical aspects, Vol 9* (Elsevier: Amsterdam) 419–25.

Price PA, Parthemore JG, Deftos LJ (1980) A new biochemical marker for bone metabolism, *J Clin Invest* **66**: 878–83.

Price PA, Williamson MK, Haba T et al (1982) Excessive mineralization with growth plate closure in rats on chronic warfarin treatment, *Proc Natl Acad Sci USA* **79**: 7734–8.

Roach H, Erenpreisa J, Aigner T (1995) Osteogenic differentiation of hypertrophic chondrocytes involves asymmetric cell division and apoptosis, *J Cell Biol* **131**: 483–94.

Rodan GA, Martin TJ (1981) Role of osteoblasts in hormonal control of bone resorption—a hypothesis, *Calcif Tissue Int* **33**: 349–51.

Scammell BE, Roach HI (1996) A new role for the chondrocyte in fracture repair: endochondral ossification includes direct bone formation by former chondrocytes, *J Bone Miner Res* **11**: 737–45.

Sela J, Schwartz Z, Swain LD et al (1992) The role of matrix vesicles in calcification. In: Bonucci E, ed, *Calcification in biological systems* (CRC Press: Florida) 73–105.

Shimomura Y, Yoneda T, Suzuki E (1975) Osteogenesis by chondrocytes from growth plate cartilage of rat rib, *Calcif Tissue Res* **19**: 179–87.

Spotila LD, Constantinou CD, Sereda L et al (1991) Mutation in a gene for type I procollagen (COL1A2) in a woman with postmenopausal osteoporosis—evidence for phenotypic and genotypic overlap with milk osteogenesis imperfecta, *Proc Natl Acad Sci USA* **88**: 5423–7.

Stacey A, Bateman J, Choi T et al (1988) Perinatal lethal osteogenesis imperfecta in transgenic mice bearing an engineered mutant pro-alpha1(I) collagen gene, *Nature* **332**: 131–6.

Strauss PG, Closs EI, Schmidt J, Erfle V (1990) Gene expression during osteogenic differentiation in mandibular condyles in vitro, *J Cell Biol* **110**: 1369–78.

Tanaka H, Hruska KA, Seino Y et al (1991) Disassociation of the macrophage-maturational effects of vitamin D from respiratory burst priming, *J Biol Chem* **266**: 10 888–92.

Termine JD, Kleinman HK, Whitson SW (1981) Osteonectin, a bone-specific protein linking mineral to collagen, *Cell* **26**: 99–105.

Thesingh CW, Groot CG, Wassenaar AM (1991) Transdifferentiation of hypertrophic chondrocytes in murine metatarsal bones, induced by co-cultured cerebrum, *Bone Miner* **25**: 40.

Tikka L, Pihlajaniemi T, Henttu P et al (1988) Gene structure for the alpha 1 chain of a human short chain collagen (Type XIII) with alternatively spliced transcripts and translation termination codon at the 5′ end of the last exon, *Proc Natl Acad Sci USA* **85**: 7491–5.

Udagawa N, Takahashi N, Akatsu T et al (1989) The bone marrow-derived stromal cell lines MC3T3-G2/PA6 and ST2 support osteoclast-cocultures with mouse spleen cells, *Endocrinology* **125**: 1805–13.

Vortkamp A, Lee K, Lanske B et al (1996) Regulation of rate of cartilage differentiation by Indian hedgehog and PTH-related protein, *Science* **273**: 613–22.

Weiss RE, Reddi AH (1980) Synthesis and localization of fibronectin during collagenous matrix–mesenchymal cell interaction and differentiation of cartilage and bone in vivo, *Proc Natl Acad Sci USA* **77**: 2074–8.

Wong G, Cohn DV (1974) Separation of parathyroid hormone and calcitonin-sensitive cells from non-responsive bone cells, *Nature* **252**: 713–15.

CHAPTER 4

Factors regulating bone resorbing and bone forming cells

The activity of osteoclasts and osteoblasts is under the control of both systemic hormones and cytokines generated in the bone cell microenvironment. The systemic hormones are parathyroid hormone, 1,25-dihydroxyvitamin D_3 and calcitonin, which are under negative feedback control and are regulated by extracellular fluid calcium concentrations. These hormones are primarily responsible for the maintenance of extracellular fluid calcium concentrations. Their effects on bone cells are in part responsible for calcium homeostasis, but their effects on the kidney and gut are probably more important. Control of calcium homeostasis is reviewed in Chapter 6. There are other systemic hormones that influence bone cell function but are not under negative feedback control by extracellular fluid calcium. These include estrogen and androgens, glucocorticoids, thyroid hormones, and growth hormone and growth regulatory factors such as insulin-like growth factor I. Bone cell formation is also controlled by cytokines and growth regulatory factors that are produced locally in bone by bone cells and marrow cells, and in some cases are even stored in the matrix and released in an active form when bone is resorbed. They are not controlled by extracellular fluid calcium concentrations, but how their production is regulated by other mechanisms is not clear. Although these factors have powerful local effects, they may also circulate when produced in sufficient amounts in pathologic situations and cause systemic effects.

Parathyroid hormone (PTH)

PTH acts on both bone resorbing cells and bone forming cells, but can have differing effects depending on whether it is administered continuously or intermittently. When administered continuously, it increases osteoclastic bone resorption and suppresses bone formation. However, when administered in low doses intermittently, it stimulates bone formation without major effects on resorption, a response which has been referred to as the so-called "anabolic" response to PTH.

In recent years there has been a marked increase in our understanding of the synthesis and secretion of parathyroid hormone, the domains in the hormone necessary for binding to and activation of the PTH receptor, and the sequence, structure and signaling mechanisms of its receptor.

Effects of PTH on bone resorption

PTH has been known to stimulate osteoclasts to resorb bone since the in vivo studies of Barnicot (1948) showed that when parathyroid glands were grafted into subcutaneous tissue over the calvariae of rats, there was a marked increase in adjacent osteoclast activity. This confirmed the observations that had been made by Albright et al

(1940) and others in patients with primary hyperparathyroidism over the preceding 30 years. They described a profound loss of bone associated with increased osteoclastic bone resorption accompanied by marrow fibrosis (the bone disease referred to in those times as "osteitis fibrosa cystica"). Understanding the effects of PTH on cells in the osteoclast lineage has mainly relied on in vitro studies. The organ culture experiments of Gaillard (1961) and Raisz (1965) using fetal rat long bones showed that PTH increased osteoclast activity to cause degradation of the bone matrix and release of bone mineral. In these systems, PTH is effective at concentrations of 10^{-7}-10^{-9}M (Figure 4.1). One of the characteristic effects of PTH in these organ culture systems is the phenomenon of "induction" (Raisz et al 1972a) whereby parathyroid hormone caused a prolonged resorptive response in the bones following a brief 4–6 hour exposure. In contrast, factors such as prostaglandins of the E series and 1,25-dihydroxyvitamin D_3 require more prolonged incubation in the bone cultures to stimulate resorption. In light of present knowledge, we suggest that agents which induce induction can do so by activating mature osteoclasts to resorb bone, whereas other factors probably exert their major effects on the formation of new osteoclasts. Bone resorption was associated with the production of lysosomal enzymes (Vaes 1968; Eilon and Raisz 1978).

Bone cells are never exposed to PTH alone in vivo (as is true for all the osteotropic hormones and cytokines), since other local and systemic hormones are always present. The effects of PTH on osteoclastic bone resorption may be modulated by these other factors. Garabedian et al (1974) showed that PTH and 1,25-dihydroxyvitamin D_3 work in concert on bone to increase the serum calcium concentration. Since PTH stimulates the production of 1,25-dihydroxyvitamin D_3 in the renal tubules, bone cells are exposed to a combination of both these hormones in vivo in states of PTH excess. The effects of PTH on renal tubular cells may be enhanced by 1,25-dihydroxyvitamin D_3 (Raisz 1970; Yamamoto et al 1984). Other factors may also influence the effects of PTH on renal tubular function and bone resorption. Interleukin-1 enhances the effects of PTH to stimulate bone resorption in vitro (Stashenko et al 1987) or provoke hypercalcemia in vivo (Sato et al 1989). Transforming growth factor α (TGFα) and epidermal growth factor have synergistic effects with PTH on bone resorption in vitro (Lorenzo and Quinton 1984; Sabatini et al 1990a,b) and hypercalcemia in vivo (Yates et al 1992). The effects of PTH and PTH-rP on bone cells and on renal tubular cells may be modulated by other factors such as TGFα, tumor necrosis factor, transforming growth factor β (TGFβ) and interleukin-1 (Gutierrez et al 1987; Gutierrez et al 1990; Katz et al 1992). It is important to recognize that although most of the information on the renal tubular effects of PTH in vitro has been described with PTH alone, PTH may cause increased production of other factors which may modulate its activity. For example, it has been shown that PTH increases the production of other factors such as 1,25-dihydroxyvitamin D_3 and interleukin-6 (Feyen et al 1989).

The morphologic effects of PTH on osteoclasts have been studied both in vitro and in vivo. In response to PTH, increased numbers of large

Figure 4.1

Effects of human PTH and human PTH-rP on bone resorption in organ cultures of fetal rat long bones. (Reproduced from Yates et al (1988).)

multinucleated osteoclasts are formed which have large active ruffled borders (Holtrop et al 1974). There is considerable question as to how PTH increases osteoclast formation and activity. PTH clearly stimulates the formation of new osteoclasts from their precursors. However, it is not possible at the present time to determine definitively at which steps in their lineage that osteoclasts respond to PTH, since these steps have not been clearly defined. It is likely that PTH acts later in the osteoclast lineage than factors such as transforming growth factor α and epidermal growth factor. Another unanswered question is whether or not PTH acts directly on cells in the osteoclast lineage, or whether its effects are indirect. The current dogma is that mature osteoclasts do not have PTH receptors and that the effects of PTH on formed osteoclasts are mediated indirectly. These data come from in vitro experiments in which mature cells are co-cultured with freshly isolated calvarial osteoblasts or osteosarcoma cells to enhance their bone resorbing capacity (McSheehy and Chambers 1986). However, these data do not exclude the possibility that PTH stimulates osteoclastic bone resorption without any important direct effect on the mature cells. It is possible that the major effect of PTH is to increase the formation of new osteoclasts, rather than acting on the mature cell to stimulate bone resorption. Moreover, there have been several recent reports suggesting that there may in fact be PTH receptors on mature osteoclasts (Teti et al 1991; Agarwala and Gay 1992). However, most workers have found that PTH receptors are not obvious in osteoclasts, but rather probably belong to the osteoblast lineage (Rouleau et al 1988). Whether PTH acts directly on earlier cells in the osteoclast lineage is also unknown. The experiments of Hakeda et al (1989) and Kurihara et al (1989) on cultures of cells with the osteoclast phenotype suggest there may be a direct effect. However, this does not exclude the possibility that there may also be additional indirect effects mediated through other cells which enhance the capacity of cells in the osteoclast lineage to form mature multinucleated osteoclasts.

Although it has not been definitively resolved that PTH does not have direct effects on osteoclasts, it is true that PTH does have indirect effects. However, whether PTH mediates indirect effects on osteoclastic bone resorption by cell–cell contact or by production of soluble mediators is unknown. A number of soluble mediators have been proposed and these include prostaglandins of the E series, cytokines such as interleukin-6, TGFβ and more recently direct cell–cell contact. Cell–cell contact is likely to be at least partly responsible. Cells in the osteoblast lineage may form cell membrane channels through direct interactions with osteoclasts, and this could be a mechanism whereby a signal for bone resorption could be transferred from accessory cells to the osteoclast.

The effects of PTH on bone formation

PTH has direct effects in vitro on cells in the osteoblast lineage to inhibit differentiated function. This has been shown in isolated osteoblasts, osteosarcoma cells and in organ cultures. However, the predominant effect of PTH in vivo is to stimulate bone formation. Thus, it is possible that the in vivo response of PTH on bone formation is indirect and is mediated by other factors that are generated in the bone cell microenvironment. Such factors may be insulin-like growth factor I (IGF-I) and TGFβ. PTH stimulates the production of IGF-I both in isolated bone cells and in rodent calvarial organ cultures (Canalis et al 1989). This occurs following transient exposure to PTH. PTH also increases the production of active TGFβ in bone organ cultures (Pfeilschifter and Mundy 1987). Both these factors either alone or in concert are powerful bone growth stimulators and may be responsible for the bone formation response to PTH as well as for an anabolic response to PTH.

The mechanism responsible for the anabolic effect of PTH is unknown. This is one of the major issues in PTH research. There is a preferential effect of PTH on vertebral bone whereas cortical bone seems to be relatively spared. The reason for this is unclear. Nephrologists have been aware of this response for many years in some patients with secondary hyperparathyroidism associated with renal failure. Some of these patients develop changes in the radiological appearance of the vertebrae which are known as "rugger jersey" spine. It remains unclear whether this is entirely due to an anabolic effect of PTH on bone surfaces that have not previously undergone resorption, or whether this is an exaggerated coupling response following stimulation of osteoclastic resorption. PTH-rP has identical anabolic effects in comparable doses (Stewart 1996). Recently, Zhang et al (1995) observed that in some bone cell lines PTH has specific effects on cyclins, which regulate cell cycle progression, and it is possible that this may explain in part the proliferative effect of PTH on osteoblasts that leads to the anabolic response. There is an obvious need for in vitro systems in which the anabolic effect of PTH can be observed. It is not known what this means physiologically, the receptor mechanism which is mediated remains unclear, and it is not known which signal transduction pathway is necessary to mediate the anabolic effect of PTH. It is probable that PTH-rP, which also causes anabolic effects on bone (Vickery et al 1996), works through similar mechanisms (Stewart 1996).

For some years, it was thought that PTH increases the type of bone resorption known as osteocytic osteolysis. This is characterized by an increase in size of the lacunae in which osteocytes form. This is noted particularly in patients with primary hyperparathyroidism. However, Boyde (1981) has suggested from scanning electron microscopy studies that osteocytic osteolysis is in fact a fixation artefact in rapidly growing woven bone, and that in fact bone resorption is mediated only by osteoclasts. PTH is known now to be secreted in pulsatile bursts. Careful observations of PTH secretion in normal adults shows that it is secreted in a basal manner with additional pulsatile bursts that contribute about 30% to the total PTH secretion (Samuels et al 1993). This pulsatile secretion of PTH may be very important for determining the biological effects of PTH. It has long been noted that PTH produces different effects on bone depending on whether it is delivered in an intermittent or constant manner. When bone cells are exposed to PTH continuously, the primary effect is a resorptive or catabolic effect. However, when PTH is given in lower doses intermittently, the primary effect is an increase is bone formation. Further exploration of the role of pulsatile PTH secretion in various disease states and correlations with the effects on bone, whether it be pulsatile or continuous PTH, may be very important for our understanding of some phenomena associated with abnormal states of bone remodeling.

Effects of PTH on calcium homeostasis

PTH is clearly the most important acute regulator of calcium homeostasis. PTH causes acute effects on the renal tubules to enhance renal tubular calcium reabsorption and increase the serum calcium (Figure 4.2). As noted earlier, PTH also increases osteoclastic bone resorption, an effect which is slower, and in addition enhances calcium absorption from the gut indirectly through increased production of 1,25-dihydroxyvitamin D_3, an effect which is likely to take 24–48 hours. Effects on the renal tubules may be the most important acute short-term effects. In contrast, in states of calcium excess caused by increased bone destruction or by excess dietary calcium fluxes, PTH secretion by the parathyroid glands is suppressed. This will lead to a fall in the serum calcium because of impaired renal tubular calcium reabsorption and other effects on bone and gut calcium absorption. The synthesis and secretion of PTH are under the primary control of the extracellular fluid calcium concentration in a long negative feedback loop. However, it is important to realize that PTH secretion from the parathyroid

Figure 4.2

Effects of human PTH and human PTH-rP on urinary calcium excretion and urinary excretion of cyclic AMP. (Reproduced from Yates et al (1988).)

glands is regulated by calcium concentrations around a fairly narrow range between 7.5 and 11.5 mg/dl. Outside this range, there is little effect on changes in serum calcium on PTH synthesis or secretion.

PTH receptors and signal transduction

The PTH/PTH-rP receptor was identified and molecularly cloned in 1991 (Juppner et al 1991; Abou-Samra et al 1992). It represents a classical 7 transmembrane spanning G-protein linked receptor for which both PTH and PTH-rP are ligands. It shares a remarkable homology with the calcitonin receptor. Recently, gene knockout experiments have revealed that the absence of this receptor leads to hastened cartilage differentiation, similar to that which occurs with PTH-rP gene knockout (Lanske et al 1996). It had been thought that this receptor explained all the biological effects of PTH/PTH-rP.

Recently, a second PTH receptor has been identified (Behar et al 1996; Usdin et al 1995, 1996). This G-protein coupled receptor shares 51% amino acid homology to the PTH/PTH-rP receptor, but PTH is to date the only identified active ligand. It is not known as yet what the significance of this second PTH receptor is and there are many important questions that need to be addressed. These include the effects of PTH and PTH-rP fragments on this receptor and whether these are identical to those of PTH itself, whether or not this receptor can explain some of the controversial nonbone effects of PTH that have been described for many years, such as those on the vascular system, identification of the signal transduction pathway, which is utilized by this receptor, and finally whether or not this receptor is related to the anabolic response of PTH. Early studies suggest the receptor is not as responsive to PTH-rP as it is to PTH, and that it may mediate its effects through cyclic AMP and intracellular calcium signal transduction pathways (Behar et al 1996).

The effects of PTH on bone cells are probably mediated through several distinct signal transduction mechanisms. Most information is available on the effects of PTH on osteoblasts or osteoblastic cells. No information is available on the effects of PTH on cells in the osteoclast lineage. PTH is associated with activation of cyclic AMP as well as an increase in intracellular protein phosphorylation. However, PTH also causes increased generation of inositol 1,4,5-triphosphate (IP3) in these same cellular preparations and this leads to an increase in intracellular calcium, and has been reviewed by Dunlay and Hruska (1990). This is also accompanied by increased diacylglycerol generation and activation of protein kinase C. Both these signal transduction mechanisms appear to work in concert. However, recently it has also been shown that PTH increases the nonreceptor tyrosine kinase c-src in MG-63 osteoblast-like osteosarcoma cells (Izbicka et al 1994). Thus, PTH has multiple potential molecular mechanisms to mediate signal transduction. It is likely that the precise roles of these different signal transduction mechanisms can be unraveled with the availability of the cloned PTH receptor, together with recombinant receptor mutants.

PTH-rP

PTH-rP—discovery and physiological role

PTH-rP was discovered in a search for the systemic factors involved in humoral hypercalcemia of malignancy (HHM). This search was based on the original observations of Albright which were reported in the case records of the Massachusetts General Hospital. Albright noted that a patient with a renal carcinoma and skeletal involvement had a hypercalcemic syndrome which resembled that of primary hyperparathyroidism, and suggested that the tumor produced a PTH-like factor. The primitive assays of PTH-like biological activity which were available at the time were negative. With the advent of PTH radioimmunoassays in the 1970s, a number of studies reported increases in PTH radioimmunoassayable material (Benson et al 1974). This was clearly not identical chemically to native PTH produced by the parathyroid glands, and at that time it was thought that an altered form of PTH was responsible.

Stewart et al (1980) showed with careful measurements of nephrogenous cyclic AMP that in patients with the humoral hypercalcemia of malignancy, there was an increase in this parameter suggesting a PTH-like syndrome. The PTH radioimmunoassays had improved by this time, but circulating PTH by radioimmunoassay was negative in these patients. These authors concluded that a PTH-like peptide rather than PTH itself was responsible for hypercalcemia.

An additional argument against the PTH hypothesis for HHM was provided by Simpson et al (1983), who showed that in a series of hypercalcemic patients there was no detectable PTH messenger RNA in the tumor extracts. Thus, a number of groups embarked on using an adenylate cyclase assay in renal tubular cells or slices in an effort to identify the mediator with PTH-like biological activity.

Attempts at purification of the PTH-like activity led to the discovery of a peptide with similarities to parathyroid hormone in the N-terminal sequence. Although first reported by Moseley et al (1987), there were also two other almost simultaneous reports of identical findings by Stewart et al (1987) and by Strewler et al (1987). These three groups identified this activity in lung cancer, a renal cancer and interestingly in a breast cancer extract. This peptide was soon cloned and expressed and its biological effects were studied in detail. It was found to have very similar properties to those of PTH.

Over the following few years, there were multiple studies on this new peptide, either using the recombinant molecule or N-terminal synthetic peptides. It was found to share identical effects with those of PTH on bone cells and on renal tubular cells. In other words, it seemed to be a perfect mimic of parathyroid hormone. A number of possibilities were raised for a physiological role including potential effects in calcium translocation between the fetus and placenta, calcium translocation in breast milk, a role in parturition, and a role in the keratinocyte and skin physiology. However, its role in mammalian physiology became much better clarified with identification of a unique phenotype in null-mutant mice in which the PTH-rP gene is not expressed (Karaplis et al 1994). These mice die at birth from abnormalities in endochondral bone formation which result in increased cartilage cell differentiation. This leads to disturbances in skeletal development and abnormalities in the rib cage. More recently, Weir et al (1996) showed that in transgenic mice in which PTH-rP was targeted to chondrocytes, there was marked impairment of cartilage differentiation and endochondral bone formation. The production of PTH-rP by perichondral cells in bone that regulate cartilage cell differentiation has been linked to expression of the Indian hedgehog gene by Vortkamp et al (1996). These workers found that Indian hedgehog protein expressed by prehypertrophic cartilage cells inhibited cartilage cell differentiation, and this inhibitory effect was mediated by PTH-rP produced by perichondral cells.

PTH-rP has 70% homology to the first 13 amino acids of the N-terminal portion of PTH (Suva et al 1987), binds to PTH receptors (Abou-Samra et al 1992) and mimics the biologic effects of PTH (Horiuchi et al 1987; Yates et al 1988). Specifically, it stimulates adenylate cyclase in renal and bone systems (Burtis et al 1987; Horiuchi et al 1987; Kemp et al 1987; Strewler et al 1987; Yates et al 1988), increases renal tubular reabsorption of calcium and osteoclastic bone resorption (Strewler et al 1987; Yates et al 1988), enhances renal phosphate excretion by inhibiting tubular reabsorption (Horiuchi et al 1987; Kemp et al 1987; Sartori et al 1987; Yates et al 1988) and stimulates the 1α-hydroxylase enzyme in renal tubular cells responsible for production of 1,25-dihydroxyvitamin D_3 from 25-hydroxyvitamin D_3 (Horiuchi et al 1987). PTH-rP has been found in a variety of tumor types associated with hypercalcemia including squamous, renal islet cell, and even breast carcinoma (Danks et al 1989; Asa et al 1990). Although the majority of squamous cell carcinomas produce PTH-rP (Dunne et al 1993), the capacity to cause hypercalcemia may depend on the level of PTH-rP gene expression, which in turn may be determined by differential transcription of the PTH-rP gene promoter (Wysolmerski et al 1996). The regulation of PTH-rP is complex and factors such as prolactin (Thiede 1989), epidermal growth factor (EGF) (Kremer et al 1991; Ferrari et al 1994; Sebag et al 1994; Southby et al 1996), insulin (Sebag et al 1994), IGF-I (Rizzoli et al 1994; Sebag et al 1994) and II (Sebag et al 1994), TGFα (Burton and Knight 1992), TGFβ (Kiriyama et al 1992; Zakalik et al 1992; Merryman et al 1994; Southby et al 1996), angiotensin II (Pirola et al 1993) and stretch (Daifotis et al 1992) have been shown to increase expression while glucocorticoids (Glatz et al 1994; Rizzoli et al 1994; Sebag et al 1994) and 1,25-dihydroxyvitamin D_3 (Kremer et al 1991; Sebag et al 1994) decrease it. Estrogen has been shown to increase PTH-rP expression in uterine tissue and in vitro studies suggest that an estrogen response element is present in the PTH-rP gene (Lu et al 1989; Thiede et al 1991).

The human PTH-rP gene is much larger and more complex than the human PTH gene. It spans approximately 15 kilobases of genomic DNA and has nine exons and three promoters. The combination of three promoters, one 5' alternative splicing event and alternative 3' splicing produces PTH-rP isoforms of 139, 141 or 173 amino acids as well as multiple distinct PTH-rP messenger RNA species (Southby et al 1996). Although there is significant sequence homology across species up to amino acid 111, there is no interspecies sequence homology beyond that point (Martin et al 1991). Differential utilization of the promoters and of the 3' alternative splicing pathways among bone, breast, kidney and lung cell lines has been demonstrated (Southby et al 1996). Dexamethasone decreases while EGF and TGFβ increase abundance of each of the alternative mRNA species. Furthermore, EGF treatment increased transcription from promoters 1 and 2 and stabilized exon VII- and IX-containing transcripts in various cell lines (Southby et al 1996).

Similar to PTH, PTH-rP undergoes endoproteolytic post-translational processing that results in several secretory forms: (1) an amino-terminal PTH-rP (1–36); (2) a mid-region species that begins at amino acid 38 and has an undefined carboxyl terminus (Burtis et al 1992; Soifer et al 1992), and (3) a carboxyl-terminal species that is recognized by an antibody directed against the 109–138 region (Burtis et al 1990, 1992; Orloff et al 1993). The arrangement of the abundant basic residues in the protein sequence suggests that members of the subtilisin family of endoproteases such as furin (Liu et al 1995), PC 1–3, PC-2, PACE-4 and PACE-8 (Bruzzaniti 1996) are responsible for post-translational processing (Soifer et al 1992; Orloff et al 1994; Plawner et al 1995). Glycosylation of an amino-terminal PTH-rP species produced by keratinocytes has also been demonstrated (Wu et al 1991). Post-translational processing of PTH-rP as well as the receptor and signal transduction pathways employed by the mature secretory forms of PTH-rP has been extensively reviewed by Orloff et al (1994). Regulation of cell secretion of PTH-rP may be cell-specific as PTH-rP expressed in neuroendocrine cells is secreted in a regulated fashion compared with a constitutive secretion when expressed in non-neuroendocrine cell types such as squamous cell carcinoma (Plawner et al 1995).

PTH-rP is widely distributed (Danks et al 1989; Asa et al 1990) and there is accumulating evidence that it has a role in normal physiology quite distinct from that of PTH (reviewed in Strewler and Nissenson 1994; Guise and Mundy, 1996; Philbrick et al 1996). PTH-rP appears to be important in the development of the normal skeleton (Karaplis et al 1994; Lanske et al 1996), regulation of placental calcium transport (Kovacs et al 1995), establishment of bone metastasis in breast cancer (Guise et al 1996), and autocrine regulation of the growth of some tumors (Burton et al 1990). In the skeleton, null mutant PTH-rP mice have provided significant insight into the role of PTH-rP in the developing skeleton (Karaplis et al 1994). These mice died postnatally from asphyxia and exhibited widespread abnormalities of endochondral bone development, including diminished chondrocyte proliferation, associated with premature maturation and differentiation of chondrocytes and accelerated bone formation from cartilage templates. Similarly, mice homozygous for the PTH/PTH-rP receptor gene null mutation had identical skeletal pathology but many were early embryonic lethals, a finding that suggested the phenotype of receptor loss was more severe than that of only PTH-rP loss. Consistent with this, transgenic mice, in which PTH-rP was overexpressed in prehypertrophic chondrocytes by the use of a mouse collagen Type II promoter that targeted the gene to these cells, had impaired chondrocyte differentiation and endochondral ossification (Weir et al 1996) and had the similar short-limbed phenotype observed in humans with Jansen's metaphyseal chondrodysplasia (Schipani et al 1995) which is caused by activating mutations in the PTH/PTH-rP receptor.

PTH-rP appears to be important in the normal physiology of the breast (Thiede and Rodan, 1988; Ratcliffe 1992) as it is expressed in lactating mammary tissue (Thiede and Rodan 1988) and secreted into milk at concentrations 10 000–100 000 times greater than plasma concentrations of humans with malignancy-associated hypercalcemia (Budayr et al 1989). Increased plasma PTH-rP concentrations have been documented in several patients with the rare condition of lactational hypercalcemia (Khosla et al 1990; Lepre et al 1993) in addition to some breast-feeding mothers (Grill et al 1992). Thus, PTH-rP may be responsible for mobilizing calcium from maternal bone for use in milk production and it may be the implicating factor in lactation-associated bone loss.

The role of PTH-rP in the causation of local osteolysis and hypercalcemia is discussed in Chapters 6 and 7. As noted above, the physiological role of the PTH-rP remains unclear. In summary, it is produced in normal skin cells as well as in amniotic cells and it may have effects on epithelial cell replication and on smooth muscle contraction during labor. It is also expressed by lactating breast tissue and is present in large amounts in breast milk. However, most interest recently has focused on its potential local effects in cartilage differentiation. PTH-rP knockout experiments performed by introducing the null-mutation into the germ line of mice have shown that the mice have died before birth of an abnormality of the rib cage that causes impaired respiration (Karaplis et al 1994). These abnormalities are caused by an enhanced cartilage cell differentiation and normal ossification in the rib cage. Thus, PTH-rP is a naturally occurring and essential inhibitor of cartilage cell differentiation, and its absence leads to abnormalities at the growth plate. Overexpression experiments using transgenic mice in which PTH-rP expression is targeted to cartilage cells by use of the Type II collagen promoter, show a marked delay in endochondral ossification (Weir et al 1996) and also demonstrate cartilage abnormalities (Weir et al 1996). Its effects in cartilage cells seem to be mediated by Indian hedgehog protein produced by prehypertrophic cartilage cells in the growth plate (Lanske et al 1996; Vortkamp et al 1996).

Calcitonin

Calcitonin is a peptide hormone secreted by the perifollicular cells of the mammalian thyroid gland whose synthesis and secretion are regulated by extracellular fluid calcium concentrations and by gastrointestinal hormones such as gastrin. It is encoded by a complex gene that undergoes alternate gene splicing and is responsible for several other peptides including a calcitonin gene-related peptide of uncertain function, but which seems to mimic most of the biological effects of calcitonin at larger concentrations (D'Souza et al 1986).

The most interesting recent work on calcitonin involves studies on the calcitonin receptor, its molecular cloning and its relationship to the PTH/PTH-rP and secretin receptors (Lin et al 1991). The calcitonin receptor exists in a number of isoforms, and its expression seems to be influenced by ambient concentrations of calcitonin itself. This may be the reason for down-regulation in the escape phenomenon that occurs in the continued presence of calcitonin (Takahashi et al 1995).

Effects on calcium homeostasis

Calcitonin causes a short-lived fall in plasma calcium. It does that by its effects to inhibit osteoclastic bone resorption (Friedman et al 1986) and to promote renal calcium excretion (Ralston et al 1985). Its effects on calcium homeostasis are usually lost after 24–48 hours (Au 1975; Binstock and Mundy 1980). For this reason, it has been suggested that calcitonin has no chronic effects on calcium homeostasis, but rather serves as a short-term regulator to maintain normocalcemia following large calcium-containing meals. This function provides a potential explanation for its regulation by gastrointestinal hormones such as gastrin.

Effects on bone

Calcitonin inhibits osteoclastic bone resorption (Friedman et al 1986). It inhibits the formation of osteoclasts, as well as inhibiting the mature cell. Calcitonin receptors have been demonstrated at multiple steps in the osteoclast lineage (Kurihara et al 1990). Calcitonin receptors are also present on many other cells including tumor cells and monocytes and macrophages, although whether calcium has important biological effects on these cells is not known. Calcitonin acts on osteoclasts by enhancing adenylate cyclase and stimulating cyclic AMP accumulation (Nicholson et al 1987). It causes a transient contraction of the osteoclast cell membrane (Chambers and Ali 1983), an effect that has been related to its capacity to inhibit osteoclastic bone resorption.

The effects of calcitonin on osteoclastic bone resorption in vitro are also transient (Wener et al 1972) (Figure 4.3). Continued exposure of osteoclasts to calcitonin for more than 48 hours leads to tachyphylaxis. This may be due to down-regulation of calcitonin receptors on osteoclasts and their precursors, although this has never been definitively demonstrated. The loss of effectiveness of calcitonin can be inhibited by simultaneous treatment with corticosteroids. This has been shown both in vitro and in vivo (Wener et al 1972; Au et al 1975).

Over the years, there have also been suggestions that calcitonin or related peptides may have mitogenic effects on bone cells (Farley et al 1988; Burns et al 1989). However, these effects have not been found by other investigators and most workers believe that the major effects of calcitonin on bone cells are mediated directly on osteoclasts.

Effects of calcitonin as a pharmacologic agent

The potential role of calcitonin as a pharmacologic agent in the treatment of states of increased bone resorption in the hypercalcemia of malignancy, Paget's disease of bone and osteoporosis is described in Chapter 5. Osteoclasts in Paget's disease may be hyper-responsive to calcitonin. Patients with Paget's disease respond to calcitonin for longer periods than do patients with normal osteoclasts. The molecular mechanism for this hyper-responsivity of pagetic osteoclasts to calcitonin is unknown.

1,25-dihydroxyvitamin D_3

The sterol 1,25-dihydroxyvitamin D_3 is produced primarily in the proximal tubules of the kidney through a series of complex and regulated metabolic steps (Figures 4.4 and 4.5), although it is also produced by lymphoid cells as well as cells in the monocyte–macrophage series in vitro. It has important and apparently unique effects on bone cells. 1,25-Dihydroxyvitamin D_3 has complex effects on calcium homeostasis and on bone remodeling. Vitamin D deficiency due to dietary lack or malabsorption of fat soluble vitamins across the gastrointestinal mucosa leads to impaired mineralization of newly formed bone, the disease known as rickets in children or osteomalacia in adults. In this condition, the proteinaceous bone matrix forms and accumulates but does not become mineralized. In contrast, excess vitamin D ingestion leads to increases in rates of bone resorption and hypercalcemia. However, recent studies in rats suggest that the capacity of 1,25-dihydroxyvitamin D_3 to stimulate mineralization of newly formed bone matrix is due not to a direct effect of the sterol on osteoblasts but rather an indirect effect through supplying an adequate source of calcium and phosphate at the mineralization site (Underwood and DeLuca 1984).

It has been known for many years that the most active metabolites of vitamin D are potent bone resorbing factors (Raisz et al 1972a–c). These effects have been described both in fetal rat long bone cultures (Raisz et al 1972a–c) and in neonatal

Figure 4.3

Effects of calcitonin and corticosteroids on calcium release from bone in organ culture. Parathyroid hormone stimulates previously incorporated ^{45}Ca from fetal rat long bone cultures. This stimulation of bone resorption is inhibited by salmon calcitonin (100 mU/ml). However, bone resorption is inhibited only transiently, and the bones soon escape from the effects of calcitonin and the resorption increases again. When small doses of cortisol (10^{-6}M) are added with calcitonin, this escape from inhibition of bone resorption is prevented (Wener et al 1972). Similar observations are seen in vivo when patients with hypercalcemia are treated with calcitonin. (Reproduced from Raisz et al (1972b).)

54 BONE REMODELING AND ITS DISORDERS

Figure 4.4

Structure of vitamin D_3 (cholecalciferol). Cholecalciferol is formed in the skin by irradiation of 7-dehydrocholesterol. Ergocalciferol (vitamin D_2) is formed by irradiation of ergosterol, which is derived from plants and is ingested in the diet. Ergocalciferol differs from cholecalciferol by having a double bond between the C22 and 23 positions and a methyl group at C24. Dihydrotachysterol does not have a double bond between C10 and C19. This results in rotation of the ring so that the hydroxyl group at C3 corresponds to the C1 position, and dihydrotachysterol does not require renal hydroxylation for activity.

Figure 4.5

Metabolic pathway of vitamin D metabolism and activation.

mouse calvarial cultures (Reynolds et al 1976). The effects of the active vitamin D metabolites on the osteoclast may be unique. Most evidence indicates that 1,25-dihydroxyvitamin D_3 works as a fusogen or differentiation agent for committed cells in the osteoblast lineage. Studies of Ibbotson et al (1984) and Roodman et al (1985) show that marrow mononuclear cells fuse to form multinucleated cells with osteoclast characteristics when incubated with 1,25-dihydroxyvitamin D_3. Autoradiographic studies indicate that these responses are not due to proliferation of the progenitor cells (Roodman et al 1985). Similar responses are seen in cells in the monocyte–macrophage lineage. Abe et al (1981) found that 1,25-dihydroxyvitamin D_3 could act as a differentiation agent on the human leukemic cell line HL-60 as well as alveolar macrophages (Reitsma et al 1983; Miyaura et al 1986), and this was confirmed in the U937 cell line (Dodd et al 1983). Active vitamin D metabolites may also act as differentiation agents for other cells. Hosomi et al (1983) showed that vitamin D metabolites can stimulate differentiation of epidermal cells, and Morimoto et al (1986) have shown that this metabolite causes striking reduction in psoriatic lesions. The effects of 1,25-dihydroxyvitamin D_3 as a differentiation agent on osteoclasts have been supported by studies of Key and co-workers (1984), who showed that in an infant with malignant osteopetrosis, a disorder in which the osteoclasts fail to resorb bone, treatment with 1,25-dihydroxyvitamin D_3 for 3 months led to a startling improvement in the appearance of active osteoclasts in bone sections and subsequent bone resorption.

The effects of 1,25-dihydroxyvitamin D_3 on osteoclastic bone resorption may be synergistic with those of parathyroid hormone. This has been difficult to demonstrate in vitro (Stern et al 1983), but in vivo studies (Garabedian et al 1974) have shown that 1,25-dihydroxyvitamin D_3 may work in concert with PTH to stimulate bone resorption and cause an increase in the serum calcium. The effects of 1,25-dihydroxyvitamin D_3 on osteoclastic bone resorption in organ cultures are of relatively slow onset, although they may be seen at very low concentrations. Metabolites other than 1,25-dihydroxyvitamin D_3 such as 25-hydroxyvitamin D_3 and 19 nor, 10-keto 25-hydroxyvitamin D_3 (Stern et al 1985), have also been shown to stimulate bone resorption. However, whether metabolites other than 1,25-dihydroxyvitamin D_3 have any significant physiological effect on osteoclastic bone resorption is not known.

1,25-Dihydroxyvitamin D_3 probably does not act on mature osteoclasts directly. Merke et al (1986) could not find receptors for 1,25-dihydroxyvitamin D_3 in mature multinucleated osteoclasts, and McSheehy and Chambers (1987) noted that activation of isolated osteoclasts to resorb bone in vitro required the presence of cells in the osteoblast lineage. However, it is possible that 1,25-dihydroxyvitamin D_3 acts on earlier cells in the osteoclast lineage directly.

1,25-Dihydroxyvitamin D_3 may have other indirect effects on osteoclastic bone resorption. Multiple reports suggest that it is a multifunctional immunoregulatory molecule (for review, see Manolagas et al 1985). 1,25-Dihydroxyvitamin D_3 inhibits lymphocyte mitogenesis and blocks production of the cytokine interleukin-2 (IL-2) by normal activated lymphocytes (Tsoukas et al 1984). This effect on inhibition of leukocyte mitogenesis can be partially overcome by adding IL-2 back to the cultures (Rigby et al 1984). Receptors for 1,25-dihydroxyvitamin D_3 appear in activated T-lymphocytes following stimulation by mitogens (Provvedini et al 1983), and are also present in a number of lymphoid cell lines and cells of the monocyte–macrophage family (Manolagas et al 1985). 1,25-Dihydroxyvitamin D_3 can also enhance the production of stimulated interleukin-1 (IL-1) production from the leukemic cell line U937 (Amento et al 1984). It is unknown at the present time whether any of these effects on cytokine production by lymphocytes and monocytes play any role in the regulation of osteoclast activity. However, since IL-2 is known to be necessary for the production of bone resorbing activity by activated leukocytes (Horowitz et al 1984), and since IL-1 is a powerful stimulator of osteoclastic bone resorption, it appears likely that lymphocytes are involved in osteoclast activity. Moreover, since normal cord blood T-lymphocytes that have been transformed develop the capacity to convert 25-hydroxyvitamin D_3 to 1,25-dihydroxyvitamin D_3 (Fetchick et al 1986), 1,25-dihydroxyvitamin D_3 may be produced in the bone microenvironment and be a local regulator of osteoclast activity.

1,25-Dihydroxyvitamin D_3 also affects osteoblast function. In organ culture experiments, 1,25-dihydroxyvitamin D_3 inhibits bone collagen synthesis in the short term (Raisz et al 1980a).

When 1,25-dihydroxyvitamin D_3 is incubated with cultured bone cells with the osteoblast phenotype, the synthesis of the bone Gla protein is enhanced (Price and Baukol 1980). Alkaline phosphatase content in cells with the osteoblast phenotype may also be stimulated (Manolagas et al 1981; Rodan et al 1983). Incubation of cells with 1,25-dihydroxyvitamin D_3 may also alter their responsiveness to other factors such as parathyroid hormone (Catherwood et al 1985; Kubota et al 1985). In these studies, the cyclic AMP response to parathyroid hormone in cultured osteoblast-like cells was diminished by preincubation with 1,25-dihydroxyvitamin D_3. In prolonged primary cultures of fetal rat calvarial cells, 1,25-dihydroxyvitamin D_3 surprisingly impairs differentiated function and inhibits the formation of mineralized bone nodules (Ishida et al 1993).

Recently, there have been further clarifications of the receptor mechanisms and response elements in target genes for 1,25-dihydroxyvitamin D_3. The gene that has been used most for studying transcriptional effects of the vitamin D receptor is the osteocalcin gene, which has provided a wealth of information. It is apparent that the vitamin D receptor functions as a transcription factor, and causes effects on target genes by forming a heterodimer with the retinoic acid receptor (RXR), and this is responsible for the mediation of its effects on gene expression (Carlberg et al 1993).

1,25-Dihydroxyvitamin D_3 also has other effects on calcium homeostasis unrelated to bone. It increases the absorption of calcium from the gut and may, in conjunction with parathyroid hormone, stimulate renal tubular calcium reabsorption. Since it is produced in the proximal tubules of the kidney in response to parathyroid hormone and lowered phosphate concentrations, both its production and effects are intimately related with those of parathyroid hormone.

Whether 24,25-dihydroxyvitamin D_3 has effects on bone metabolism has been a controversial issue for years. Many people have believed it is biologically inert. However, recent studies in null mutant mice in which the 25-hydroxyvitamin D_3 24-hydroxylase gene is deleted throw doubt on this notion (St Arnaud et al 1996). Although the heterozygotes are apparently normal, about one-half of the homozygotes die before weaning, apparently due to hypercalcemia associated with nephrocalcinosis. Although the bone histology is normal in the first generation of homozygotes, the second generation show an accumulation of osteoid tissue at sites of intramembranous ossification, such as in the calvaria, clavicle, mandible and periosteal surface of long bones. These studies suggest that 24,25-dihydroxyvitamin D_3 plays an important role in normal intramembranous bone formation.

Vitamin D_3 analogs have been used in a variety of situations. One of the most interesting is their capacity to inhibit PTH-rP production. It is possible this effect could be used therapeutically in the treatment of patients with cancer in which PTH-rP is overexpressed, since the vitamin D_3 analog 22-oxa-1,25-dihydroxyvitamin D_3 (OCT) has been shown to reduce PTH-rP production by cancer cells (Endo et al 1994).

Prostaglandins and other arachidonic acid metabolites

Since prostaglandins have been shown to have multiple effects on bone cells, and sometimes opposite effects in different species, their role in physiologic bone resorption or bone diseases is very difficult to discern. They were first shown to resorb bone in fetal rat long bone organ cultures many years ago (Klein and Raisz 1970). They are powerful bone resorbing factors in organ culture, and are produced by monocytes in response to appropriate stimuli (Dominguez and Mundy 1980). Since monocytes are frequently found adjacent to endosteal bone surfaces, they could regulate osteoclast activity by their local production of prostaglandins. Most evidence indicates that they are locally active substances, and their effects are unlikely to be mediated systemically. However, their role has been greatly clouded recently by further examination of the multiple effects they may have on bone cells.

The observation by Klein and Raisz (1970) that prostaglandins of the E series resorb bone in organ cultures of fetal rat long bones was later confirmed in mouse calvarial organ cultures by Tashjian et al (1972) and Goodson et al (1973). The major prostaglandins are not equipotent in stimulating bone resorption. The most potent are the prostaglandins of the E series and the 13,14H_2-compounds. The endoperoxides produce a very rapid but transient increase in ^{45}Ca release from organ cultures (Raisz et al 1977). In organ cultures, prostaglandins have shallow dose-response curves and are slow in onset of action compared with parathyroid hormone and IL-1 (Dietrich et al 1976a,b). The effects on bone are associated with increased intracellular cyclic AMP (Yu et al 1976; Atkins and Martin 1977; Rao et al 1977). Resorbing bones examined histologically reveal changes in osteoclast morphology, including increases in the ruffled border area as well as in cell size and number of nuclei (Holtrop et al 1978).

The role of prostaglandins as bone resorbing factors has become unclear over recent years because of the observation of Chambers and his co-workers that when prostaglandins are applied directly to isolated osteoclasts in culture, the cells respond by a decrease in motility and contraction of cell size (Chambers and Ali 1983). Calcitonin, which is an inhibitor of bone resorption, produces a similar response. This effect of the prostaglandins is transient, and Chambers interprets it as reflecting inhibition of osteoclastic bone resorption. Thus, prostaglandins may have a bidirectional effect on osteoclasts—an immediate transient effect to slow or inhibit bone resorption but a more sustained long-lasting effect to increase osteoclastic bone resorption.

The effects of prostaglandins have also been examined on osteoclast formation. In human marrow culture systems, prostaglandins of the E series inhibit the formation of cells with osteoclast characteristics (Chenu et al 1990). In contrast, however, in mouse culture systems prostaglandins stimulate the formation of cells with osteoclast characteristics (Akastu et al 1989). Species differences may be very important in determining effects of prostaglandins on bone cell function.

Prostaglandins may also be involved in the effects of other factors on bone resorption. Raisz et al (1974) found that when complement-sufficient sera was added to bones, prostaglandins were generated endogenously by bone cultures and the bones subsequently resorbed. This bone resorption was prevented by indomethacin, a drug which inhibits prostaglandin synthesis. Later, Tashjian and co-workers found that epidermal growth factor, phorbol esters and platelet-derived growth factor (Tashjian et al 1978, 1982) all stimulated bone resorption in mouse calvariae by generating endogenous prostaglandin synthesis in the cultures. Bockman and Repo (1981) found that media harvested from activated leukocytes also stimulated endogenous prostaglandin synthesis in bone cultures. However, this phenomenon seems to be more frequently found in mouse organ culture systems than in fetal rat long bone systems. Epidermal growth factor and transforming growth factor α do not stimulate prostaglandin generation in fetal rat long bone cultures (Raisz et al 1980b; Ibbotson et al 1985a,b). The mechanism of stimulation of bone resorption is different in that system. It has now become apparent that mouse calvarial bones freshly explanted secrete endogenous prostaglandins (Lerner 1987; Garrett and Mundy 1989), and this may be confusing some of the results obtained in these cultures.

The potential role of local generation of prostaglandins in bone to mediate the effects of systemic factors was clarified with the work of Boyce et al (1989a), who showed that at least part of the effects of IL-1 on bone resorption in vivo were dependent on prostaglandin synthesis (Figure 4.6).

Prostaglandins also have effects on bone forming cells. In short-term culture, they inhibit calvarial collagen synthesis (Dietrich et al 1976a,b). However, over longer periods, bone collagen synthesis may be increased (Chyun et al 1984). In infants and in beagle dogs injected locally with high doses of prostaglandins there appears to be an increase in bone volume (Ueno et al 1985). The relevance of these findings to normal bone remodeling or bone formation still remains

Figure 4.6

Effects of interleukin-1 in vivo to stimulate bone resorption are partially inhibited by indomethacin. (Reproduced from Boyce et al (1989a).)

Figure 4.7

Pathways of arachidonic acid metabolism, showing lipoxygenase products, which have powerful stimulatory effects on isolated osteoclasts.

unclear. However, the bone formation response is quite striking, and it remains possible that the major effects of pharmacologic administration of prostaglandins of the E series on bone are on bone formation rather than bone resorption.

Prostaglandins of the E series are not the only arachidonic acid metabolites which have the capability of stimulating bone resorption. Meghji et al (1988) found that leukotrienes stimulated bone resorption in organ cultures of neonatal mouse calvariae. These compounds were compared for potency with PGE2, and were all found to be more potent in this study. The authors linked the bone resorption observed with clinical situations where there may be enhanced production of these lipoxygenase products, such as in rheumatoid arthritis and periodontal disease (Davidson et al 1983; El Attar and Lin 1983; El Attar et al 1986).

Recently, interesting studies have been performed on deletion mutants of the 5-lipoxygenase enzyme. These mutants have an increase in cortical bone growth, a defect which is similar to that seen with the osteocalcin deletion mutants. These findings suggest that the major effect of the 5-LO metabolites may not be on osteoclasts but rather on osteoblasts. The mutant mice have no evidence of an abnormality in osteoclast function or osteopetrosis (Flynn et al 1996).

We have also examined the effects of leukotrienes on osteoclastic bone resorption. We

Figure 4.8

Stimulatory effects of lipoxygenase products on isolated osteoclasts in vitro. (Reproduced from Gallwitz et al (1993).)

Figure 4.9

Lipoxygenase products were first identified as stimulators of osteoclast activity in human giant cell tumors of bone. The leukotrienes are produced by the mononuclear cells in these tumors and activate multinucleated cells with the osteoclast phenotype to stimulate bone resorption (right panel). A typical lytic lesion in the femur caused by one of these tumors is shown in the left panel.

Control   LTB4

Figure 4.10

Leukotriene B4 (LTB4) increases osteoclast formation and bone resorption when administered locally in vivo into the subcutaneous tissue of the murine calvaria. Note the increase in osteoclast number in LTB4-treated mice (Garcia et al 1996).

have found that the peptidoleukotrienes LTE-4 and LTD-4 as well as 5-HETE all stimulate isolated osteoclasts to resorb bone (Gallwitz et al 1993) (Figures 4.7 and 4.8). The role of these mediators in physiological and pathological bone resorption is unknown, but they may be important in the same situations where prostaglandins of the E series are generated, and particularly chronic inflammatory diseases involving bone. They were first identified as mediators of osteoclast activity in giant cell tumors of bone (Figure 4.9). In these tumors, the stromal cell component of the giant cell tumors produced large amounts of leukotrienes that are capable of activating the giant cells, which have many of the phenotypic characteristics of osteoclasts, to form resorption pits on bone or dentine slices. LTB-4 was found to stimulate osteoclast formation and activation of mature osteoclasts (Garcia et al 1996a,b). LTB-4 was also shown to be a powerful inducer of bone resorption in vivo when injected over the calvaria of mice (Figure 4.10).

Interleukin-1 (IL-1)

Interleukin-1 represents a multifunctional family of cytokines that have multiple effects on many target cell types. This family comprises interleukin-1α, interleukin-1β and the interleukin-1 receptor antagonist. IL-1α and IL-1β appear to have equivalent effects on bone, and are equally potent. They are very powerful and potent stimulators of osteoclastic bone resorption, and cause hypercalcemia in vivo (Figures 4.11 and 4.12). This effect to cause hypercalcemia is mediated through osteoclastic bone resorption. This has been shown by the use of osteopetrotic mice which have nonfunctional osteoclasts (Boyce et al 1992). When these mice are injected with IL-1α or IL-1β they show no increase in blood ionized calcium, compared with similar wild-type mice, which do show a hypercalcemic response, or similar osteopetrotic mice treated with PTH or PTHrP, which develop hypercalcemia because of the effects of these latter peptides on renal tubular calcium reabsorption.

IL-1α and IL-1β mediate their effects on osteoclastic bone resorption probably at multiple sites in the osteoclast lineage (Gowen et al 1983; Gowen and Mundy 1986). They are powerful growth regulatory factors for osteoclasts, stimulating their formation (Pfeilschifter et al 1989). In vivo studies show that they increase numbers of colony forming units for granulocyte–macrophage colonies (CFU-GM), which are early multipotent and uncommitted osteoclast progenitors (Uy et al 1993). However, in addition, they also influence differentiation of committed progenitors (Pfeilschifter et al 1989), and possibly also have the capacity to activate the mature cells—effects that have been ascribed to an indirect action mediated through accessory cells (Thomson et al 1986). IL-1 causes hypercalcemia whether it is administered by infusion (Sabatini et al 1988) or by repeated injections (Boyce et al 1989a). With repeated injections for several days, it stimulates increased osteoclastic bone resorption and hypercalcemia, an effect which can last for 7–10 days, and then, unless IL-1 administration is continued, a phase of new bone formation

Figure 4.11

Effects of interleukin-1 administered locally over the calvaria to stimulate osteoclastic bone resorption in normal intact mice. (Reproduced from Boyce et al (1989a).)

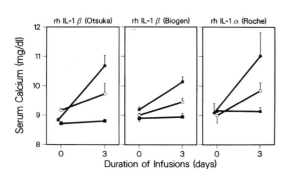

Figure 4.12

Effects of recombinant human interleukin-1 of different sources on calcium homeostasis in normal mice during 72-hour infusions. Maximal effects are seen at 2 µg/day, and intermediate effects at 1.25 µg/day. (Reproduced from Sabatini et al (1988).)

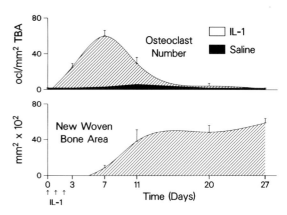

Figure 4.13

Effects of injections of interleukin-1 given for 3 days on osteoclastic bone resorption and new bone formation in the calvaria of normal mice. Osteoclast and osteoblast activity were assessed by quantitative histomorphometry. (Reproduced from Boyce et al (1989a).)

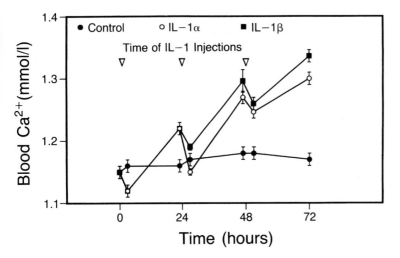

Figure 4.14

Effects of interleukin-1α and interleukin-1β, causing transient decrease in blood ionized calcium followed by more prolonged increase. The transient decrease is inhibited by treatment of the mice with indomethacin. (Reproduced from Boyce et al (1989b).)

occurs to repair the defects made by the previously stimulated osteoclasts (Boyce et al 1989a) (Figure 4.13). At least part of the effects of IL-1 in vivo are mediated through local generation of prostaglandins, and can be ameliorated by concomitant administration to rodents of indomethacin in sufficient doses to inhibit prostaglandin synthesis. It should be noted that immediately after injections of IL-1, there is a transient small decrease in blood ionized calcium, followed by a marked increase (Boyce et al 1989b). The mechanism responsible for this transient decrease is unknown, although similar effects have been described in the past with parathyroid hormone. In the case of IL-1, the transient decrease is inhibited by indomethacin (Figure 4.14).

IL-1α and IL-1β have both been implicated in various types of bone diseases. IL-1α is frequently produced by solid tumors and may work either alone or in conjunction with other factors such as PTH-rP to cause hypercalcemia (Sato et al 1989). Solid tumors have not been shown to produce IL-1β, but it has been linked to increased bone resorption associated with cultures of myeloma cells (Cozzolino et al 1989, Kawano et al 1989), and also with bone loss associated with a subset of patients with osteoporosis. In this situation, increased IL-1β production has been demonstrated in vitro by circulating peripheral blood monocytes isolated from patients with postmenopausal osteoporosis, and production of IL-1 by these cells in vitro is abrogated by the use of estrogen in these patients (Pacifici et al 1987, 1989).

IL-1 has growth stimulatory effects on osteoblastic cells, but inhibits their differentiated function (Gowen et al 1985; Smith et al 1987). Transient exposure to IL-1 and then withdrawal causes increased bone formation in vivo (Boyce et al 1989b). However, prolonged exposure to IL-1 probably causes inhibition of new bone formation in vivo.

Interleukin-1 receptor antagonist

A molecule in the IL-1 family has been identified which acts as a naturally occurring antagonist to the effects of IL-1α and IL-1β on the IL-1 receptors (Arend et al 1989; Carter et al 1990; Eisenberg et al 1990; Hannum et al 1990). This factor is known as the IL-1 receptor antagonist (IL-1 RA). It inhibits the effects of IL-1α and IL-1β to cause hypercalcemia when administered in vivo (Guise et al 1993) (Figure 4.15). This IL-1 receptor antagonist has effects that block both the 80 and 60 kilodalton IL-1 receptor molecule. It appears not to have any agonist activity, certainly as far as bone cell function is concerned. It needs to be used in large doses to inhibit the effects of IL-1 on calcium homeostasis. The major effects of the IL-1α and IL-1β molecule on bone are mediated through the 80 kilodalton receptor. This has been demonstrated with the use of neutralizing antibodies to the receptor that are specific for this receptor component (Garrett et al 1993).

Tumor necrosis factor (TNF) and lymphotoxin

Tumor necrosis factor (TNF) and lymphotoxin are two related multifunctional cytokines that share

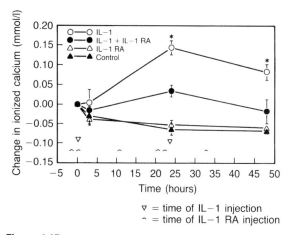

Figure 4.15

Effects of interleukin-1 receptor antagonist, lowering blood ionized calcium in mice made hypercalcemic with interleukin-1. Interleukin-1 (2 μg) was given subcutaneously at 0 and 24 hours. Interleukin-1 receptor antagonist (100 μg) was given subcutaneously 1 hour before the injections. See Guise et al (1993) for details. (Reproduced from Guise et al (1993).)

similar receptor mechanisms, but are encoded by separate genes. They seem to have identical biological effects on bone cells. Many of the activities of lymphotoxin and TNF also overlap with those of the IL-1 molecules, particularly as far as bone is concerned. TNF and lymphotoxin both stimulate osteoclastic bone resorption (Bertolini et al 1986) and cause hypercalcemia when administered in vivo (Garrett et al 1987; Tashjian et al 1987). Like IL-1, their effects on bone are mediated at least in part through local generation in bone of prostaglandin synthesis. TNF and lymphotoxin both stimulate the formation of new osteoclasts from precursors (Pfeilschifter et al 1989), but also have the capacity to activate mature osteoclasts, probably indirectly (Thomson et al 1987). TNF and lymphotoxin stimulate proliferation of osteoclast progenitors and enhance differentiation of committed progenitors to form mature multinucleated cells (Pfeilschifter et al 1989).

Recently, a member of the TNF receptor superfamily has been identified by two independent groups which inhibits bone resorption independent of the stimulus (Simonet et al, 1997; Tsuda et al, 1997). This protein has been named osteoclastogenesis inhibitory factor (OCIF) or osteoprotegerin (OPG), and represents a peptide which is a soluble secreted form of the TNF receptor and acts as an antagonist to osteoclastic bone resorption both in vitro and in vivo. Even more recently, the ligand for this endogenous antagonist has been identified as the putative osteoclastogenesis differentiation-inducing factor (ODIF) which acts directly on osteoclasts. It appears to be identical or at the very least related to RANK ligand (also called TRANCE) (Wong et al, 1997). This peptide, which has a membrane-bound form, is also a ligand for OPG/OCID (Yasuda et al, 1998) and has been shown to stimulate osteoclastic bone resorption in marrow cultures by acting directly on cells in the osteoclast lineage. This has led to the concept that osteoprotegerin or OCIF inhibits bone resorption by binding directly to TRANCE/ODIF, the final common mediator of osteoclastic bone resorption.

TNF and lymphotoxin have been implicated in the bone destruction and hypercalcemia associated with several types of malignancies. Lymphotoxin is produced by established cultures of human and animal myeloma cell lines (Garrett et al 1987). These tumor cells release lymphotoxin into the conditioned media and the majority of the biological activity in the conditioned media can be inhibited by neutralizing antibodies to lymphotoxin. These cell lines do not express either IL-1α or IL-β, or TNF. TNF is rarely if ever produced by solid tumors. However, it may be produced in patients with tumors by normal host cells stimulated by the presence of the tumor. Some solid tumors produce mediators such as

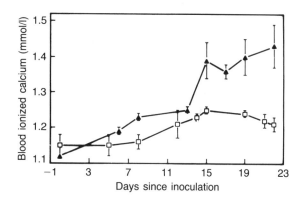

Figure 4.16

Effects of murine interleukin-6 to cause hypercalcemia in nude mice. Murine interleukin-6 was transfected into Chinese hamster ovarian cells (CHO cells), and the tumor cells expressing interleukin-6 were then inoculated into mice. The mice developed hypercalcemia, and in addition leukocytosis, thrombocytosis and cachexia. Mice carrying tumors expressing interleukin-6 are shown by triangles, and control mice by squares. (Reproduced from Black et al (1991).)

granulocyte–macrophage colony stimulating factor (GM-CSF) and other mediators, which can stimulate normal immune cells such as monocytes and macrophages to enhance production of TNF and cause hypercalcemia (Sabatini et al 1990a,b; Yoneda et al 1991a–f). This has been demonstrated in several models of the hypercalcemia of malignancy, namely the A375 human melanoma (Sabatini et al 1990a,b), the rat Leydig cell tumor (Sabatini et al 1990a,b) and the MH-85 tumor (Yoneda et al 1991a–f). In each of these cases, tumor-bearing rodents develop hypercalcemia. In the case of the A375 human melanoma, the tumor cells release GM-CSF which is responsible for provoking immune cells to release TNF. In the case of the MH-85 tumor, the mediator that is responsible for stimulating TNF production is unknown, but is distinct from GM-CSF. In this tumor, hypercalcemia can be abrogated by treatment of nude mice carrying this human tumor with neutralizing antibodies to TNF.

TNF may be also involved in bone destruction associated with some other conditions. For example, it is likely to be important in the bone destruction associated with chronic inflammatory diseases where accumulations of inflammatory cells occur adjacent to bone surfaces. This occurs in patients with periodontal disease, rheumatoid arthritis and cholesteatoma of the ear. TNF may be also involved in bone loss associated with the postmenopausal period, since circulating monocytes derived from postmenopausal patients produce increased amounts of TNF compared with similar cells from nonmenopausal controls, or postmenopausal patients treated with estrogen. TNF may also be responsible for some of the other paraneoplastic syndromes associated with malignancy, such as cachexia, hypertriglyceridemia, the anemia of chronic disease and, in some patients, leukocytosis.

Osteoprotegerin (OPG)

Osteoprotegerin (OPG) is a secreted member of the TNF superfamily. This molecule is a powerful inhibitor of bone resorption in vivo (Simonet et al 1997). It is a 401 amino acid-secreted glycoprotein, but does not have a typical transmembrane domain. It causes osteopetrosis when overexpressed in transgenic mice, but with normal tooth eruption. Its effects on bone appear to be to inhibit both osteoclast formation and osteoclast action. It reduces the bone loss associated with ovariectomy. Whether this factor will turn out to be as important as has been suggested awaits further study.

Interleukin-6 (IL-6)

Interleukin-6 (IL-6) is an extremely interesting cytokine which appears to have novel effects on bone distinct from those of other cytokines such as interleukin-1 (IL-1) and tumor necrosis factor (TNF) (Mundy 1996). In fact, it represents a family of cytokines that includes Oncostatin M and leukocyte inhibitory factor (LIF). All these cytokines mediate their effects through the GP-130 signal transduction mechanism. GP-130 is a transmembrane protein that interacts with the IL-6 receptor (either membrane bound or soluble) for intracellular signaling to occur. Until recently, it was thought that signal transduction is mediated through the JAK/STAT pathway, although it is now realized that it is much more complicated. For example, IL-6 influences not just the JAK/STAT pathway but also the MAP kinase pathway in bone cells. It has recently been demonstrated that interference with the JAK/STAT pathway leads to impaired MAP kinase expression. Interference with the JAK/STAT pathway also leads to decreased phosphorylation of GP-130, and interference with the MAP kinase pathway impairs STAT-3 binding to response elements in target genes such as alkaline phosphatase. Clarification of these molecular mechanisms involved in IL-6 signal transduction may provide potential molecular targets for interfering with these pathways and ultimately with bone cell function.

IL-6 has unusual effects on bone resorption. Unlike other known cytokines, IL-6 production in bone cells is enhanced by osteotropic hormones such as PTH, 1,25-dihydroxyvitamin D_3 and IL-1 (Feyen et al 1989). It causes hypercalcemia in vivo (Black et al 1991) (Figure 4.16), as does TNF and IL-1, but its effects on osteoclastic bone resorption are different. IL-6 appears to increase the formation of new osteoclasts from precursors and in combination with 1,25-dihydroxyvitamin D_3

increases the number of multinucleated cells in human marrow cultures from 50% to 90% (Ishimi et al 1990; Kurihara et al 1990). IL-6 also has complex effects on the mature osteoclasts. It appears that IL-6 is expressed by human cells with the osteoclast phenotype (giant cell tumors of bone), as well as osteoclast-like cells generated from marrow cultures derived from cells obtained from patients with Paget's disease. The capacity of these giant cells to form resorption pits on sperm whale dentine is inhibited both by neutralizing antibodies to IL-6 as well as antisense oligonucleotides (Reddy et al 1994). Thus, IL-6 appears to be required for these osteoclast-like cells to resorb.

IL-6 has been implicated in the bone resorption and hypercalcemia associated with several different types of bone diseases. As already noted, it seems to be expressed excessively by cells in the osteoclast lineage from patients with Paget's disease of bone (Roodman et al 1991), and may act as an autocrine growth factor for osteoclast-like cells or their precursors. IL-6 is produced by osteoblasts (Feyen et al 1989) and its production by osteoblasts is suppressed by estrogen in vitro (Girasole et al 1992). This information has been used by Manolagas and colleagues to show that in oophorectomized mice, increased osteoclastic resorption can be inhibited by treatment with neutralizing antibodies to IL-6, suggesting that at least part of the bone loss associated with estrogen withdrawal may be related to excess IL-6 production (Jilka et al 1992). IL-6 has also been implicated in the hypercalcemia associated with myeloma and with solid tumors associated with bone destruction. In myeloma, several patients with plasma cell leukemia have been found to have increased circulating concentrations of IL-6, which is also known to be a B-cell growth factor (Klein and Bataille 1991a,b). Treatment with neutralizing antibodies to IL-6 has reduced the serum calcium of these hypercalcemic patients (Klein et al 1991). Treatment of nude mice carrying a human tumor that produced IL-6 and was responsible for hypercalcemia in the donor patient, with neutralizing antibodies to IL-6, lowers their serum calcium (Yoneda et al 1993). Thus, it appears that IL-6 may play an important subsidiary and in some cases even primary role in the pathophysiology of bone loss and disturbance of calcium homeostasis associated with a number of disease states.

IL-6 can also be associated with other paraneoplastic syndromes such as leukocytosis and thrombocytosis associated with malignancy. This has been demonstrated in murine models injected with Chinese hamster ovarian cells transfected with the IL-6 gene. When these tumor cells are inoculated into nude mice, the nude mice develop the paraneoplastic syndromes of hypercalcemia, leukocytosis and thrombocytosis (Black et al 1991).

An important question is the role of IL-6 in bone remodeling. Manolagas and Jilka (1995) have postulated that IL-6, and more particularly its signal transduction target GP 130, play a critical and central role in normal bone remodeling influencing not just bone resorption but also bone formation. In fact, IL-6 alone is a weak bone resorbing factor. It is probably responsible for having important effects on generation of osteoclast precursors and maintaining a pool of committed precursors, but has little effect on osteoclast differentiation on its own. Alternatively, it may be a very powerful synergistic factor and potentiate the effects of systemic hormones such as PTH and PTH-rP on osteoclastic resorption. This has been demonstrated in vivo by De La Mata et al (1995), who showed that IL-6 has synergistic effects with PTH-rP on bone resorption and on hypercalcemia in vivo. There is little direct evidence at the present time that IL-6 has direct effects on bone forming cells.

Interleukin-4 (IL-4)

Interleukin-4 (IL-4) is a multifunctional cytokine (Paul 1991), which inhibits bone resorption in organ cultures in vitro (Watanabe et al 1990). Recently, it has also been shown to inhibit the formation of osteoclasts from precursors. An interesting recent finding is that transgenic mice overexpressing IL-4 developed an osteopenic syndrome that has been likened to osteoporosis (Lewis et al 1992). Whether IL-4 will have important pathophysiologic effects that can be used therapeutically remains to be determined.

γ-Interferon

Gamma interferon is a powerful inhibitor of osteoclastic bone resorption. It inhibits both the formation and differentiation of osteoclasts from their precursors. It does not have any morphologic effects on mature preformed osteoclasts. We have not found it to be very useful in vivo to lower serum calcium because of its toxicity. The effects of γ-interferon on bone resorbing cells to oppose those of IL-1 and TNF are surprising, since in most other in vitro systems it enhances the effects of these other cytokines. Gamma-interferon appears to be a more effective inhibitor of bone resorption mediated by IL-1 and TNF rather than bone resorption stimulated by parathyroid hormone or 1,25-dihydroxyvitamin D_3 (Gowen et al 1986).

Colony-stimulating factors (CSFs)

The osteoclast is derived from a hematopoietic precursor it shares with the formed elements of the blood. The growth regulatory factors that regulate the formation of blood cells, as well as the continued survival of their precursors, also affect cells in the osteoclast lineage. The best documented of the effects of these factors on cells in the osteoclast lineages is that for monocyte–macrophage colony stimulating factor (M-CSF) (also known as CSF-1). M-CSF is responsible for osteoclast formation in neonatal mice, as demonstrated by the op/op variant of murine osteopetrosis. In this mouse model of osteopetrosis there is a defect in the coding region of M-CSF (Yoshida et al 1990), and as a consequence osteoclasts are not formed in early life (Wiktor-Jedzrejczak et al 1982). The mice are born with osteopetrosis, the disease characterized by impaired osteoclast function. This particular variant of osteopetrosis can be cured by treatment with M-CSF (Felix et al 1990), but not by transplantation of osteoclast precursors, indicating that it is caused by abnormal production of M-CSF by accessory cells required for osteoclast formation, but not for activation of preformed osteoclasts. Recent information suggests that the M-CSF receptor (the c-fms oncogene) is present on cells in the osteoclast lineage, confirming this concept (Hofstetter et al 1992). M-CSF also increases the formation of cells with the osteoclast phenotype in vitro, as demonstrated by human marrow cell culture systems in which cells with the osteoclast phenotype form (MacDonald et al 1986). However, M-CSF does not stimulate bone resorption in organ cultures of neonatal mouse calvaria or fetal rat long bones, suggesting that its primary effect on osteoclasts occurs early in the osteoclast lineage.

The effects of other colony stimulating factors such as granulocyte–macrophage colony-stimulating factor (GM-CSF) or granulocyte colony-stimulating factor (G-CSF) on osteoclasts are not as well documented as those for M-CSF. G-CSF seems to have no effect in any system. There are controversial data with GM-CSF. GM-CSF enhances osteoclast formation in human marrow cultures, although it does not have any effect on osteoclastic bone resorption in organ culture models.

Colony-stimulating factors for granulocytes and macrophages are frequently produced by tumors which cause leukocytosis and hypercalcemia (Yoneda et al 1991a–f). It is not clear whether the colony-stimulating factors are directly associated with the development of increased osteoclastic bone resorption and hypercalcemia, or whether they merely represent concomitant expression of related growth factors. It appears more likely that the latter is the case. In many of these tumors there is enhanced production of a factor distinct from the known colony-stimulating factors that enhances osteoclast formation in vitro. This has been tentatively called the osteoclastpoietic factor (OPF) and will be described in more detail below.

Osteoclastpoietic factor (OPF)

Osteoclasts share a common precursor with formed elements of the blood, and it is has always seemed likely that there are relatively specific growth regulatory factors for cells in the osteoclast lineage which are analogous to the colony-stimulating factors for blood cells. We and others have looked for such factors using assays that affect osteoclast formation in vitro. A potential source for such factors has been tumor cells associated with increased osteoclastic activity in vivo, hypercalcemia, as well as the production of other colony-stimulating factors. We have identified a peptide produced by a human tumor which we call osteoclastpoietic factor (OPF). This tumor also produces colony-stimulating factor for the granulocyte macrophage series (GM-CSF), monocyte–macrophage colony–stimulating factor

(M-CSF), granulocyte colony-stimulating factor (G-CSF) and IL-6 (Yoneda et al 1991a–f). Others have detected a similar factor of the same size from a murine tumor associated with the same types of activity both for colony-stimulating factor activity and hypercalcemia (Lee et al 1991). This factor also appears to be produced by activated leukocytes. Its complete amino acid sequence and molecular cloning have not yet been reported.

Bone matrix-derived growth regulatory factors

The bone matrix contains a number of powerful bone growth regulatory factors, in addition to structural proteins such as Type-I collagen and osteocalcin. These growth regulatory factors include the transforming growth factor β (TGFβ) molecules, the bone morphogenetic proteins, the heparin-binding fibroblast growth factors, the insulin-like growth factors and platelet-derived growth factor. All these growth regulatory factors have powerful effects on cells in the osteoblast lineage. The most powerful effects appear to be produced by TGFβ, but the other bone-derived growth factors also have very prominent effects on bone in vivo, either alone or in combination. These growth regulatory factors are potential mediators of the coupling response, which links bone formation with previous bone resorption, and they are also potentially important in fracture repair as well as the repair of bone defects and bone grafts.

Transforming growth factor β (TGFβ)

Transforming growth factor β1 (TGFβ1) and TGFβ2 are homologous disulfide-linked homodimers of 25 kilodaltons that have powerful effects on bone. These growth regulatory factors are present in the bone matrix in concentrations of 0.1 mg/kg dry weight, indicating that they are among the most abundant of the known growth regulatory factors in bone. Moreover, bone is the major storage site in the body for these growth regulatory factors. Both TGFβ1 and TGFβ2 have similar effects on bone cells. They are powerful stimulators of bone formation. When injected subcutaneously adjacent to bone surfaces they cause a profound increase in new bone formation (Noda and Camilliere 1989; Mackie and Trechsel 1990; Marcelli et al 1990). In the calvarium of the mouse, 1 µg TGFβ administered by injection once daily for 3 days can lead to a 40% increase in the width of the calvarial bone over a period of 1 month (Marcelli et al 1990). This bone is initially woven bone but it is later replaced by lamellar bone. TGFβ2 produces identical responses. Similar effects are seen when TGFβ is injected or infused into the marrow cavity of the femur. These effects in vivo can be replicated in vitro in prolonged cultures of primary fetal rat calvarial cells. When these cells are exposed to active TGFβ, they respond by increased proliferation. However, continued exposure to TGFβ impairs bone cell differentiation and the formation of mineralized nodules. Thus for TGFβ to exert its stimulatory effects on bone formation, it is possible that active TGFβ needs to be exposed to bone cells for only transient periods. TGFβ also increases the capacity of osteoblasts to migrate unidirectionally (Pfeilschifter et al 1990), suggesting that it may have an important chemotactic function in normal bone remodeling, attracting osteoblast precursors to sites of active bone resorption. Overexpression of TGFβ targeted to cells in the osteoblast lineage by using promoters such as osteocalcin has led to marked increases in bone turnover similar to those seen in primary hyperparathyroidism (Erlebacher and Derynck 1996). These are obviously pharmacologic effects of TGFβ and the physiological significance remains unclear.

TGFβ has complex effects on osteoclasts that still need to be clarified to determine their significance. TGFβ has no apparent effects on osteoclast precursors in the periosteum (Marcelli et al 1990). However, when injected subcutaneously over the calvarium of the rodent, it increases the size of the marrow spaces by increased osteoclast activity. This effect is inhibited by indomethacin, suggesting that it is mediated by prostaglandins of the E series. When incubated with fetal rat long bone cultures in vitro, TGFβ inhibits osteoclast formation and bone resorption (Chenu et al 1988; Pfeilschifter et al 1988). However, in neonatal mouse calvarial organ cultures, it increases bone resorption because of its effects on stimulation of prostaglandin generation.

The activation of latent TGFβ in the bone microenvironment may be a very important regulatory step for control of the events involved in bone remodeling (Bonewald and Mundy 1989, 1990). TGFβ is present in bone as a latent complex. This latent complex is of several forms. In one form, it contains the active TGFβ moiety together with the precursor molecule also known as the latency associated peptide. In another form, TGFβ is bound to α2 macroglobulin to form a large molecular weight complex, and in yet another form it is bound to the latent TGFβ binding protein 135–190 kilodaltons. All these latent forms can be activated by exposure to acid, and possibly by proteolytic enzymes. The acidic microenvironment under the osteoclast is an ideal site for activation of TGFβ, but it is also a site where enzymes could be involved in the activation process.

There have been considerable recent advances in our knowledge of the biological effects of TGFβ and related molecules, and in particular mechanisms by which they mediate their effects. In the last few years, the receptor molecules responsible for recognizing active TGFβ have been identified. These consist of a complex system that involves separate molecules known as Type I and Type II receptors. Type I receptors are responsible for signal transduction, and Type II receptors for ligand binding. Thus, this general receptor mechanism is reminiscent of the IL-6 receptor mechanism. Dominant negative Type I receptors interfere with biological effects of TGFβ.

The signal transduction mechanism for TGFβ is a rapidly developing field. A complex group of important signal transduction molecules belonging to the MAD (mothers against drosophila) family are responsible for signal transduction in the TGFβ superfamily (including TGFβ, BMPs and activin). This family of signal transduction molecules was first recognized in drosophila as targets for BMP-like molecules (dpp). The corresponding vertebrate genes are now referred to as smad genes, five of which are currently identified (Derynck et al 1996). The precise molecules which are responsible for TGFβ signal transduction still remain to be identified, but should be apparent very soon.

There has also been further clarification of the binding proteins that TGFβ utilizes. The major binding protein is LTBP-1 (latent transforming growth factor β binding protein 1), which is an extracellular matrix protein of the fibrillin family. It binds to latent TGFβ via the precursor or latency-associated protein and is laid down in bone matrix in fibrillar form. It is now apparent that latent TGFβ is released from matrix by a sequence of events that involves plasmin-mediated cleavage of the LTBP-1 molecule to release latent TGFβ from the bone matrix, and ultimate release of the active TGFβ moiety from the precursor LTBP-1 subunit complex. This may be hormone-regulated. PTH, for example, increases plasminogen activator activity in bone cells (Hamilton et al 1985). Moreover, osteoclasts may produce enzymes responsible for this cleavage, and also are rich producers of protons. An acidic microenvironment is also responsible for the unfolding of the latent complex by either making it more susceptible to enzymatic cleavage, or assisting in other ways in release of active TGFβ. The association between TGFβ active moiety and its precursor and binding proteins may be critical in understanding the important part that this molecule plays in normal bone remodeling.

Recently, Erlebacher and Derynck (1996) have performed interesting experiments in which they have studied transgenic mice in which TGFβ2 is targeted to the osteoblast lineage by the use of the osteocalcin promoter. They found in the mice there was a state of increased bone turnover that they likened to that seen in hyperparathyroidism and osteoporosis. The findings are very interesting but difficult to interpret. First, morphologic abnormalities in bone in human hyperparathyroidism and osteoporosis are quite clearly distinct. Secondly, it is difficult to determine whether these gains of function experiments are indicative of any physiological state. TGFβ2 is present in approximately one-tenth the amounts of TGFβ1 in bone. Finally, in no condition or disease state have such high levels of active TGFβ been described. Alternatively, it clearly shows the powerful effects that TGFβ-like molecules might have on bone turnover. In these mice, a high level of TGFβ2 overexpression caused marked loss of trabecular bone and severe hypoplasia of the clavicles, which the authors likened to cleidocranial dysplasia.

Fibroblast growth factors (FGFs)

The mineralized bone matrix also contains heparin-binding fibroblast growth factors (FGFs) (Hauschka et al 1986). These factors are powerful mitogenic stimulants for osteoblasts (Rodan et al 1987; Globus et al 1988). FGF may mediate some of its effects indirectly, since it may enhance the expression of TGFβ in cells with the osteoblast phenotype (Rodan et al 1989). Recently, we have found that both acidic and basic fibroblast growth factors have profound stimulatory effects on bone formation in vivo, possibly even more potent and powerful than those of TGFβ (Dunstan et al 1993).

There are nine currently known members of the FGF family in mammals. Although encoded by nine distinct genes (FGFs 1–9), these are all structurally related and probably arose from a common ancestral gene. Despite the fact that FGFs-1, -2 and -9 lack classical leader sequences for secretion, current evidence suggests that probably all members of this family can be secreted (Jackson et al 1992). The FGFs act on their target cells in a tertiary complex that includes the ligand, at least one of four high affinity receptors, and at least one of three heparin sulfate proteoglycans (Klagsbrun and Baird 1991; Mason 1994). There are four distinct high affinity mammalian receptors (reviewed by Givol and Yayon 1992; Johnson and Williams 1993). However, since different isoforms of both the ligands (of which there are nine) and of the receptors (of which there are four) are well described, either through the use of alternative initiation codons for translation (Acland et al 1990; Powell and Klagsbrun 1991) or alternative splicing, the potential for diversity is enormous. There is still little understanding of the utilization of this diversity in biological responses and specific tissues such as bone.

The FGF superfamily represents potent mitogens for mesenchymal cells which have importance to diverse fields of biology. There has recently been an explosive increase in findings which indicate their importance in normal skeletal development, including chondrogenesis and osteogenesis. This has led to a situation where we now have the basic knowledge and tools to utilize this information to apply it to our understanding of the normal regulation of bone formation and the treatment of osteopenia.

Effects of FGFs on bone cells in vitro

For some years it has been known that bone cells synthesize members of the fibroblast growth factor family and secrete them into the extracellular bone matrix (Globus et al 1989). It is also possible that other cells present in bone synthesize members of the FGF family. One such possibility is the endothelial cell, which is a known source of FGF-2 (Vlodavsky et al 1987). However, little is known about the regulation of expression of the FGFs by bone cells. FGF production by bone cells may represent an example of autocrine secretion, since FGFs are powerful mitogenic stimulants for osteoblasts (Rodan et al 1987; Globus et al 1988; Canalis et al 1989). Fibroblast growth factors may mediate some of these effects indirectly, since they may enhance expression of other growth regulatory factors such as TGFβ in cells with the osteoblast phenotype (Rodan et al 1989). Both FGF-1 and FGF-2 cause a dose-dependent stimulation of DNA synthesis and cell replication in cultures of isolated osteoblastic cells as well as in organ cultures of intact calvaria. Subsequent to this mitogenic effect, there is also an increase in collagen and noncollagen protein synthesis in the bone organ cultures. The effect of FGF-1 on bone cells in vitro is enhanced by heparin. The mitogenic effects of FGFs on osteoblastic cells may not be the only effects in bone tissues. They also stimulate endothelial cell replication, which may be important in normal bone formation (Montesano et al 1986). The FGFs are also potent mitogens for chondrocytes, and thus they may also be important in cartilage repair.

Effects on bone formation in vivo

The FGFs, which are present in stored form in the bone matrix, have recently been shown to stimulate bone formation in vivo when injected locally or systemically in mice (Dunstan et al 1993; Mayahara et al 1993; Nakamura et al 1995). They have profound effects on bone, similar in magnitude to those of TGFβ, but possibly even greater (Dunstan et al 1993). Moreover, unlike TGFβ, they appear not to have deleterious effects of simultaneously stimulating bone resorption. Their therapeutic potential is still under investigation.

The effects of FGF-2 on bone formation have also been described by others. Mayahara et al (1993) showed that intravenous administration of human FGF-1 and -2 for 2 weeks caused profound new bone formation in young and aged rats. More recently, Nakamura et al (1995) showed that FGF-2 could enhance wound repair and also stimulate endosteal bone formation when administered systemically.

Effects on limb formation during embryogenesis

Recently, it has been shown by Cohn et al (1995) that FGF-4 is important in initiating accessory limb generation in chicks. Beads soaked in FGF-1, FGF-2, or FGF-4 and placed in the flank of chick embryos induce formation of ectopic limb buds, which eventually develop into complete limbs (Cohn et al 1995). In addition, it has also been shown that FGF-8 is expressed in the prospective limb bud region and apical ectodermal ridge (AER) (Mahmood et al 1995). Purified FGF-8 will substitute for the inductive action of the AER and sustain limb bud outgrowth in mice from which the AER has been removed. The results of these experiments suggest that local production of a member of the FGF family may initiate limb development, and that FGF is responsible for activation of other genes (sonic hedgehog and Hoxd-13) that ensure complete limb development.

Role in inherited disorders of skeletal development

During the past several years, several inherited disorders of skeletal development have been shown to be associated with point mutations in FGF receptors.

Achondroplasia

Achondroplasia occurs in 1 in 15 000 live births and is a disorder of limb development in those bones that develop by endochondral ossification, but not in intramembranous bones. It results in short-limbed dwarfism and macrocephaly. More than 90% of cases are sporadic and it is inherited as an autosomal dominant. In this disorder, single point mutations have been found in the transmembrane domain of FGF receptor 3 (Rousseau et al 1994; Shiang et al 1994). FGFR-3 mutations have also been identified in hypochondroplasia, an autosomal dominant disorder with features similar to, but milder than, achondroplasia (Bellus et al 1995). In several patients with hypochondroplasia, a single point mutation in the tyrosine kinase domain of FGFR-3 has been identified. Null mutations in FGFR-3 cause enhanced and prolonged endochondral bone growth (Deng et al 1996), suggesting that the naturally occurring mutations in achondroplasia represent ligand-independent activating mutations.

Crouzon syndrome

This rare syndrome of craniosynostosis (premature fusion of the cranial sutures) is associated with several mutations in the extracellular domain of FGFR-2, presumably altering binding of the ligand to this receptor (Reardon et al 1994). Recently, it has been shown that one of the mutations associated with Crouzon syndrome, Cys342Tyr, results in constitutive activation of FGFR-2 in oocytes. This mutation also abrogates the ability of this mutant receptor to bind FGF (Neilson and Friesel 1995).

Pfeiffer syndrome and Jackson–Weiss syndrome

Craniosynostoses with defects in intramembranous ossification occur in addition to abnormalities in limb bud development. Individuals with Pfeiffer syndrome have broad thumbs and big toes. In Jackson–Weiss syndrome, foot anomalies distinguish the clinical phenotype from Crouzon syndrome. There are similar mutations in these two disorders in FGFR-1 and FGFR-2 respectively (Jabs et al 1994; Muenke et al 1994). These results indicate the importance of these ligand–receptor interactions for normal bone development in both intramembranous bones as well as bones which develop based on a cartilage template.

FGF receptors and signal transduction

The bioavailability of FGFs, and subsequent specificity of effects on specific target tissues, could be explained at a number of levels (Klagsbrun and Baird 1991; Mason 1994). Cell surface interactions between FGF receptors and ligands are extremely complex. There are four known genes that encode for high affinity receptors for FGF-1 and FGF-2, which are tyrosine kinases and represent extracellular domains of molecules related to the immunoglobulin family. Alternative splicing of these genes occurs and makes possible a number of forms of potential high affinity receptors encoded by any one gene. However, there are also low affinity proteoglycan FGF receptors that may play an important role in the regulation of FGF action. These low affinity FGF receptors are of three types: syndecans, β-glycan and glycipan. All these heparan sulfate proteoglycans are likely to bind FGF, and are probably involved in delivering FGF to the high affinity receptors. Thus there are several mechanisms by which FGF activity at the cell surface may be regulated. The low affinity receptors may serve to sequester FGF and under some circumstances deliver it to its high affinity receptor. These low affinity receptors may also have multiple patterns of complexity, which are dependent on the extent of heparan sulfate glycosylation and sulfation. Interactions with low affinity receptors may be the reason that some mutants are more potent in bone than others. In general, we have found that there is a rough correlation between the heparin affinity of various FGF mutant ligands and their mitogenic properties on target cells. Earlier studies on mutants indicate that binding to and activation of the high affinity tyrosine kinase receptors is not sufficient to elicit a mitogenic response to exogenous FGF-1 (Burgess et al 1990, 1991, 1994). Although the sequence of events between ligand binding and tyrosine phosphorylation with mitogenesis is not clearly established, it is likely to involve tyrosine phosphorylation of PLC-γ, Shc and MAP kinase, and increased immediate-early gene and delayed-early gene expression and late (i.e., 8 hours) increases in the tyrosine phosphorylation of cortactin. However, our data with various mutants indicate that transcription of early response genes such as c-fos and c-jun is not sufficient for biological responses in indicator cells. An analogous situation has been demonstrated with IL-1β, where a point mutation uncouples biological activity and receptor binding (Gehrke et al 1990; Conca et al 1991). Thus there are multiple potential levels where the specificity of FGFs on target tissues could be regulated, including at the level of gene expression, at the level of export from cells, at the level of the cell surface where interactions with the cell associated proteoglycans in addition to high affinity tyrosine kinase receptors are involved, and at the level of signal transduction within target cells, where it is possible that there are different signal transduction pathways mediating specific biological effects.

Bone morphogenetic proteins (BMPs)

The bone morphogenetic proteins are members of the extended TGFβ family which have the unique capability of stimulating the formation of ectopic bone when injected intramuscularly or subcutaneously into rodents (Urist 1965). An ossicle of bone forms in the subcutaneous tissue, preceded by a cartilage phase. Thus this process is similar to endochondral bone formation and fracture repair. At least six distinct bone morphogenetic proteins have been identified. These peptides have sequence homology with TGFβ. Whether they have different effects one from another is unknown but it appears that subtle differences will almost certainly be present. Their effects on bone are clearly different from those of TGFβ. Unlike TGFβ, they enhance differentiated function in cultured osteoblasts (Harris et al 1992). Osteogenin (BMP-3) has been shown to inhibit osteoclastic bone resorption, and is chemotactic for monocytes (Cunningham et al 1992). Since they are presumably released from the bone matrix when bone is resorbed, they are available locally to stimulate all the events involved in bone formation. However, their precise role in the bone remodeling process is yet to be determined. However, recent data suggest they may be extremely effective in enhancing repair in segmental bone defects (Wozney and Rosen 1993).

BMPs have a similar receptor mechanism to that of TGFβ, with the exception that BMPs may bind not just to Type I but also to Type II receptors. Type I BMP receptors can be further divided into Type IA and Type IB receptors, and these clearly possess separate functions (Chen et al 1996). Dominant negative mutants of the Type IA receptor cause impaired osteoblast differentiation and decreased bone formation, whereas in contrast, dominant negative mutants of the Type IB receptor increase bone mineralization and osteoblast differentiation. There is great interest in identifying the MAD protein or other signaling proteins which the BMP receptor complex receptor utilizes in bone cells.

Insulin-like growth factors (IGFs) I and II

The insulin-like growth factors have long been associated with bone growth, since it was realized that they are responsible for mediating many of the effects of growth hormone on bone cells. It has been known for some years that IGF-I stimulates bone cell mitogenesis as well as collagen synthesis in bone organ cultures (Canalis 1980a,b), and in addition the enhancement of bone formation in vivo (Spencer et al 1991). The anabolic effect of intermittent PTH on bone has been ascribed to expression of IGF-I, since Canalis and co-workers (1989) showed that transient exposure by organ cultures to PTH leads to enhanced production of IGF-I. Moreover, by extrapolation, IGF-I has been linked to the coupling phenomenon, since if it is indeed the mediator of the anabolic response to PTH, then it is likely to be released following bone resorption locally at the bone resorption site and could lead to events involved in subsequent bone formation. IGF-I is unlikely to be a useful therapy for enhancing bone growth when administered systemically, since it causes hypoglycemia. IGF-II is present in the bone matrix and has been known for some years to be mitogenic for cells with the osteoblast phenotype. Baylink and colleagues purified the mitogenic activity they ascribed to skeletal growth factor from bone and found that it was identical to IGF-II (Mohan et al 1988).

Results on experiments of targeted mutations of IGF-I, IGF-II and the IGF receptor I remain extremely difficult to interpret. It seems likely that IGF-I and IGF-II are important in embryogenesis, since the knockout experiments showed decreased size at birth (DeChiara et al 1990; Baker et al 1993; Liu et al 1993). There is delayed ossification and hypertrophy of the proliferative zone at the growth plate in these animals. These are effects opposite to those seen with PTH-rP knockout mice (Karaplis et al 1994). There is a marked reduction in the appearance of ossification centers also in the Type I IGF receptor deletion mutants. A complicating factor may be the effects of the IGF binding proteins, whose biological roles have not been entirely clarified but may be very complex (Jones and Clemmons 1995).

Platelet-derived growth factor (PDGF)

Platelet-derived growth factor is a powerful bone cell mitogen. PDGF stimulates osteoblast proliferation, which can presumably lead to a sufficient team of osteoblasts to enhance differentiated function including collagen synthesis in organ culture (Canalis 1980a,b). For many years it has been known that PDGFs are produced by cells with the osteoblast phenotype including osteosarcoma cells (Graves et al 1983, 1984), and that these cells also surprisingly have receptors for PDGF. PDGF has been shown to have dramatic effects by filling in periodontal defects when used in conjunction with IGF-I (Lynch et al 1989). PDGF may also be a regulator of osteoclastic bone resorption. PDGF stimulates bone resorption in neonatal mouse calvariae (Tashjian et al 1982), but not in fetal rat long bones. Recently, we have found that it enhances c-src expression in osteoclast cultures, and that the PDGF receptor co-localizes with pp60[c-src] in these cultures (Niewolna et al 1993). This suggests a potential mechanism for a factor directly regulating c-src activity in mature osteoclasts.

References

Abe E, Miyaura C, Sakagami H et al (1981) Differentiation of mouse myeloid leukemia cells induced by 1 alpha,25-dihydroxyvitamin D_3, *Proc Natl Acad Sci USA* **78**: 4990–4.

Abou-Samra AB, Juppner H, Force T et al (1992) Expression cloning of a common receptor for parathyroid hormone and parathyroid hormone-related peptide from rat osteoblast-like cells: a single receptor stimulates intracellular accumulation of both cAMP and inositol triphosphates and increases intracellular free calcium, *Proc Natl Acad Sci USA* **89**: 2732–6.

Acland P, Dixon M, Peters G et al (1990) Subcellular fate of the int-2 oncoprotein is determined by choice of initiation codon, *Nature* **343**: 662–5.

Agarwala N, Gay CV (1992) Specific binding of parathyroid hormone on living osteoclasts, *J Bone Miner Res* **7**: 531–9.

Akatsu T, Takahashi N, Debari K et al (1989) Prostaglandins promote osteoclast like cell formation by a mechanism involving cyclic adenosine 3′,5′-monophosphate in mouse bone marrow cell cultures, *J Bone Miner Res* **4**: 29–35.

Albright F, Bloomberg F, Smith PH (1940) Postmenopausal osteoporosis, *Trans Assoc Am Physicians* **55**: 298–305.

Amento EP, Bhalla AK, Kurnick JT et al (1984) 1 alpha 25-dihydroxyvitamin D_3 induces maturation of the human monocyte cell line U937, and, in association with a factor from human T lymphocytes, augments production of the monokine, mononuclear cell factor, *J Clin Invest* **73**: 731–9.

Arend WP, Joslin FG, Thompson RC et al (1989) An IL-1 inhibitor from human monocytes. Production and characterization of biologic properties, *J Immunol* **15**: 1851–8.

Asa SL, Henderson J, Goltzman D et al (1990) Parathyroid hormone-like peptide in normal and neoplastic human endocrine tissues, *J Clin Endocrinol Metab* **71**: 1112–18.

Atkins D, Martin TJ (1977) Rat osteosarcogenic sarcoma cells: effects of some prostaglandins, their metabolites, and analogues on cyclic AMP production, *Prostaglandins* **13**: 861–71.

Au WYW (1975) Calcitonin treatment of hypercalcemia due to parathyroid carcinoma: synergistic effect of prednisone on long term treatment of hypercalcemia, *Arch Intern Med* **135**: 1594–7.

Baker J, Liu JP, Robertson EJ et al (1993) Role of insulin-like growth factors in embryonic and postnatal growth, *Cell* **75**: 73–82.

Barnicot NA (1948) The local action of the parathyroid and other tissues on the bone in intracerebral grafts, *J Anat* **82**: 233–48.

Behar V, Pines M, Nakamoto C et al (1996) The human PTH-2 receptor: binding and signal transduction properties of the stably expressed recombinant receptor, *Endocrinology* **137**: 2748–57.

Bellus GA, McIntosh I, Smith EA et al (1995) A recurrent mutation in the tyrosine kinase domain of fibroblast growth factor receptor 3 causes hypochondroplasia, *Nat Genet* **10**: 357–9.

Benson RC, Riggs BL, Pickard BM et al (1974) Radioimmunoassay of parathyroid hormone in hypercalcemic patients with malignant disease, *Am J Med* **56**: 821–6.

Bertolini DR, Nedwin GE, Bringman TS et al (1986) Stimulation of bone resorption and inhibition of bone formation in vitro by human tumour necrosis factors, *Nature* **319**: 516–18.

Binstock ML, Mundy GR (1980) Effect of calcitonin and glucocorticoids in combination in malignant hypercalcemia, *Ann Intern Med* **93**: 269–72.

Black K, Garrett IR, Mundy GR (1991) Chinese hamster ovarian cells transfected with the murine interleukin-6 gene cause hypercalcemia as well as cachexia, leukocytosis and thrombocytosis in tumor-bearing nude mice, *Endocrinology* **128**: 2657–9.

Bockman RS, Repo MA (1981) Lymphokine-mediated bone resorption requires endogenous prostaglandin synthesis, *J Exp Med* **154**: 529–34.

Bonewald LF, Mundy GR (1989) Role of transforming growth factor beta on bone remodeling: a review, *Connect Tissue Res* **19**: 201–8.

Bonewald LF, Mundy GR (1990) Role of transforming growth factor beta in bone remodeling, *Clin Orthop Rel Res* **250**: 261–76.

Boyce BF, Aufdemorte TB, Garrett IR et al (1989a) Effects of interleukin-1 on bone turnover in normal mice, *Endocrinology* **125**: 1142–50.

Boyce BF, Yates AJP, Mundy GR (1989b) Bolus injections of recombinant human interleukin-1 cause transient hypocalcemia in normal mice, *Endocrinology* **125**: 2780–3.

Boyce BF, Yoneda T, Lowe C et al (1992) Requirement of pp60[c-src] expression of osteoclasts to form ruffled borders and resorb bone, *J Clin Invest* **90**: 1622–7.

Boyde A (1981) Electron microscopy of the mineralizing front. In: Jee WS, Parfitt AM, eds, *Bone histomorphometry. Third International Workshop* (Société Nouvelle de Publications Médicales et Dentaires: Paris) 69–78.

Bruzzaniti A, Goodge K, Jay P et al (1996) C8, a new member of the convertase family, *Biochem J* **314**: 727–31.

Budayr AA, Halloran BP, King JC et al (1989) High levels of parathyroid hormone-like protein in milk, *Proc Natl Acad Sci USA* **86**: 7183–5.

Burgess WH, Friesel R, Winkles JA (1994) Structure-function studies of FGF-1: dissociation and partial reconstitution of certain of its biological activities, *Mol Reprod Dev* **39**: 56–60.

Burgess WH, Shaheen AM, Ravera M et al (1990) Possible dissociation of the heparin-binding and mitogenic activities of heparin-binding (acidic fibroblast) growth factor-1 from its receptor-binding activities by site-directed mutagenesis of a single lysine residue, *J Cell Biol* **111**: 2129–38.

Burgess WH, Shaheen AM, Hampton B et al (1991) Structure-function studies of heparin-binding (acidic fibroblast) growth factor-I using site-directed mutagenesis, *J Cell Biochem* **45**: 131–8.

Burns DM, Forstrom JM, Friday KE et al (1989) Procalcitonin's amino-terminal cleavage peptide is a bone-cell mitogen, *Proc Natl Acad Sci USA* **86**: 9519–23.

Burtis WJ, Wu T, Bunch C et al (1987) Identification of a novel 17,000-dalton parathyroid hormone-like adenylate cyclase-stimulating protein from a tumor associated with humoral hypercalcemia of malignancy, *J Biol Chem* **262**: 7151–6.

Burtis WJ, Bady TF, Orloff JJ et al (1990) Immunochemical characterization of circulating parathyroid hormone-related protein in patients with humoral hypercalcemia of cancer, *N Engl J Med* **322**: 1106–12.

Burtis WJ, Fodero JP, Gaich G et al (1992) Preliminary characterization of circulating amino- and carboxyl-terminal fragments of parathyroid hormone-related peptide in humoral hypercalcemia of malignancy, *J Clin Endocrinol Metab* **75**: 1110–14.

Burton PBJ, Knight DE (1992) Parathyroid hormone-related peptide can regulate growth of human lung cancer cells, *FEBS Lett* **305**: 228–32.

Burton PBJ, Moniz C, Knight D (1990) Parathyroid hormone-related peptide can function as an autocrine growth factor in human renal cell carcinoma, *Biochem Biophys Res Commun* **167**: 1134–8.

Canalis E (1980a) Platelet derived growth factor stimulates DNA and protein synthesis in cultured fetal rat calvaria, *Metabolism* **30**: 970–5.

Canalis E (1980b) Effect of insulin-like growth factor I on DNA and protein synthesis in cultured rat calvaria, *J Clin Invest* **66**: 709–19.

Canalis E, Centrella M, Burch W et al (1989) Insulin-like growth factor I mediates selective anabolic effects of parathyroid hormone in bone cultures, *J Clin Invest* **83**: 60–5.

Carlberg C, Bendik I, Wyss A et al (1993) Two nuclear signalling pathways for vitamin D, *Nature* **361**: 657–60.

Carter DB, Deibel MR, Dunn CJ et al (1990) Purification, cloning, expression and biological characterization of an interleukin-1 receptor antagonist protein, *Nature* **344**: 633–8.

Catherwood BD (1985) 1,25-Dihydroxycholecalciferol and glucocorticosteroid regulation of adenylate cyclase in an osteoblast-like cells line, *J Biol Chem* **260**: 736–43.

Chambers TJ, Ali HN (1983) Inhibition of osteoclastic motility by prostaglandins I_2, E_1E_2 and 6-oxoE_1, *J Pathol* **139**: 383–97.

Chen D, Feng JQ, Ji X et al (1996) Differentiation of roles of type 1A and 1B BMP receptors in osteoblasts, *J Bone Miner Res* **11** (Suppl 1): no 58.

Chenu C, Pfeilschifter J, Mundy GR et al (1988) Transforming growth factor beta inhibits formation of osteoclast-like cells in long-term human marrow cultures, *Proc Natl Acad Sci USA* **85**: 5683–7.

Chenu C, Kukita T, Mundy GR et al (1990) Prostaglandin E_2 inhibits formation of osteoclast-like cells in long-term human marrow cultures but is not a mediator of the inhibitory effects of transforming growth factor β, *J Bone Miner Res* **5**: 677–81.

Chyun YS, Kream BE, Raisz LG (1984) Cortisol decreases bone formation by inhibiting periosteal cell proliferation, *Endocrinology* **114**: 477–80.

Cohn MJ, Izpisua-Belmonte JC, Abud H et al (1995) Fibroblast growth factors induce additional limb development from the flank of chick embryos, *Cell* **80**: 739–46.

Conca W, Auron PE, Aoun-Wathne M et al (1991) An interleukin-1β point mutant demonstrates that jun/fos expression is not sufficient for fibroblast metalloproteinase expression, *J Biol Chem* **266**: 16 265–8.

Cozzolino F, Torcia M, Aldinucci D et al (1989) Production of interleukin-1 by bone marrow myeloma cells, *Blood* **74**: 380–7.

Cunningham NS, Paralkar V, Reddi AH (1992) Osteogenin and recombinant bone morphogenetic protein 2B are chemotactic for human monocytes and stimulate transforming growth factor β1 messenger RNA expression, *Proc Natl Acad Sci USA* **89**: 11 740–4.

Daifotis AG, Weir EC, Dreyer BE et al (1992) Stretch-induced parathyroid hormone-related protein gene expression in the rat uterus, *J Biol Chem* **33**: 23 455–8.

Danks JA, Ebeling PR, Hayman J et al (1989) Parathyroid hormone-related protein: immunohistochemical localization in cancers and in normal skin, *J Bone Miner Res* **4**: 273–8.

Davidson EM, Rae SA, Smith MJ (1983) Leukotriene B_4, a mediator of inflammation present in synovial fluid in rheumatoid arthritis, *Ann Rheum Dis* **43**: 677–9.

DeChiara TM, Efstratiadis A, Robertson EJ (1990) A growth-deficiency phenotype in heterozygous mice carrying an insulin-like growth factor II gene disrupted by targeting, *Nature* **345**: 78–80.

De La Mata J, Uy H, Guise TA et al (1995) IL-6 enhances hypercalcemia and bone resorption mediated by PTH-rP in vivo, *J Clin Invest* **95**: 2846–52.

Deng C, Wynshaw-Boris A, Zhou F et al (1996) Fibroblast growth factor receptor 3 is a negative regulator of bone growth, *Cell* **84**: 911–21.

Derynck R, Gelbart WM, Harland RMI (1996) Nomenclature: vertebrate mediators of TGFβ family signals, *Cell* **87**: 173.

Dietrich JW, Canalis EM, Maina DM et al (1976a) Hormonal control of bone collagen synthesis in vitro: effects of parathyroid hormone and calcitonin, *Endocrinology* **98**: 943–9.

Dietrich JW, Canalis EM, Maiina DM et al (1976b) Dual effect of glucocorticoids on bone collagen synthesis, *Pharmacology* **18**: 234–40.

Dodd RC, Cohen MS, Newman SL et al (1983) Vitamin D metabolites change the phenotype of monoblastic U937 cells, *Proc Natl Acad Sci USA* **80**: 7538–41.

Dominguez JH, Mundy GR (1980) Monocytes mediate osteoclastic bone resorption by prostaglandin production, *Calcif Tissue Int* **31**: 29–34.

D'Souza SM, MacIntyre I, Girgis SI et al (1986) Human synthetic calcitonin-gene related peptide inhibits bone resorption in vitro, *Endocrinology* **119**: 58–61.

Dunlay R, Hruska K (1990) PTH receptor coupling to phospholipase-C is an alternate pathway of signal transduction in bone and kidney, *Am J Physiol* **258**: F223–F231.

Dunne FP, Lee S, Ratcliffe WA et al (1993) Parathyroid hormone-related protein (PTH-rP) gene expression in solid tumors associated with normocalcemia and hypercalcemia, *J Pathol* **171**: 215–21.

Dunstan CR, Boyce BF, Izbicka E et al (1993) Acidic and basic fibroblast growth factors promote bone growth *in vivo* comparable to that of TGFβ, *J Bone Miner Res* **8** (Suppl 1): no 250.

Eilon G, Raisz LG (1978) Comparison of the effects of stimulators and inhibitors of resorption on the release of lysosomal enzymes and radioactive calcium from fetal bone in organ culture, *Endocrinology* **103**: 1969–75.

Eisenberg SP, Evans RJ, Arend WP et al (1990) Primary structure and functional expression from complementary DNA of a human interleukin-1 receptor antagonist, *Nature* **343**: 341–6.

El Attar TMA, Lin HS (1983) Relative conversion of arachidonic acid through lipoxygenase and cyclooxygenase pathways by homogenates of diseased periodontal tissues, *J Oral Pathol* **12**: 7–10.

El Attar TMA, Lin HS, Killoy WJ et al (1986) Hydroxy fatty acids and prostaglandin formation in diseased human periodontal pocket tissue, *J Periodontal Res* **21**: 169–76.

Endo K, Ichikawa F, Uchiyama Y et al (1994) Evidence for the uptake of a vitamin D analogue (OCT) by a human carcinoma and its effect of suppressing the transcription of parathyroid hormone-related peptide gene in vivo, *J Biol Chem* **269**: 32 693–9.

Erlebacher A, Derynck R (1996) Increased expression of TGFβ2 in osteoblasts results in an osteoporosis-like phenotype, *J Cell Biol* **132**: 195–210.

Farley JR, Tarbaux NM, Hall SL et al (1988) The anti-bone resorptive agent calcitonin also acts in vitro to directly increase bone formation and bone cell proliferation, *Endocrinology* **123**: 159–67.

Felix R, Cecchini MG, Fleisch H (1990) Macrophage colony stimulating factor restores in vivo bone resorption in the op/op osteopetrotic mouse, *Endocrinology* **127**: 2592–4.

Ferrari SL, Rizzoli R, Bonjour JP (1994) Effects of epidermal growth factor on parathyroid hormone-related protein production by mammary epithelial cells, *J Bone Miner Res* **9**: 639–44.

Fetchick DA, Bertolini DR, Sarin P et al (1986) Production of 1,25-dihydroxyvitamin D_3 by human T-cell lymphotrophic virus-I transformed lymphocytes, *J Clin Invest* **78**: 592–6.

Feyen JHM, Elford P, Dipadova FE et al (1989) Interleukin-6 is produced by bone and modulated by parathyroid hormone, *J Bone Miner Res* **4**: 633–8.

Flynn MA, Qiao M, Dallas M et al (1996) Mice lacking the gene for 5-lipoxygenase have increased cortical bone thickness, *J Bone Miner Res* **11** (Suppl 1): no 53.

Friedman J, Au WYW, Raisz LG (1986) Responses of fetal rat bone to thyrocalcitonin in tissue culture, *Endocrinology* **82**: 149–56.

Gaillard PJ (1961) Parathyroid and bone tissue in culture. In: Greep RO, Talmage RV, eds, *The parathyroids* (Charles C Thomas: Springfield, IL) 20.

Gallwitz WE, Mundy GR, Lee CH et al (1993) 5-Lipoxygenase metabolites of a stromal cell line (C433) activate osteoclasts and giant cells from human giant cell tumors of bone, *J Biol Chem* **368**: 10 087–94.

Garabedian M, Tanaka Y, Holick MF et al (1974) Response of intestinal calcium transport and bone calcium mobilization to 1,25-dihydroxyvitamin D_3 in thyroparathyroidectomised rats, *Endocrinology* **94**: 1022–7.

Garcia C, Qiao M, Gallwitz W et al (1996a) Effects of synthetic peptido-leukotrienes on bone resorption in vitro, *J Bone Miner Res* **11**: 521–9.

Garcia C, Boyce B, Gilles J et al (1996b) Leukotriene B4 stimulates osteoclastic bone resorption both in vitro and in vivo, *J Bone Miner Res* **11**: 1619–27.

Garrett IR, Mundy GR (1989) Relationship between interleukin-1 and prostaglandins in resorbing neonatal calvariae, *J Bone Miner Res* **4**: 789–94.

Garrett IR, Durie BGM, Nedwin GE et al (1987) Production of the bone resorbing cytokine lymphotoxin by cultured human myeloma cells, *N Engl J Med* **317**: 526–32.

Garrett IR, Guise TA, Bonewald LF et al (1993) Evidence that interleukin-1 mediates its effects on bone resorption via the 80 kilodalton interleukin-1 receptor, *Calcif Tissue Int* **52**: 438–41.

Gehrke L, Jobling SA, Paik LS et al (1990) A point mutation uncouples human interleukin-1β biological activity and receptor binding, *J Biol Chem* **265**: 5922–5.

Girasole G, Jilka RL, Passeri G et al (1992) 17β-Estradiol inhibits interleukin-6 production by bone marrow derived stromal cells and osteoblasts in vitro. A potential mechanism for the antiosteoporotic effect of estrogens, *J Clin Invest* **89**: 883–91.

Givol D, Yayon A (1992) Complexity of FGF receptors—genetic basis for structural diversity and functional specificity, *FASEB J* **6**: 3362–9.

Glatz JA, Heath JK, Southby J et al (1994) Dexamethasone regulation of parathyroid hormone-related protein (PTH-rP) expression in a squamous cancer cell line, *Mol Cell Endocrinol* **101**: 295–306.

Globus RK, Patterson-Buckendahl P, Gospodarowicz D (1988) Regulation of bovine bone cell proliferation by fibroblast growth factor and transforming growth factor alpha, *Endocrinology* **123**: 98–105.

Globus RK, Plouet J, Gospodarowicz D (1989) Cultured bovine bone cells synthesize basic fibroblast growth factor and store it in their extracellular matrix, *Endocrinology* **124**: 1539–47.

Goodson JM, Dewhirst A, Brunitti J (1973) Prostaglandin E2 levels in human gingival tissue, *J Dent Res* **52**: 182.

Gowen M, Mundy GR (1986) Actions of recombinant interleukin-1, interleukin-2 and interferon gamma on bone resorption in vitro, *J Immunol* **136**: 2478–82.

Gowen M, Wood DD, Russell RGG (1985) Stimulation of the proliferation of human bone cells in vitro by human monocyte products with interleukin-1 activity, *J Clin Invest* **75**: 1223–9.

Gowen M, Nedwin G, Mundy GR (1986) Preferential inhibition of cytokine stimulated bone resorption by recombinant interferon gamma, *J Bone Miner Res* **1**: 469–74.

Gowen M, Wood DD, Ihrie EJ et al (1983) An interleukin-1 like factor stimulates bone resorption in vitro, *Nature* **306**: 378–80.

Graves DT, Owen AJ, Antoniades HN (1983) Evidence that a human osteosarcoma cell line which secretes a mitogen similar to platelet-derived growth factor requires growth factors present in platelet-poor plasma, *Cancer Res* **43**: 83–7.

Graves DT, Owen AJ, Barth RK et al (1984) Detection of c-sis transcripts and synthesis of PDGF-like proteins by human osteosarcoma cells, *Science* **226**: 972–4.

Grill V, Hillary J, Ho PMW et al (1992) Parathyroid hormone-related protein: a possible endocrine function in lactation, *Clin Endocrinol* **37**: 405–10.

Guise TA, Mundy GR (1996) Pathologic and physiologic roles of PTH-rP, *Curr Opin Nephrol Hypertens* **5**: 307–15.

Guise TA, Garrett IR, Bonewald LF et al (1993) The interleukin-1 receptor antagonist inhibits hypercalcemia mediated by interleukin-1, *J Bone Miner Res* **8**: 583–8.

Guise TA, Yin JJ, Taylor SD et al (1996) Evidence for a causal role of parathyroid hormone-related protein in the pathogenesis of human breast cancer-mediated osteolysis, *J Clin Invest* **98**: 1544–9.

Gutierrez GE, Mundy GR, Derynck R et al (1987) Inhibition of parathyroid hormone-responsive adenylate cyclase in clonal osteoblast-like cells by transforming growth factor alpha and epidermal growth factor, *J Biol Chem* **262**: 15 845–50.

Gutierrez GE, Mundy GR, Manning DR et al (1990) Transforming growth factor β enhances parathyroid hormone stimulation of adenylate cyclase in clonal osteoblast-like cells, *J Cell Physiol* **144**: 438–47.

Hakeda Y, Hiura K, Sato T et al (1989) Existence of parathyroid hormone binding sites on murine hemopoietic blast cells, *Biochem Biophys Res Commun* **163**: 1481–6.

Hamilton JA, Lingelbach S, Partridge NC et al (1985) Regulation of plasminogen activator production by bone-resorbing hormones in normal and malignant osteoblasts, *Endocrinology* **116**: 2186–91.

Hannum CH, Wilcox CJ, Arend WP et al (1990) Interleukin-1 receptor antagonist activity of a human interleukin-1 inhibitor, *Nature* **343**: 336–40.

Harris SE, Harris MA, Feng JW et al (1992) Expression of bone morphogenetic proteins (BMPs) during differentiation of fetal rat calvarial osteoblasts in vitro, *J Bone Miner Res* **7** (Suppl 1): no 112.

Hauschka PV, Mavrakos AE, Iafrati MD et al (1986) Growth factors in bone matrix, *J Biol Chem* **261**: 12 665–74.

Hofstetter W, Wetterwald A, Cecchini MC et al (1992) Detection of transcripts for the receptor for macrophage colony-stimulating factor, c-fms, in murine osteoclasts, *Proc Natl Acad Sci USA* **89**: 9637–41.

Holtrop ME, Raisz LG, Simmons HA (1974) The effects of parathyroid hormone, colchicine and calcitonin on the ultrastructure and the activity of osteoclasts in organ culture, *J Cell Biol* **60**: 346–55.

Holtrop ME, King GJ, Raisz LG (1978) Factors influencing osteoclast activity as measured by ultrastructural morphometry. In: Copp DH, Talmage AR, eds, *Endocrinology of calcium metabolism* (Excerpta Medica: Amsterdam) 91–6.

Horiuchi N, Caulfield M, Fisher JE et al (1987) Similarity of synthetic peptide from human tumor to parathyroid hormone in vivo and in vitro, *Science* **238**: 1566–7.

Horowitz M, Vignery A, Gershon RK et al (1984) Thymus derived lymphocytes and their interactions with macrophages are required for the production of osteoclast activating factor in the mouse, *Proc Natl Acad Sci USA* **81**: 2181–5.

Hosomi J, Hosoi J, Abe E et al (1983) Regulation of terminal differentiation of cultured mouse epidermal cells by $1\alpha,25$-dihydroxyvitamin D_3, *Endocrinology* **3**: 1950–7.

Ibbotson KJ, Roodman GD, McManus LM et al (1984) Identification and characterization of osteoclast-like cells and their progenitors in cultures of feline marrow mononuclear cells, *J Cell Biol* **99**: 471–80.

Ibbotson KJ, D'Souza SM, Smith DD et al (1985a) EGF receptor antiserum inhibits bone resorbing activity produced by a rat Leydig cell tumor associated with the humoral hypercalcemia of malignancy, *Endocrinology* **116**: 469–71.

Ibbotson KJ, Twardzik DR, D'Souza SM et al (1985b) Stimulation of bone resorption in vitro by synthetic transforming growth factor alpha, *Science* **228**: 1007–9.

Ishida H, Bellows CG, Aubin JE et al (1993) Characterization of the $1,25$-$(OH)_2D_3$-induced inhibition of bone nodule formation in long-term cultures of fetal rat calvaria cells, *Endocrinology* **132**: 61–6.

Ishimi Y, Miyaura C, Jin CH et al (1990) IL-6 is produced by osteoblasts and induces bone resorption, *J Immunol* **145**: 3297–303.

Izbicka E, Niewolna M, Yoneda T et al (1994) pp60 c-src expression and activity in MG-63 osteoblastic cells is modulated by PTH, but is not required for PTH-mediated adenylate cyclase response, *J Bone Miner Res* **9**: 127–32.

Jabs EW, Li X, Scott AF et al (1994) Jackson–Weiss and Crouzon syndromes are allelic with mutations in fibroblast growth factor receptor 2, *Nat Genet* **8**: 275–9.

Jackson A, Friedman S, Zhan X et al (1992) Heat shock induces the release of fibroblast growth factor-1 from NIH 3T3 cells, *Proc Natl Acad Sci USA* **89**: 10 691–5.

Jilka RL, Hangoc G, Girasole G et al (1992) Increased osteoclast development after estrogen loss—mediation by interleukin-6, *Science* **257**: 88–91.

Johnson DE, Williams LT (1993) Structural and functional diversity in the FGF receptor multigene family, *Adv Cancer Res* **60**: 1–41.

Jones JI, Clemmons DR (1995) Insulin-like growth factors and their binding proteins: biological actions, *Endocrinol Rev* **16**: 3–34.

Juppner H, Abou-Samra AB, Freeman M et al (1991) A G protein-linked receptor for parathyroid hormone and parathyroid hormone-related peptide, *Science* **254**: 1024–6.

Karaplis AC, Luz A, Glowacki J et al (1994) Lethal skeletal dysplasia from targeted disruption of the parathyroid hormone-related peptide gene, *Genes Dev* **8**: 277–89.

Katz MS, Gutierrez GE, Mundy GR et al (1992) Tumor necrosis factor and interleukin-1 inhibit parathyroid hormone-responsive adenylate cyclase in clonal osteoblast-like cells by down-regulating parathyroid hormone receptors, *J Cell Physiol* **153**: 206–13.

Kawano M, Tanaka H, Ishikawa H et al (1989) Interleukin-1 accelerates autocrine growth of myeloma cells through interleukin-6 in human myeloma, *Blood* **73**: 2145–8.

Kemp BE, Moseley JM, Rodda CP et al (1987) Parathyroid hormone-related protein of malignancy: active synthetic fragments, *Science* **238**: 1568–70.

Key L, Carnes D, Cole S et al (1984) Treatment of congenital osteopetrosis with high dose calcitriol, *N Engl J Med* **310**: 410–15.

Khosla S, van Heerden JA, Gharib H et al (1990) Parathyroid hormone-related protein and hypercalcemia secondary to massive mammary hyperplasia, *N Engl J Med* **322**: 1157.

Kiriyama T, Gillespie MT, Glatz JA et al (1992) Transforming growth factor β stimulation of parathyroid hormone-related protein (PTH-rP): a paracrine regulator? *Mol Cell Endocrinol* **92**: 55–62.

Klagsbrun M, Baird A (1991) A dual receptor system is required for basic fibroblast growth factor activity, *Cell* **67**: 229–31.

Klein B, Bataille R (1991a) Recent advantages in the biology of IL-6 in multiple myeloma, *Cancer J* **4**: 81–2.

Klein B, Bataille R (1991b) Interleukin-6 in human multiple myeloma, *M S Med Sci* **7**: 937–43.

Klein B, Wijdene J, Zhang XG et al (1991) Murine anti-interleukin-6 monoclonal antibody therapy for a patient with plasma cell leukemia, *Blood* **78**: 1198–204.

Klein DC, Raisz LG (1970) Prostaglandins: stimulation of bone resorption in tissue culture, *Endocrinology* **86**: 1436–40.

Kovacs CS, Lanske B, Karaplis A et al (1995) PTH-rP-knockout mice have reduced ionized calcium, fetal-maternal calcium gradient and 45-calcium transport in utero, *J Bone Miner Res* **10** (Suppl 1): S157.

Kremer R, Karaplis AC, Henderson J et al (1991) Regulation of parathyroid hormone-like peptide in cultured normal human keratinocytes, *J Clin Invest* **87**: 884–93.

Kubota M, Ng KW, Martin TJ (1985) Effect of 1,25-dihydroxyvitamin D_3 on cyclic AMP responses to hormones in clonal osteogenic sarcoma cells, *Biochem J* **231**: 11–17.

Kurihara N, Civin C, Roodman GD (1989) Identification of a pure population of committed osteoclast precursors, *J Bone Miner Res* **4**: 324.

Kurihara N, Bertolini D, Suda T et al (1990) Interleukin-6 stimulates osteoclast-like multinucleated cell formation in long term human marrow cultures by inducing IL-1 release, *J Immunol* **144**: 426–30.

Lanske B, Karaplis AC, Lee K et al (1996) PTH/PTH-rP receptor in early development and Indian hedgehog-regulated bone growth, *Science* **273**: 653–66.

Lee MY, Eyre DR, Osborne WRA (1991) Isolation of a murine osteoclast colony-stimulating factor, *Proc Natl Acad Sci USA* **88**: 8500–4.

Lepre F, Grill V, Ho PWM et al (1993) Hypercalcemia in pregnancy and lactation associated with parathyroid hormone-related protein, *N Engl J Med* **328**: 666–7.

Lerner UH (1987) Modifications of the mouse calvarial technique improve the responsiveness to stimulators of bone resorption, *J Bone Miner Res* **2**: 375–83.

Lewis DB, Liggit D, Teitelbaum S et al (1992) Mechanism of osteoporosis in IL-4 transgenic mice, *J Bone Miner Res* **7** (Suppl 1): no 20.

Lin HY, Harris TL, Flannery MS et al (1991) Expression cloning of an adenylate cyclase-coupled calcitonin receptor, *Science* **254**: 1022–4.

Liu B, Amizuka N, Goltzman D et al (1995) Inhibition of processing of parathyroid hormone-related peptide by antisense furin: effect in vitro and in vivo on rat Leydig (H500) tumor cells, *Int J Cancer* **63**: 276–81.

Liu JP, Baker J, Perkins AS et al (1993) Mice carrying null mutations of the genes encoding insulin-like growth factor I (Igf-I) and type I IGF receptor (Igflr), *Cell* **75**: 59–72.

Lorenzo JA, Quinton J (1984) Epidermal growth factor enhances the resorptive response to parathyroid hormone, *Calcif Tissue Int* **36**: 465.

Lu C, Ikeda K, Deftos LJ et al (1989) Glucocorticoid regulation of parathyroid hormone-related peptide gene transcription in a human neuroendocrine cell line, *Mol Endocrinol* **3**: 2034–40.

Lynch SE, Williams RC, Polson AM et al (1989) A combination of platelet-derived and insulin-like growth factors enhances periodontal regeneration, *J Clin Periodontol* **16**: 545–8.

MacDonald BR, Mundy GR, Clark S et al (1986) Effects of human recombinant CSF-GM and highly purified CSF-1 on the formation of multinucleated cells with osteoclast characteristics in long term bone marrow cultures, *J Bone Miner Res* **1**: 227–33.

Mackie EJ, Trechsel U (1990) Stimulation of bone formation in vivo by transforming growth factor β—remodeling of woven bone and lack of inhibition by indomethacin, *Bone* **11**: 295–300.

Mahmood R, Bresnick J, Hornbruch A et al (1995) A role for FGF-8 in the initiation and maintenance of vertebrate limb bud outgrowth, *Curr Biol* **5**: 797–806.

Manolagas SC, Jilka RL (1995) Mechanisms of disease: bone marrow, cytokines, and bone remodeling—emerging insights into the pathophysiology of osteoporosis, *N Engl J Med* **332**: 305–11.

Manolagas SC, Burton DW, Deftos LJ (1981) 1,25-dihydroxyvitamin D_3 stimulates the alkaline phosphatase activity of osteoblast-like cells, *J Biol Chem* **256**: 7115–17.

Manolagas SC, Provvedini DM, Tsoukas C (1985) Interactions of 1,25-dihydroxyvitamin D_3 and the immune system, *Mol Cell Endocrinol* **43**: 113–22.

Marcelli C, Yates AJP, Mundy GR (1990) In vivo effects of human recombinant transforming growth factor beta on bone turnover in normal mice, *J Bone Miner Res* **5**: 1087–96.

Martin TJ, Moseley JM, Gillespie MT (1991) Parathyroid hormone-related protein: biochemistry and molecular biology, *Crit Rev Biochem Mol Biol* **26**: 377–95.

Mason IJ (1994) The ins and outs of fibroblast growth factors, *Cell* **78**: 547–52.

Mayahara H, Ito T, Nagai H et al (1993) In vivo stimulation of endosteal bone formation by basic fibroblast growth factor in rats, *Growth Factors* **9**: 73–80.

McSheehy PMJ, Chambers TJ (1986) Osteoblastic cells mediate osteoclastic responsiveness to parathyroid hormone, *Endocrinology* **118**: 824–8.

McSheehy PMJ, Chambers TJ (1987) 1,25-dihydroxyvitamin D_3 stimulates rat osteoblastic cells to release a soluble factor that increases osteoclastic bone resorption, *J Clin Invest* **80**: 425–9.

Meghji S, Sandy JR, Scutt AM et al (1988) Stimulation of bone resorption by lipoxygenase metabolites of arachidonic acid, *Prostaglandins* **36**: 139–47.

Merke J, Klaus G, Hugel U et al (1986) No 1,25-dihydroxyvitamin D_3 receptors on osteoclasts of calcium-deficient chicken despite demonstrable receptors on circulating monocytes, *J Clin Invest* **77**: 312–14.

Merryman JI, DeWille JW, Werkmeister JR et al (1994) Effects of transforming growth factor β on parathyroid hormone-related protein production and ribonucleic acid expression by a squamous carcinoma cell line in vitro, *Endocrinology* **134**: 2424–30.

Miyaura C, Segawa A, Nagasawa H et al (1986) Effects of retinoic acid on the activation and fusion of mouse alveolar macrophages induced by 1 alpha,25-dihydroxyvitamin D_3, *J Bone Miner Res* **1**: 359–68.

Mohan S, Jennings TA, Linkhardt JE et al (1988) Primary structure of human skeletal growth factor (SGF): homology with IGF-II, *J Bone Miner Res* **3**: 598.

Montesano R, Vassalli JD, Baird A et al (1986) Basic fibroblast growth factor induces angiogenesis in vitro, *Proc Natl Acad Sci USA* **83**: 7297–301.

Morimoto S, Onishi T, Imanaka S et al (1986) Topical administration of 1,25-dihydroxyvitamin D_3 for psoriasis: report of five cases, *Calcif Tissue Int* **38**: 119–22.

Moseley JM, Jubota M, Diefenbach-Jagger H et al (1987) Parathyroid hormone-related protein purified from a human lung cancer cell line, *Proc Natl Acad Sci USA* **84**: 5048–52.

Muenke M, Schell U, Hehr A et al (1994) A common mutation in the fibroblast growth factor receptor 1 gene in Pfeiffer syndrome, *Nat Genet* **8**: 269–74.

Mundy GR (1996) Editorial: an OAF by any other name, *Endocrinology* **137**: 1149–50.

Nakamura T, Hanada K, Tamura M et al (1995) Stimulation of endosteal bone formation by systemic injections of recombinant basic fibroblast growth factor in rats, *Endocrinology* **136**: 1276–84.

Neilson KN, Friesel RE (1995) Constitutive activation of fibroblast growth factor receptor-2 by a point mutation associated with Crouzon syndrome, *J Biol Chem* **270**: 26 037–40.

Nicholson GC, Moseley JM, Sexton PM et al (1987) Chicken osteoclasts do not possess calcitonin receptors, *J Bone Miner Res* **2**: 53–9.

Niewolna M, Yoneda T, Izbicka E et al (1993) Direct regulation of src tyrosine kinase activity and bone resorption in mature osteoclasts by a soluble mediator, platelet-derived growth factor (PDGF), *J Bone Miner Res* **8** (Suppl 1): no 6.

Noda M, Camilliere JJ (1989) In vivo stimulation of bone formation by transforming growth factor β, *Endocrinology* **124**: 2991–4.

Orloff JJ, Reddy D, de Papp A (1994) Parathyroid hormone-related protein as a prohormone: posttranslational processing and receptor interactions, *Endocrinol Rev* **15**: 40–60.

Orloff JJ, Soifer NE, Fodero JP et al (1993) Accumulation of carboxyl-terminal fragments of parathyroid hormone-related protein in renal failure, *Kidney Int* **43**: 1371–6.

Pacifici R, Rifas L, Teitelbaum S et al (1987) Spontaneous release of interleukin-1 from human blood monocytes reflects bone formation in idiopathic osteoporosis, *Proc Natl Acad Sci USA* **84**: 4616–20.

Pacifici R, Rifas L, McCracken R et al (1989) Ovarian steroid treatment blocks a postmenopausal increase in blood monocyte interleukin-1 release, *Proc Natl Acad Sci USA* **86**: 2398–402.

Paul WE (1991) Interleukin-4: a prototypic immunoregulatory lymphokine, *Blood* **77**: 1859–70.

Pfeilschifter J, Mundy GR (1987) Modulation of transforming growth factor beta activity in bone cultures by osteotropic hormones, *Proc Natl Acad Sci USA* **84**: 2024–8.

Pfeilschifter JP, Seyedin S, Mundy GR (1988) Transforming growth factor β inhibits bone resorption in fetal rat long bone cultures, *J Clin Invest* **82**: 680–5.

Pfeilschifter J, Chenu C, Bird A et al (1989) Interleukin-1 and tumor necrosis factor stimulate the formation of human osteoclast-like cells in vitro, *J Bone Miner Res* **4**: 113–18.

Pfeilschifter J, Wolf O, Naumann A et al (1990) Chemotactic response of osteoblast-like cells to transforming growth factor β, *J Bone Miner Res* **5**: 825–30.

Philbrick WM, Wysolmerski JJ, Galbraith S et al (1996) Defining the roles of parathyroid hormone-related protein in normal physiology, *Physiological Rev* **76**: 127–73.

Pirola CJ, Wang HM, Kamyar A et al (1993) Angiotensin II regulates parathyroid hormone-related protein expression in cultured rat aortic smooth muscle cells through both transcriptional and posttranscriptional mechanisms, *J Biol Chem* **268**: 1987–94.

Plawner LL, Philbrick WM, Burtis WJ et al (1995) Cell type-specific secretion of parathyroid hormone-related protein via the regulated versus the constitutive secretory pathway, *J Biol Chem* **270**: 14 078–84.

Powell PP, Klagsbrun M (1991) Three forms of rat basic fibroblast growth factor are made from a single mRNA and localize to the nucleus, *J Cell Physiol* **148**: 202–10.

Price PA, Baukol SA (1980) 1,25-Dihydroxyvitamin D_3 increases synthesis of the vitamin K-dependent bone protein by osteosarcoma cells, *J Biol Chem* **255**: 11 660–3.

Provvedini DM, Tsoukas CD, Deftos LJ et al (1983) 1,25-Dihydroxyvitamin D_3 receptors in human leukocytes, *Science* **221**: 1181–3.

Raisz LG (1965) Bone resorption in tissue culture. Factors influencing the response to parathyroid hormone, *J Clin Invest* **44**: 103–16.

Raisz LG (1970) Physiologic and pharmacologic regulation of bone resorption, *N Eng J Med* **282**: 909–16.

Raisz LG, Trummel CL, Simmons H (1972a) Induction of bone resorption in tissue culture: prolonged response after brief exposure to parathyroid hormone or 25-hydroxycholecalciferol, *Endocrinology* **90**: 744–51.

Raisz LG, Trummel CL, Wener JA et al (1972b) Effect of glucocorticoids on bone resorption in tissue culture, *Endocrinology* **90**: 961–7.

Raisz LG, Trummel CL, Holick MF et al (1972c) 1,25 Dihydroxycholecalciferol: a potent stimulator of bone resorption in tissue culture, *Science* **175**: 768–9.

Raisz LG, Sandberg AL, Goodson JM et al (1974) Complement-dependent stimulation of prostaglandin synthesis and bone resorption, *Science* **185**: 789–91.

Raisz LG, Dietrich JW, Simmons HA et al (1977) Effects of prostaglandin endoperoxides and metabolites and bone resorption in vitro, *Nature* **267**: 532–5.

Raisz LG, Kream BE, Smith MD et al (1980a) Comparison of the effects of vitamin D metabolites on collagen synthesis and resorption of fetal rat bone in organ culture, *Calcif Tissue Int* **32**: 135–8.

Raisz LG, Simmons HA, Sandberg AL et al (1980b) Direct stimulation of bone resorption by epidermal growth factor, *Endocrinology* **107**: 270–3.

Ralston SH, Gardner MD, Jenkins AS et al (1985) Comparison of aminohydroxypropylidene diphosphonate, mithramycin and corticosteroids/calcitonin in treatment of cancer associated hypercalcaemia, *Lancet* **ii**: 207–10.

Rao LG, Ng B, Brunette DM et al (1977) Parathyroid hormone and prostaglandin E1 response in a selected population of bone cells after repeated sub-culture and storage at $-80°$ C, *Endocrinology* **100**: 1233–41.

Ratcliffe WA (1992) Role of parathyroid hormone-related protein in lactation, *Clin Endocrinol* **37**: 402–4.

Reardon W, Winter RM, Rutland P et al (1994) Mutations in the fibroblast growth factor receptor 2 gene cause Crouzon syndrome, *Nat Genet* **8**: 98–103.

Reddy SV, Takahashi S, Dallas M et al (1994) IL-6 antisense deoxyoligonucleotides inhibit bone resorption by giant cells from human giant cell tumors of bone, *J Bone Miner Res* **9**: 753–7.

Reitsma PH, Rothbert PG, Astria SM et al (1983) Regulation of myc gene expression in HL-50 leukaemia cells by a vitamin D metabolite, *Nature* **306**: 492–4.

Reynolds JJ, Pavlovitch H, Balsan S (1976) 1,25-dihydroxycholecalciferol increases bone resorption in thyroparathyroidectomized mice, *Calcif Tissue Res* **21**: 207–12.

Rigby WFC, Stacy T, Fanger MW (1984) Inhibition of T lymphocyte mitogenesis by 1,25-dihydroxyvitamin D_3 (calcitriol), *J Clin Invest* **74**: 1451–5.

Rizzoli R, Feyen JHM, Grau G et al (1994) Regulation of parathyroid hormone-related protein production in a human lung squamous cell carcinoma line, *J Endocrinol* **143**: 333–41.

Rodan SB, Insogna KL, Vignery AM et al (1983) Factors associated with humoral hypercalcemia of malignancy stimulate adenylate cyclase in osteoblastic cells, *J Clin Invest* **72**: 1511–15.

Rodan SB, Wesolowski G, Thomas K et al (1987) Growth stimulation of rat calvaria osteoblastic cells by acidic fibroblast growth factor, *Endocrinology* **121**: 1917–23.

Rodan SB, Wesolowski G, Thomas KA et al (1989) Effects of acidic and basic fibroblast growth factors on osteoblastic cells, *Connect Tissue Res* **20**: 283–8.

Roodman GD, Ibbotson KJ, MacDonald BR et al (1985) 1,25-Dihydroxyvitamin D_3 causes formation of multinucleated cells with several osteoclast characteristics in cultures of primate marrow, *Proc Natl Acad Sci USA* **82**: 8213–17.

Roodman GD, Kurihara N, Ohsaki Y et al (1991) Interleukin-6 a potential autocrine/paracrine factor in Paget's disease of bone, *J Clin Invest* **89**: 46–52.

Rouleau MF, Mitchell J, Goltzman D (1988) In vivo distribution of parathyroid hormone receptors in bone: evidence that a predominant osseous target cell is not the mature osteoblast, *Endocrinology* **123**: 187–91.

Rousseau F, Bonaventure J, Legeal-Mallet L et al (1994) Mutations in the gene encoding fibroblast growth factor receptor 3 in achondroplasia, *Nature* **371**: 252–4.

Sabatini M, Boyce B, Aufdemorte T et al (1988) Infusions of recombinant human interleukin-1 α and β cause hypercalcemia in normal mice, *Proc Natl Acad Sci USA* **85**: 5235–9.

Sabatini M, Chavez J, Mundy GR et al (1990) Stimulation of tumor necrosis factor release from monocytic cells by the A375 human melanoma via granulocyte–macrophage colony stimulating factor, *Cancer Res* **50**: 2673–8.

Sabatini M, Yates AJ, Garrett R et al (1990) Increased production of tumor necrosis factor by normal immune cells in a model of the humoral hypercalcemia of malignancy, *Lab Invest* **63**: 676–81.

Samuels MH, Veldhuis J, Cawley C et al (1993) Pulsatile secretion of parathyroid hormone in normal young subjects: assessment by deconvolution analysis, *J Clin Endocrinol Metab* **77**: 399–403.

Sartori L, Weir EC, Stewart AF et al (1987) Synthetic and partially-purified adenylate cyclase-stimulating proteins from tumors associated with humoral hypercalcemia of malignancy inhibit phosphate transport in a PTH-responsive renal cell line, *J Clin Endocrinol Metab* **66**: 459–61.

Sato K, Fujii Y, Kasono K et al (1989) Parathyroid hormone-related protein and interleukin-1α synergistically stimulate bone resorption in vitro and increase the serum calcium concentration in mice in vivo, *Endocrinology* **124**: 2172–8.

Schipani E, Krese K, Juppner H (1995) A constitutively active mutant PTH-PTH-rP receptor in Jansen-type metaphyseal chondrodysplasia, *Science* **268**: 98–100.

Sebag M, Henderson J, Goltzman D et al (1994) Regulation of parathyroid hormone-related peptide production in normal human mammary epithelial cells in vitro, *Am J Physiol* **267**: C723–30.

Shiang R, Thomspon LM, Zhu Y-Z et al (1994) Mutations in the transmembrane domain of FGFR3 cause the most common genetic form of dwarfism, achondroplasia, *Cell* **78**: 335–42.

Simonet WS, Lacey DL, Dunstan CR et al (1997) Osteoprotegerin: a novel secreted protein involved in the regulation of bone density, *Cell* **89**: 309–19.

Simpson EL, Mundy GR, D'Souza SM et al (1983) Absence of parathyroid hormone messenger RNA in nonparathyroid tumors associated with hypercalcemia, *N Engl J Med* **309**: 325–30.

Smith D, Gowen M, Mundy GR (1987) Effects of interferon gamma and other cytokines on collagen synthesis in fetal rat bone cultures, *Endocrinology* **120**: 2494–9.

Soifer NE, Dee KE, Insogna KL et al (1992) Parathyroid hormone-related protein. Evidence for secretion of a novel mid-region fragment by three different cell types, *J Biol Chem* **367**: 18 236–43.

Southby J, Murphy LM, Martin TJ et al (1996) Cell-specific and regulator-induced promoter usage and messenger ribonucleic acid splicing for parathyroid hormone-related protein, *Endocrinology* **137**: 1349–57.

Spencer EM, Liu CC, Si ECC et al (1991) In vivo actions of insulin-like growth factor-I (IGF-I) on bone formation and resorption in rats, *Bone* **12**: 21–6.

St Arnaud R, Arabian A, Glorieux FH (1996) Abnormal bone development in mice deficient for the vitamin D 24-hydroxylase gene, *J Bone Miner Res* **11** (abstract): no 127.

Stashenko P, Dewhirst FE, Peros WJ et al (1987) Synergistic interactions between interleukin-1, tumor necrosis factor, and lymphotoxin in bone resorption, *J Immunol* **138**: 1464–8.

Stern PH, Halloran BP, DeLuca HF et al (1983) Responsiveness of vitamin D deficient fetal rat limb bones to parathyroid hormone in culture, *Am J Physiol* **224**: E421.

Stern PH, Horst RL, Gardner R et al (1985) 10-Keto or 25-hydroxy substitution confer equivalent in vitro bone resorbing activity to vitamin D_3, *Arch Biochem Biophys* **236**: 555–8.

Stewart AF (1996) PTHrP (1–36) as a skeletal anabolic agent for the treatment of osteoporosis, *Bone* **19**: 303–6.

Stewart AF, Horst R, Deftos LJ et al (1980) Biochemical evaluation of patients with cancer-associated hypercalcemia: evidence for humoral and nonhumoral groups, *N Engl J Med* **303**: 1377–83.

Stewart AF, Wu T, Goumas D et al (1987) N-terminal amino acid sequence of two novel tumor-derived adenylate cyclase-stimulating proteins: identification of parathyroid hormone-like and parathyroid hormone-unlike domains, *Biochem Biophys Res Commun* **146**: 672–8.

Strewler GJ, Nissenson RA (1994) The parathyroid hormone-related protein as a regulator of normal tissue function, *Curr Opin Endocrinol Diab* 286–92.

Strewler GJ, Stern PH, Jacobs JW et al (1987) Parathyroid hormone-like proteins from human renal carcinoma cells: structural and functional homology with parathyroid hormone, *J Clin Invest* **80**: 1803–7.

Suva LJ, Winslow GA, Wettenhall REH et al (1987) A parathyroid hormone-related protein implicated in malignant hypercalcemia: cloning and expression, *Science* **237**: 893–6.

Takahashi S, Goldring S, Katz M et al (1995) Down regulation of calcitonin receptor mRNA expression by calcitonin during human osteoclast-like cell differentiation, *J Clin Invest* **95**: 167–71.

Tashjian AH, Voelkel EF, Levine L et al (1972) Evidence that the bone resorption-stimulating factor produced by mouse fibrosarcoma cells is prostaglandin E2: a new model for the hypercalcemia of cancer, *J Exp Med* **136**: 1329–43.

Tashjian AH, Wright DR, Ivey JL et al (1978) Calcitonin binding sites in bone: relationships to biological response and "escape", *Recent Prog Horm Res* **34**: 285–334.

Tashjian AH, Hohmann EL, Antoniades HN et al (1982) Platelet-derived growth factor stimulates bone resorption via a prostaglandin mediated mechanism, *Endocrinology* **111**: 118–24.

Tashjian AH, Voelkel EF, Lazzaro M et al (1987) Tumor necrosis factor (cachectin) stimulates bone resorption in mouse calvaria via a prostaglandin-mediated mechanism, *Endocrinology* **120**: 2029–36.

Teti A, Rizzoli R, Zambonin-Zallone A (1991) Parathyroid hormone binding to cultured avian osteoclasts, *Biochem Biophys Res Commun* **174**: 1217–22.

Thiede MA (1989) The mRNA encoding a parathyroid hormone-like peptide is produced in mammary tissue in response to elevations in serum prolactin, *Mol Endocrinol* **3**: 1443–7.

Thiede MA, Rodan GA (1988) Expression of a calcium-mobilizing parathyroid hormone-related like peptide in lactating mammary tissue, *Science* **242**: 278–80.

Thiede MA, Harm SC, Hasson DM et al (1991) In vivo regulation of parathyroid hormone-related peptide messenger ribonucleic acid in the rat uterus by 17 β-estradiol, *Endocrinology* **128**: 2317–23.

Thomson BM, Saklatvala J, Chambers TJ (1986) Osteoblasts mediate interleukin-1 stimulation of bone resorption by rat osteoclasts, *J Exp Med* **164**: 104–12.

Thomson BM, Mundy GR, Chambers TJ (1987) Tumor necrosis factors alpha and beta induce osteoblastic cells to stimulate osteoclastic bone resorption, *J Immunol* **138**: 775–9.

Tsoukas CD, Provvedini DM, Manolagas SC (1984) 1,25 Dihydroxyvitamin D_3: a novel immunoregulatory hormone, *Science* **224**: 1438–40.

Tsuda E, Goto M, Mochizuki S et al (1997) Isolation of a novel cytokine from human fibroblasts that specifically inhibits osteoclastogenesis, *Biochem Biophys Res Commun* **234**: 137–42.

Ueno K, Haba T, Woodbury D et al (1985) The effects of prostaglandin E2 in rapidly growing rats: depressed longitudinal and radial growth and increased metaphyseal hard tissue mass, *Bone* **6**: 79–86.

Underwood JL, DeLuca HF (1984) Vitamin D is not directly necessary for bone growth and mineralization, *Am J Physiol* **246**: E493–E498.

Urist MR (1965) Bone: formation by autoinduction, *Science* **150**: 893.

Usdin TB, Gruber C, Bonner TI (1995) Identification and functional expression of a receptor selectively recognizing parathyroid hormone, the PTH2 receptor, *J Biol Chem* **270**: 15 455–8.

Usdin TB, Bonner TI, Harta G et al (1996) Distribution of parathyroid hormone-2 receptor messenger ribonucleic acid in rat, *Endocrinology* **137**: 4285–97.

Uy HL, Dallas M, Wright K et al (1993) Multipotent hematopoietic osteoclast precursors are increased by interleukin-1 in vivo, *J Bone Miner Res* **8** (Suppl 1): no 1084.

Vaes G (1968) On the mechanism of bone resorption. The action of parathyroid hormone on the excretion and synthesis on the lysosomal enzymes and on the extracellular release of acid by bone cells, *J Cell Biol* **39**: 676–97.

Vickery BH, Avnur A, Cheng Y et al (1996) RS-66271, a C-terminally substituted analog of human parathyroid hormone-related protein (1–34), increases trabecular and cortical bone in ovariectomized, osteopenic rats, *J Bone Miner Res* **11**: 1943–51.

Vlodavsky I, Folkman J, Sullivan R et al (1987) Endothelial cell-derived basic fibroblast growth factor: synthesis and deposition into subendothelial extracellular matrix, *Proc Natl Acad Sci USA* **84**: 2292–6.

Vortkamp A, Lee K, Lanske B et al (1996) Regulation of rate of cartilage differentiation by Indian hedgehog and PTH-related protein, *Science* **273**: 613–22.

Watanabe K, Tanaka Y, Morimoto I et al (1990) Interleukin-4 as a potent inhibitor of bone resorption, *Biochem Biophys Res Commun* **172**: 1035–41.

Weir EC, Philbrick WM, Amling M et al (1996) Targeted overexpression of parathyroid hormone-related peptide in chondrocytes causes chondrodysplasia and delayed endochondral bone formation, *Proc Natl Acad Sci USA* **93**: 10 240–5.

Wener JA, Gorton SJ, Raisz LG (1972) Escape from inhibition of resorption in cultures of fetal bone treated with calcitonin and parathyroid hormone, *Endocrinology* **90**: 752–9.

Wiktor-Jedzrejcak W, Ahmed A, Szczylik C et al (1982)

Hematological characterization of congenital osteopetrosis in op/op mouse, *J Exp Med* **156**: 1516–27.

Wong BR, Josien R, Lee SY et al (1997) TRANCE (tumor necrosis factor (TNF)-related activation induced cytokine, a new TNF family member predominantly expressed in T cells, is a dendritic cell-specific survival factor, *J Exp Med* **186**: 2075–80.

Wozney JM, Rosen V (1993) Bone morphogenetic proteins. In: Mundy GR, Martin TJ, eds, *Physiology and pharmacology of bone* (Springer Verlag: Berlin) 725–48.

Wu TL, Soifer NE, Burtis WJ et al (1991) Glycosylation of parathyroid hormone-related peptide secreted by human epidermal keratinocytes, *J Clin Endocrinol Metab* **73**: 1002–7.

Wysolmerski JJ, Vasavada R, Foley J et al (1996) Transactivation of the PTH-rP gene in squamous carcinomas predicts the occurrence of hypercalcemia in athymic mice, *Cancer Res* **56**: 1043–9.

Yamamoto M, Kawanobe Y, Takahashi H et al (1984) Vitamin D deficiency and renal calcium transport in the rat, *J Clin Invest* **74**: 507–13.

Yasuda H, Shima N, Nakagawa N et al (1998) Osteoclast differentiation factor is a ligand for osteoprotegerin/osteoclastogenesis-inhibitory factor and is identical to TRANCE/RANKL, *Proc Natl Acad Sci* **95**: 3597–602.

Yates AJP, Gutierrez GE, Smolens P et al (1988) Effects of a synthetic peptide of a parathyroid hormone-related protein on calcium homeostasis, renal tubular calcium reabsorption and bone metabolism, *J Clin Invest* **81**: 932–8.

Yates AJP, Favarato G, Aufdemorte TB et al (1992) Expression of human transforming growth factor α by Chinese hamster ovarian tumors in nude mice causes hypercalcemia and increase osteoclastic bone resorption, *J Bone Miner Res* **7**: 847–53.

Yoneda T, Alsina MM, Chavez JB et al (1991) Evidence that tumor necrosis factor plays a pathogenetic role in the paraneoplastic syndromes of cachexia, hypercalcemia, and leukocytosis in a human tumor in nude mice, *J Clin Invest* **87**: 977–85.

Yoneda T, Alsina MM, Garcia JL et al (1991) Differentiation of HL-60 cells into cells with the osteoclast phenotype, *Endocrinology* **129**: 683–9.

Yoneda Y, Aufdemorte TB, Nishimura R et al (1991) Occurrence of hypercalcemia and leukocytosis with cachexia in a human squamous cell carcinoma of the maxilla in athymic nude mice. A novel experimental model of three concomitant paraneoplastic syndromes, *J Clin Oncol* **9**: 468–77.

Yoneda T, Takaoka Y, Alsina MM et al (1991) Porcine pancreas extract decreases blood ionized calcium in mice and inhibits osteoclast formation and bone resorption in culture, *FEBS Lett* **278**: 171–4.

Yoneda T, Alsina MM, Watatani K et al (1991) Dependence of a human squamous carcinoma and associated paraneoplastic syndromes on ambient epidermal growth factor concentrations and its receptors in nude mice, *Cancer Res* **51**: 2438–43.

Yoneda T, Nishimura R, Kato I et al (1991) Frequency of hypercalcemia-leukocytosis syndrome in oral malignancies, *Cancer* **68**: 617–22.

Yoneda T, Nakai M, Moriyama K et al (1993) Neutralizing antibodies to human interleukin-6 reverse hypercalcemia associated with a human squamous carcinoma, *Cancer Res* **53**: 737–40.

Yoshida H, Hayashi SI, Kunisada T et al (1990) The murine mutation osteopetrosis is in the coding region of the macrophage colony stimulating factor gene, *Nature* **345**: 442–4.

Yu JH, Wells H, Ryan WJ et al (1976) Effects of prostaglandins and other drugs on the cyclic AMP content of cultured bone cells, *Prostaglandins* **12**: 501–13.

Zakalik D, Diep D, Hooks MA et al (1992) Transforming growth factor β increases stability of parathyroid hormone-related protein messenger RNA, *J Bone Miner Res* **7**: 104.

Zhang WY, Cao X, Onishi T et al (1995) The osteoblast proliferative action of parathyroid hormone is mediated by increased expression and activity of cdc2, *J Bone Miner Res* **10** (Suppl 1): no T525.

CHAPTER 5

Pharmacologic treatment for diseases of bone remodeling

The pharmacologic therapies available for the treatment of bone disease have expanded within the last 10 years, although not as dramatically as they may in the next 10 years. Effective (albeit imperfect) drugs to inhibit osteoclastic bone resorption are available. Paget's disease of bone and the hypercalcemia of malignancy can be readily treated. Estrogen therapy is useful both in the prevention and treatment of osteoporosis. Unfortunately, the treatment of established osteoporosis is still a major problem. During the last 10 years, most attention has centered on the bisphosphonate compounds, and the new generation bisphosphonates that can be administered orally as well as parenterally clearly have great potential. Much less success has been achieved so far in the development of drugs to stimulate bone formation.

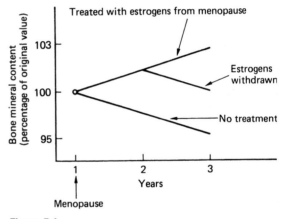

Figure 5.1

Effects of estrogens in slowing the rate of bone loss after the menopause. In normal women, bone mineral content begins to decrease following the menopause. This loss in bone mineral content is prevented by estrogen therapy.

Estrogen

Although Albright first suggested 50 years ago that estrogen may be useful therapy for postmenopausal osteoporosis, it was not documented until approximately 15 years ago that estrogen is a very effective inhibitor of the rapid bone loss associated with the postmenopausal period (Figure 5.1). It is one of the few areas in osteoporosis research where there is little controversy. However, there is still much to be learned about the mode of action of estrogen, and whether knowledge of this mode of action will lead to more useful drugs with the beneficial effects of estrogen but without the unwanted effects.

Indications

The indications for estrogen therapy for osteoporosis are the following:

- For the prevention of menopause-associated bone loss in women who are at risk of the later development of osteoporosis (because of the presence of osteoporosis-associated risk factors such as low bone mineral density or early menopause).
- For women with established osteoporosis within 20 years of the menopause, and in whom there is no contraindication.
- For postmenopausal women with primary hyperparathyroidism in whom surgical therapy is contraindicated.

For each of these indications, the minimal effective dose is 0.625 mg of premarin each day. Generic compounds have not been well studied and should be avoided until equivalent bio-availability has been documented. In women with an intact uterus, medroxyprogesterone is prescribed (5–10 mg per day) for the first 14 days of each calendar month, and premarin should be taken daily year round. All patients on this regimen should undergo yearly mammography, frequent breast examination and thorough investigation of abnormal vaginal bleeding.

Mechanism of action

Estrogen therapy reduces the rapid phase of bone loss that occurs in all postmenopausal adult women. A number of studies dating back over many years have shown that enhanced bone loss associated with increased bone turnover occurs for 5–10 years following the menopause (Aitken et al 1973; Heaney et al 1978; Christiansen and Lindsay 1990). Estrogen inhibits the activation frequency of osteoclasts on bone resorbing surfaces (Parfitt 1979). The mechanism by which estrogen inhibits bone resorption remains unknown. Estrogen deficiency is associated with hyperactive or "killer" osteoclasts as described by Parfitt (1979), which appear to have increased capacity to perforate trabecular bone plates. One possibility is that estrogen deficiency increases osteoclast lifespan. Hughes et al (1996) have shown that estrogen enhances programmed cell death in osteoclasts and that in states of estrogen withdrawal, osteoclast apoptosis is reduced and osteoclasts live longer. This may be the explanation for the "killer" osteoclasts described by Parfitt (1979). The effects of estrogen on bone are likely indirect, and there is data to suggest that the effect of estrogen on apoptosis is mediated by transforming growth factor β (TGFβ) (Hughes et al 1996). Estrogens do not inhibit all forms of osteoclastic bone resorption. For example, they are not effective in the treatment of the hypercalcemia of malignancy or in Paget's disease. However, they do reduce osteoclastic bone resorption in the postmenopausal period, and they do lower the serum calcium in postmenopausal patients with primary hyperparathyroidism (Marcus et al 1984; Selby and Peacock 1986). Early studies suggested that there is decreased sensitivity of bone cells to parathyroid hormone (PTH) in the presence of estrogen (Heaney 1965). Recently, it has been shown that there are relatively small numbers of estrogen receptors in bone cells, both osteoblasts and osteoclasts (Eriksen et al 1988; Komm et al 1988; Oursler et al 1991). Osteoblasts release factors that influence osteoclast activity such as TGFβ and bone resorbing cytokines such as interleukin-6, interleukin-1 and tumor necrosis factor. It is possible that estrogens exert their effects by modulating the production of these local factors in bone.

Much attention recently has been focused on the potential role of IL-1 and IL-6 in bone loss associated with the menopause. Pacifici et al (1987, 1989) have shown data that circulating monocytes produced enhanced amounts of IL-1 in vitro in the postmenopausal period, and this can be reduced by treating patients with estrogen. Enhanced production of IL-1 as the mediator of the effects of estrogen withdrawal is potentially useful information, since IL-1 receptor antagonists could be used for the treatment of postmenopausal bone loss. A review of the role of these cytokines has recently been published (Pacifici et al 1996). An alternative viewpoint is that of Jilka et al (1992) who have suggested that IL-6 may be responsible, at least in part, for the bone loss secondary to estrogen withdrawal in mice that had been ovariectomized. These workers showed that neutralizing antibodies to IL-6 blocked the bone loss associated with ovariectomy. IL-1 and IL-6 are not the only cytokines influenced by estrogen. Pacifici (1996) has implicated a number of others. One cytokine in the bone microenvironment that may be responsible for some of the estrogen effects on bone cells is

TGFβ. TGFβ production by bone cells is enhanced by estrogen and anti-estrogens (Komm et al 1988; Oursler et al 1994; Yang et al 1996).

Available compounds and mode of administration

The pharmacokinetics and pharmacodynamics of estrogen therapy have not been thoroughly and systematically studied. In the treatment of osteoporosis, most information is available for the use of premarin (conjugated equine estrogen). However, it is likely that all forms of estrogen are effective in equivalent doses. Dose-response studies have shown that 0.625 mg premarin daily is the minimal effective dose (Christiansen et al 1982; Lindsay et al 1983). This is equivalent to 0.2 mg ethinyl estradiol or 0.625 mg estrone sulfate. Transdermal estrogen patches or gels applied to the skin are effective (Riis et al 1987; Ludkin et al 1992). Equivalent doses of estrace and estraderm (transdermal 17β-estradiol) are 1 mg and 0.05 mg respectively. It is hoped that these modes of administration may avoid some of the side effects associated with oral estrogen therapy.

Efficacy

Estrogen therapy is very effective in preventing the rapid phase of bone loss associated with the menopause. Epidemiologic studies show that estrogen provides protection against the risk of later development of osteoporotic fractures (Weiss et al 1980; Ettinger et al 1985). Estrogen reduces the hip fracture rate by at least 50%, and probably has similar or even greater effects on vertebral fracture rates (Lindsay 1996). Retrospective case–control studies and prospective clinical trials have confirmed the long-term efficacy of estrogen (Ettinger et al 1985; Cauley et al 1995). Thus, its effects on bone are comparable to those of the available bisphosphonate, alendronate. Maximal effects are produced when estrogens are used from menopause until old age. Estrogen therapy clearly produces a beneficial effect during the first 10 years after the menopause, but most physicians in this field now prescribe estrogens even up to 20 years after the menopause. Although there is emerging evidence that estrogens may decrease fracture rate in these older patients, responses are probably more modest in patients aged over 60. Concomitant use of progestins as 19-nor-testosterone derivatives may enhance the effects of estrogen on bone mineral density (Lindsay 1996).

There are other important indications for estrogen therapy in women after menopause. These include beneficial effects of estrogen on the cardiovascular system and blood lipid profiles as well as effects on general well being and possible effects on preventing or at least slowing the progression of dementia.

Adverse drug reactions

There are no immediate serious adverse drug reactions. The major long-term concerns associated with estrogen therapy have been the development of uterine cancer or risk of breast cancer. The risk of endometrial cancer (about 1% per year) can be prevented by adding sequential progestin to the estrogen therapy. This is only necessary in patients who have an intact uterus. There is arguably a slight risk of development of breast cancer, or of acceleration of already existing occult breast cancer, but the risk is small and most of the studies so far reported that have indicated a significant risk have had methodological problems. There continue to be conflicting and confusing reports on this issue (Colditz et al 1995; Couzi et al 1995; McPherson 1995; Newcomb et al 1995; Schneider et al 1995; Speroff 1996). Each one tends to receive publicity in the lay press and increases the anxiety of patients who are considering or taking estrogen therapy. If there is increased risk, it requires 10–15 years of estrogen use. It is not known if this potential slight risk is dependent on the type of estrogen used or whether the addition of progestin has any effect. Other adverse effects of estrogen therapy include the development of hypertension because of increased production of renin substrate, gall stones associated with increased hepatic production of bile acids and thromboembolic phenomena, possibly associated with the increased hepatic production of coagulation factors, but these are associated more often with oral contraceptive preparations containing higher doses of estrogen. Estrogen therapy likely has a beneficial effect on serum lipids and decreases the likelihood of later development of coronary artery disease. If progestin is added, the beneficial effect on serum lipids may be reduced. The effects of added progestin on the risk of later cardiovascular disease are still not clear.

The most common reasons why women will not take estrogen therapy are not related to these severe toxicities, but rather to withdrawal bleeding and unpleasant premenstrual symptoms.

Bisphosphonates

Description

Bisphosphonates are synthetic analogs of pyrophosphate (Fleisch et al 1969; Francis et al 1969). Their chemical structure is shown in Figure 5.2. They were originally developed as agents that would prevent plaque formation on teeth and calcification. However, it was soon discovered that they also inhibited osteoclastic bone resorption (Russell et al 1970) and their current therapeutic uses are based on this effect. There are now three generations of compounds. Only etidronate, pamidronate, tiludronate and alendronate are currently available in the United States. However, other second and third generation bisphosphonates of high potency (Table 5.1) are also available in other countries. The current agents most widely used world-wide are etidronate, clodronate and pamidronate, and alendronate (Fosamax). Others such as risedronate, tiludronate, zoledronate and ibandronate are likely to become widely available in the next few years.

Etidronate was the only bisphosphonate available in the United States until 1992. This is clearly a transitional drug that will eventually be replaced by other more effective, less toxic and more potent bisphosphonates. Treatment of Paget's disease with etidronate is associated with impairment of mineralization in doses that inhibit bone resorption. Patients with the hypercalcemia of malignancy do not respond to oral etidronate without a previous course of intravenous etidronate, and the response is not as reliable as with the newer bisphosphonates.

Of the other widely used bisphosphonates, two

Pyrophosphate

$$PO_3H_2 - O - PO_3H_2$$

EHDP (ethane-1-hydroxy-1,1-bisphosphonate)

$$PO_3H_2 - \underset{\underset{OH}{|}}{\overset{\overset{CH_3}{|}}{C}} - PO_3H_2$$

APD (3-amino-1-hydroxy propane-1,1-bisphosphonate)

$$PO_3H_2 - \underset{\underset{CH_2CH_2NH_2}{|}}{\overset{\overset{OH}{|}}{C}} - PO_3H_2$$

Cl$_2$MDP (dichloromethane bisphosphonate)

$$PO_3H_2 - \underset{\underset{Cl}{|}}{\overset{\overset{Cl}{|}}{C}} - PO_3H_2$$

Figure 5.2

Structures of commonly used bisphosphonate compounds compared with pyrophosphate.

(alendronate and pamidronate) are amino bisphosphonates. Because of the amino group, these bisphosphonates are associated with acute phase reactions in vivo. These are probably less common with alendronate. Currently, no oral formulation for pamidronate is used outside South America. Both these drugs are extremely effective inhibitors of bone resorption when used in appropriate doses and modes of administration. They are used exclusively in osteoporosis (alendronate), Paget's disease (alendronate and pamidronate, IV. infusion) and cancer which involves the skeleton with or without hypercalcemia (pamidronate, IV. infusion). Tiludronate and clodronate are also very effective, but are less potent. An oral preparation of clodronate is available and widely used in western Europe. There are no problems with mineralization at the doses used for inhibition of bone resorption. It has not been released in the United States because several patients treated in investigative studies over

Table 5.1 Antiresorbing potency of various bisphosphonates in the rat (Fleisch 1995).

Bisphosphonate	Relative potency
Etidronate	1
Clodronate	10
Tiludronate	10
Pamidronate	100
Alendronate	1000
Risedronate	5000
Zoledronate	10 000

15 years ago developed acute leukemia. However, in retrospect, it seems most likely that this was an unrelated event.

Mechanism of action

Bisphosphonates are effective inhibitors of osteoclastic bone resorption (Russell et al 1970). However, it is still not known how they inhibit osteoclast activity. In bones treated with bisphosphonates, osteoclasts are not reduced in number, and may even be increased, although their capacity to resorb bone is clearly impaired. One postulate is that bisphosphonates coat bone surfaces, and thereby prevent osteoclasts from resorbing bone (Carano et al 1990; Sato et al 1991). However, it is not clear whether their affinity for bone surfaces correlates with their anti-osteoclastic activity. It is also not clear whether there is any relationship between their capacity to inhibit mineralization and their antiresorptive activity. They have many effects on osteoblastic cells, and these effects have been related directly to their capacity to inhibit osteoclastic bone resorption (Sahni et al 1993). Some workers believe that some of these compounds also have additional effects on osteoclastic bone resorption that are mediated through the immune system (Lowik et al 1986).

Several newer ideas of bisphosphonate action have been postulated (Rodan and Fleisch 1996). Hughes et al (1996) have suggested that bisphosphonates enhance apoptosis in osteoclasts, thereby reducing their lifespan and reducing bone resorption. Bisphosphonates increase morphologic appearances of osteoclast apoptosis both in vitro and in vivo. The relative importance of apoptosis in the mode of action of bisphosphonates remains unclear. Sahni et al (1993) have suggested that bisphosphonates may act through a cellular mechanism where the primary target is the osteoblast, which in turn inhibits osteoclast activity. These studies, based on cell culture effects, show a good relationship with the in vivo potency of the bisphosphonates (Sahni et al 1993). More recently, Schmidt et al (1996) have suggested that bisphosphonates act by specifically targeting a protein tyrosine phosphatase in the osteoclast called PTP epsilon. Although it is important to determine if there is a molecular target for bisphosphonates in the osteoclast, it is not clear whether the bisphosphonates bind to this phosphatase, or whether this is a specific effect of the bisphosphonates and not one common to other agents that inhibit bone resorption. Rogers et al (1994) have suggested that the target for bisphosphonates may be similar to a protein they have studied in the slime mold *Dictostelium discoideum*, which binds bisphosphonates and which is related to an increase in cell proliferation. It will be interesting to see if this protein or its homologue is also expressed in osteoclasts. These workers have recently suggested that this effect is mediated by inhibitory effects on enzymes in the cholesterol biosynthesis pathway (Rogers et al 1997).

Mode of administration

All the bisphosphonate compounds are poorly absorbed from the gastrointestinal tract. Less than 10% of an ingested dose of any of these compounds is absorbed, and with many it is probably between 1% and 5%. This has led to problems in assessing toxicity and therapeutic effects, and in comparing potency of individual agents. Of the total amount of bisphosphonate that is absorbed, 50% goes rapidly to bone (within minutes), and 50% appears unmetabolized and unchanged in the urine. With all bisphosphonates there is prolonged skeletal retention. This is greater than one year in the rat and is probably the same or even longer in humans. This has led to concerns of potential skeletal toxicity of long-term treatment with bisphosphonates. In particular, it has been questioned whether bisphosphonate retention in the skeleton may cause prolonged inhibition of normal bone remodeling (that is, may "freeze" the skeleton).

Since all bisphosphonates are poorly absorbed, parenteral administration by the intravenous route is most desirable when an urgent response is required. Although oral therapy is preferred for long-term therapy, some bisphosphonates such as pamidronate are not available in oral formulations for general use. The amino-bisphosphonates are associated with mucosal ulcerations when taken orally (De Groen et al 1996). Drugs such as alendronate should be given one hour before breakfast with a large amount of water and the patient is advised to stand upright. This serves to enhance absorption and prevent mucosal alterations in the gastrointestinal tract (Harris et al 1993). When clodronate is given orally, gastrointestinal irritation can be limited by giving the drug in divided doses throughout the day. Mucosal ulcerations have not been described with clodronate.

When used in the treatment of hypercalcemia of malignancy, all the bisphosphonates have a relatively slow onset of action. Serum calcium is unlikely to return to normal range until about 4–5 days after institution of therapy. For these reasons, calcitonin should be administered at the same time as bisphosphonate therapy is commenced if an urgent response is required (Ralston et al 1986).

Efficacy

Bisphosphonates have now been approved by the Food and Drug Administration (FDA) for the treatment of established osteoporosis (alendronate), Paget's disease of bone (alendronate, tiludronate, pamidronate, etidronate), the hypercalcemia of malignancy (etidronate, pamidronate), and osteolytic bone disease due to solid tumors and myeloma (pamidronate).

All the bisphosphonates probably have efficacy in the treatment of established osteoporosis when used in appropriate doses (Storm et al 1990; Liberman et al 1995, 1996). Alendronate has been shown to decrease both vertebral and hip fracture rates, probably by about 50% (Black 1996; Liberman et al 1995, 1996). Ibandronate and risedronate are in phase III clinical trials. Bisphosphonates are also efficacious in Paget's disease of bone (Frijlink et al 1979; Meunier et al 1979), hypercalcemia of malignancy (Mundy et al 1983; Sleeboom et al 1983; Singer and Fernandez 1987), osteolytic bone disease due to tumor metastasis (Van Breukelen et al 1979; Siris et al 1980, 1983; Berenson et al 1996; Hortobagyi et al 1996), and in primary hyperparathyroidism (Shane et al 1981) (Figures 5.3–5.5). Longer-term studies have confirmed that pamidronate, particularly when given in a monthly intravenous infusion, is effective in osteolytic bone disease due to solid tumors and myeloma (Berenson, 1998; Hortobagyi, 1998; Lipton, 1998). Bisphosphonates have also been used in the treatment of Sudek's osteodystrophy, heterotopic ossification and calcification, and renal stones, although their beneficial effects in these latter conditions are not well documented.

One contentious issue frequently raised with the bisphosphonates, and most recently with alendronate, is whether they have a true anabolic effect on bone. The reported data are that alendronate increases bone mineral density about 9% over 3 years in the spine, with more modest increases at the hip (Liberman et al 1995, 1996). It is important to recognize that this does not necessarily mean new bone formation. It could readily be explained by several other mechanisms, for example, hypermineralization of pre-existing bone or filling in of the remodeling space. Until there is histomorphometric evidence of new bone formation, this cannot be claimed as a true anabolic effect.

We have used new generation bisphosphonates such as risedronate and ibandronate in animal models of human metastatic breast cancer to bone. We have found that these agents effectively reduce osteoclastic bone resorption, prevent the development of osteolytic bone lesions, prevent the progression of osteolytic bone lesions, and even more importantly, decrease tumor burden in bone (Sasaki et al 1995). Although these studies are more difficult to perform in patients with metastatic bone disease because of many confounding variables, there is now accumulating evidence that bisphosphonates of the new generation are also very effective in preventing skeletal events associated with metastatic solid tumors (Hortobagyi et al 1996). The general use of new generation bisphosphonates in patients with osteolytic bone disease should soon be widespread, particularly following their recent approval by the FDA for this purpose.

Bisphosphonates are also used as targeting agents for technetium bone scans. They direct the scanning agent to sites of increased bone turnover.

Adverse reactions

The major adverse effect of etidronate is impairment of mineralization when the drug is used in

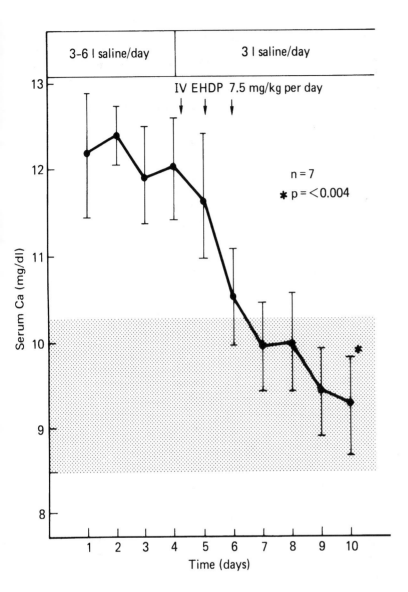

Figure 5.3

Effects of intravenous etidronate on serum calcium in patients with hypercalcemia of malignancy. (Conversion of traditional units to SI units: serum calcium 1 mmol/l = 4 mg/dl.) (Reproduced from Singer and Fernandez (1987).)

large doses for prolonged periods of time (for example, 20 mg/kg body weight for more than 3 months). However, even when it is used in lower doses in patients with Paget's disease of bone, etidronate has been associated with progression of osteolytic lesions (Krane 1982; Singer and Krane 1990) and osteomalacia (Boyce et al 1984). The impairment of mineralization is not as apparent with the second and third generation bisphosphonates in doses that inhibit osteoclastic bone resorption, although this may need to be investigated more closely since focal osteomalacia has been noted in association with pamidronate (Adamson et al 1993).

The aminobisphosphonates (pamidronate and alendronate) have been associated with acute phase responses including transient fever and leukocytosis (Frijlink et al 1979; Bijvoet et al 1980). Oral administration of pamidronate and alendronate has also been associated with ulceration of the mouth and esophagus (De Groen et al 1996). This is not as frequent with alendronate,

Figure 5.4

Effects of APD (pamidronate) on serum calcium in patients with hypercalcemia of malignancy. (Reproduced from Mundy et al (1983).)

and should not frequently occur in patients with normal gastrointestinal tracts who take the medication according to the instructions provided in the package insert, namely before breakfast with a large amount of water and with the patient standing upright. If less potent bisphosphonates such as etidronate are administered too rapidly intravenously, then they may cause precipitation in the bloodstream and subsequent renal failure (Bounameaux et al 1983).

Indications

Bisphosphonates are currently indicated in those conditions associated with increased osteoclastic bone resorption. They are effective in the treatment of established osteoporosis (Liberman et al 1996), Paget's disease of bone (Frijlink et al 1979; Meunier et al 1979), hypercalcemia of malignancy (Mundy et al 1983; Sleeboom et al 1983; Singer and Fernandez 1987; Nussbaum et al 1993), osteolytic bone disease due to tumor metastasis (Van Breukelen et al 1979; Siris et al 1980, 1983; Berenson et al 1996; Hortobagyi et al 1996), and in primary hyperparathyroidism (Shane et al

Figure 5.5

Effects of different bisphosphonates on serum calcium in patients with hypercalcemia of malignancy. Patients treated with pamidronate received a single intravenous infusion of 30 mg in 0.9% saline over 4 hours. Patients treated with clodronate received a single intravenous infusion of 600 mg in 500 ml 0.9% saline over 6 hours. Patients treated with etidronate received 7.5 mg/kg body weight in 500 ml 0.9% saline over 2 hours for 3 consecutive days. (Reproduced from Ralston et al (1989).)

1981). They have also been used in the treatment of Sudek'sosteodystrophy, heterotopic ossification and calcification, and renal stones, although their beneficial effects in these latter conditions are not well documented.

Calcitonin

Description

Calcitonin is one of the most widely prescribed drugs for diseases of bone. The world market in 1991 was well over $500 million, although this has fallen dramatically in the last few years because of reduced government reimbursement for calcitonin use in Europe, combined with more widespread use of new therapies such as the bisphosphonates. However, there are great regional prescribing differences. Calcitonin has been very popular in Italy and Japan, but is less popular in the United States.

Available compounds and mode of administration

Calcitonin preparations are currently available in different countries as derivatives of salmon, human, porcine or eel calcitonin. In the United States, only salmon and human forms are available. Salmon is the most widely used and most potent, although all are probably equally effective. Calcitonin can be administered intramuscularly, subcutaneously or intranasally. It has a rapid onset of action within 30 minutes, but loss of effectiveness occurs within 48 hours due to the "escape" phenomenon, which is associated with decreased expression of calcitonin receptor mRNA (Takahashi et al 1995). Several alternative modes of administration are now being utilized. These include the use of intranasal aerosol sprays, aerosols for oral inhalation and suppositories. These latter preparations may eventually prove more suitable modes of administration for chronic therapy with possibly fewer side effects. Their absorption may be less reliable, but there is accumulating evidence for their efficacy (Reginster et al 1987; Overgaard et al 1989; Rizzato et al 1989; Overgaard et al 1992; Ellerington et al 1996). Calcitonin has not been compared side-by-side with alendronate or estrogen-related compounds, so it is difficult to compare. Intranasal calcitonin has been approved by the FDA to be used in doses of 200 IU daily in women more than 5 years postmenopausal and with low bone mass.

Indications

- Osteoporosis – in particular, patients with evidence of high bone turnover and patients with immobilization osteoporosis. Data suggest that patients with high turnover forms of osteoporosis respond best to calcitonin treatment (Civitelli et al 1988). Calcitonin is a suitable alternative to estrogen or bisphosphonates as an inhibitor of resorption.
- Paget's disease of bone – may stop progression of lytic lesions and promote healing.
- Hypercalcemia of malignancy, particularly if a rapid effect is desired and the patient has poor renal function.

Mechanism of action

Calcitonin is an effective inhibitor of osteoclastic bone resorption. It has direct effects on osteoclasts, increasing cyclic AMP content, causing contraction of cytoplasmic membranes, a decrease in area of the osteoclast ruffled border and inhibiting the osteoclast's capacity to resorb bone (Friedman et al 1968; Heersche et al 1974; Chambers and Magnus 1982). Osteoclasts may "escape" from the inhibitory effects of calcitonin by down-regulation of cell surface receptors (Wener et al 1972). Osteoclast responsivity to calcitonin may be prolonged by concomitant corticosteroid therapy (Binstock and Mundy 1980). Calcitonin also lowers plasma calcium by increasing renal calcium excretion (Ralston et al 1985). The relative contribution of inhibiting bone resorption and increasing renal calcium excretion to the lowering of the serum calcium remains unclear. Calcitonin also has a direct central analgesic effect that may be mediated through increases in β-endorphin secretion.

The target cells in the osteoclast lineage for calcitonin are shown in Figure 5.6.

Adverse effects

Calcitonin has no major side effects. Some patients may suffer transient nausea or anorexia associated with administration. This effect is dose-dependent and occurs in about 10–20% of patients. Some patients experience facial flushing following administration especially of the parenteral form. The development of antibodies to calcitonin does not appear to be a significant clinical problem. Systemic allergic reactions are very rare, although intradermal administration of a test dose before beginning therapy is recommended.

Efficacy

Calcitonin has been shown to be modestly effective in the treatment of osteoporosis for periods up to 2 years. These early results were obtained by Gruber et al (1984) using neutron activation analysis to follow changes in total body calcium content and by Civitelli et al (1988) who used bone mineral density measurements. In the latter study, calcitonin was shown to be most effective in patients with high turnover osteoporosis. Whether calcitonin will be shown to be effective in longer-term studies remains to be demonstrated since the short-term 2-year effects to increase bone mass have been attributed to filling in of the bone remodeling space following inhibition of resorption. Other studies with salmon calcitonin have also shown a significant reduction of risk of vertebral fracture (Overgaard et al 1992; Kanis et al 1992; Rico et al 1992). Calcitonin is effective in the treatment of patients with hypercalcemia of malignancy, and particularly patients with hematologic malignancies (Binstock and Mundy 1980). It is most useful in this situation when it is used with concomitant corticosteroids (Figures 5.7–5.9). It is less useful in primary hyperparathyroidism or in patients with solid tumors and hypercalcemia (Mundy et al 1983). Calcitonin is extremely effective in the treatment of Paget's disease of bone (Bijvoet et al 1968). Approximately 70% of patients will achieve a good therapeutic response. There have been suggestions that it may be even more effective when used in combination with bisphosphonates such as etidronate.

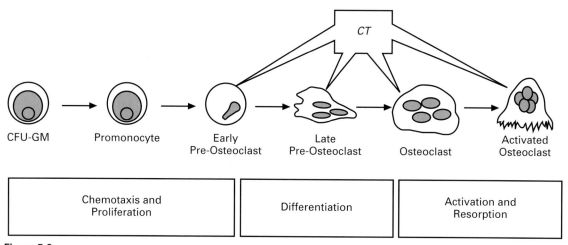

Figure 5.6

Sites in the osteoclast lineage at which calcitonin exerts effects. Note that calcitonin inhibits both formation of new osteoclasts as well as activity of pre-existing osteoclasts.

PHARMACOLOGIC TREATMENT FOR DISEASES OF BONE REMODELING   93

Figure 5.7

Effects of calcitonin alone and the combination of calcitonin and glucocorticoids in patients with hypercalcemia of malignancy. (A) Patients treated with calcitonin alone. (B) Patients with lymphoproliferative disorders treated with the combination of calcitonin and glucocorticoids. (C) Patients with solid tumors treated with a combination of calcitonin and glucocorticoids. (Conversion of traditional units to SI units: serum calcium 4 mg/dl = 1 mmol/l.) (Reproduced from Binstock and Mundy (1980) with permission from the *Annals of Internal Medicine*.)

Figure 5.8

Effects of calcitonin and glucocorticoids compared with calcitonin alone in the treatment of patients with the hypercalcemia of malignancy. The combination produced a prolonged beneficial effect where calcitonin alone produced only a transient effect followed by rapid relapse to the pre-treatment level of serum calcium. These patients had not responded to glucocorticoids alone. (Conversion of traditional units to SI units: 4 mg/dl = 1 mmol/l.) (Reproduced from Binstock and Mundy (1980) with permission from the *Annals of Internal Medicine*.)

Figure 5.9

Effects of calcitonin and glucocorticoids in the long-term management of a patient with renal failure and the hypercalcemia of malignancy due to myeloma. Calcitonin was withdrawn for 2 days out of every 7, and the serum calcium was maintained in an acceptable range that did not cause symptoms. (Conversion of traditional units to SI units: 4 mg/dl = 1 mmol/l.) (Reproduced from Binstock and Mundy (1980) with permission from the *Annals of Internal Medicine*.)

Oral calcium

Description

Oral calcium has been widely used in the prevention and treatment of osteoporosis for many years. Its use reached a peak in the mid-1980s. Since negative calcium balance associated with dietary calcium deficiency is present in many patients with osteoporosis (Heaney et al 1982), it has been thought reasonable to correct this deficiency. Although the place of oral calcium therapy in the treatment of established osteoporosis is controversial, it is well accepted that oral calcium intake sufficient to maintain normal calcium balance is necessary during adolescence to ensure development of optimal peak bone mass, and that calcium-deficient diets can aggravate bone loss associated with the menopause and aging (Heaney 1991; Johnston et al 1992). It has been found that people who ingest diets that contain less than enough calcium to ensure normal calcium balance have increased incidence of hip fractures in later life (Matkovic et al 1979).

Available compounds

Many forms of oral calcium preparations are available. Since the amount of elemental calcium in these calcium salts differs widely, the total amount of calcium (and the number of tablets) that need to be ingested to receive 1 g of elemental calcium varies. The commonly used preparations include calcium gluconate, calcium carbonate, calcium lactate and calcium citrate (Table 5.2). The bioavailability of each of these forms of oral calcium varies. The dose that is required for maximal beneficial effects in the postmenopausal period is controversial.

Mechanism of action

Aging and low dietary calcium intakes are associated with secondary hyperthyroidism. Oral calcium therapy suppresses parathyroid hormone (PTH) secretion and increases calcitonin secretion in patients with postmenopausal osteoporosis (Riggs et al 1976). It leads to an improvement in

Table 5.2 Table of comparisons of various calcium supplement preparations.

Salt	Tablet size (mg)	Elemental Ca (%)	Required[a] dose/day (tablets)
Calcium gluconate	500	9	22
Calcium lactate	325	13	24
Calcium carbonate	1250	40	2
Calcium citrate	1000	24	4

[a] For 1 g elemental calcium.

calcium balance, which is presumably beneficial since many patients with osteoporosis are in negative calcium balance due to impaired calcium absorption from the gut. It may also increase the availability of mineral at sites of bone formation.

Efficacy

Oral calcium therapy may be most important for the development of peak bone mass (Heaney 1991). Adolescent teenage girls are the segment of the population most deficient in dietary calcium. However, adult women are also in negative calcium balance, which can be corrected by calcium supplements, particularly in patients in the later age groups with Type II osteoporosis who suffer hip fracture. Negative calcium balance is also present in the postmenopausal period, but recent data suggest that oral calcium cannot replace estrogen as a form of therapy to reduce the accelerated bone loss associated with the menopause. However, increasing dietary calcium intake to 1000–1500 mg per day lowers PTH secretion and reduces bone loss in postmenopausal women.

Adverse drug reactions

The potential risks of oral calcium therapy include development of renal calculi, nephrocalcinosis, milk–alkali syndrome and hypercalcemia. All these are very unlikely if less than 1500 mg/day of elemental calcium is used and the patient is monitored. Some forms of calcium therapy, and particularly calcium gluconate, may be associated with gastrointestinal upset such as nausea, constipation or diarrhea.

Mode of administration and indications

Everyone agrees that calcium deficiency should be corrected. However, it is more controversial how much calcium is required. This is made more difficult by the absence of any satisfactory test to monitor calcium deficiency, and the variable bioavailability of calcium preparations. If the diet is deficient in milk, as is frequently the case in women, or in green leafy vegetables, then it should be supplemented with calcium. Calcium supplementation of the diet either in the form of calcium salts or of calcium-rich foods to achieve a calcium intake of 1000–1500 mg/day is recommended. Assuming that the dietary calcium intake is 300–500 mg per day (unless the patients history suggests otherwise), it is reasonable to prescribe 1000 mg elemental calcium for teenagers and 1500 mg for women in the postmenopausal years.

Although calcium carbonate is probably the most widely used calcium supplement, calcium citrate is a reasonable alternative, particularly in elderly patients who may be achlorhydric, since it has better bioavailability in this situation.

Fluoride

Fluoride has been widely used in the treatment of postmenopausal osteoporosis for many years. It has always been a controversial drug because many physicians have doubted its efficacy and have been concerned by the frequency of side effects, and particularly the risk of increased bone fragility. This issue remains unresolved. New preparations of fluoride such as monofluorophosphate and slow release sodium fluoride may reduce some of these side effects, although not all these studies are positive, and some investigators remain unconvinced that fluoride therapy reduces vertebral fracture rates in nontoxic doses.

Mechanism of action

Fluoride therapy increases bone formation. These effects are seen in spinal trabecular bone, not cortical bone. The mechanism by which fluoride stimulates bone formation is not clear. One group has suggested that fluoride acts directly on bone cells to inhibit the activity of an osteoblast acid phosphatase that is responsible for the dephosphorylation of tyrosine kinases (Farley et al 1983; Lau et al 1989). Such an effect would lead to enhanced tyrosine kinase activity, and potentially enhance the effects of growth factor to cause proliferation of bone cells. An alternative theory proposed by Burgener et al (1995) is that fluoride increases tyrosine kinase activity in osteoblasts, and this effect is potentiated by small amounts of aluminum (Caverzasio et al 1996). Although there is a dramatic increase in bone formation in response to fluoride therapy, the new bone may be structurally abnormal when higher doses are used. Fluoride is incorporated into the mineral phase of bone and newly formed bone frequently shows evidence of mineralization defects. The bone tends to be spongy and irregular and mineralizes poorly. If supplemental oral calcium and vitamin D are given with fluoride, this mineralization defect does not occur.

Mode of administration

Three different types of preparation of fluoride are used: sodium fluoride, sodium monoflourophosphate, and now slow-release sodium fluoride. The latter two are associated with fewer gastrointestinal side effects and are much safer compounds than plain sodium chloride. This is very important because the therapeutic window for fluoride is very narrow. Following therapy with sodium fluoride, serum concentrations of 10 µM/l may lead to maximal beneficial effects, but 15 µM/l may be toxic. The importance of the bioavailability of the preparation has recently been emphasized in view of the narrow therapeutic window (Pak et al 1989; Nagant et al 1990). The use of concomitant oral calcium and vitamin D is necessary to prevent osteomalacia.

Efficacy

Fluoride therapy increases bone mass in the vertebrae in approximately 70% of osteoporotic patients. Bone mass is increased by 10% per year as measured by bone mineral density. The increase is progressive without a plateau, and is dramatic. Similar effects are not produced with any other current form of therapy. The responses may be even greater when assessed by quantitative computerized tomography. Many uncontrolled studies have reported the benefits of fluoride therapy. However, recent randomized controlled studies show there may be an increased risk of fractures in the appendicular skeleton (Riggs et al 1990). Fracture rates are unchanged in the vertebrae.

The problem with fluoride therapy was apparent with several NIH-sponsored studies in the US during the 1980s (Riggs et al 1990; Kleerekoper et al 1991). Although there was an impressive increase in bone mineral density in the vertebral spine, there was not a concomitant improvement found in vertebral fracture rates. This led to considerable skepticism regarding the benefits of fluoride. Some investigators felt that these negative results were due to the dose of fluoride being too high in these studies and considered lower doses or alternative forms of therapy, including slow-release sodium fluoride and sodium monofluorophosphate. These have been shown to be effective in some studies (Pak et al 1996a,b), but not in others, as reported by Meunier for the FAVOS study in patients at the World Osteoporosis Congress in May 1996.

Adverse reactions

There is an increased risk of fracture in patients treated with fluoride, which is presumably related to structurally abnormal bone and the mineralization defect caused by excessive fluoride administration. In uncontrolled studies, increases in spinal fracture rates have not been observed (Farley et al 1990). In addition, there are other less serious side effects that occur in 30–40% of patients treated with this form of therapy. These include synovitis, anemia, gastric irritation (discomfort, nausea, vomiting), and a periarticular pain syndrome in the lower extremities associated with stress microfractures. These dose-related side effects may be so irritating that approximately 30% of patients will not continue to take this therapy. The nonskeletal side effects can be reduced by discontinuation of therapy for one month and then resumption at a lower dose. They can also be limited by using slow-release or enteric-coated preparations. The critical factor, however, may be careful selection of dose with measurement of serum fluoride levels.

Indications

At the current time, fluoride should probably not be used except in investigational studies until clearer information is available on doses that decrease bone fragility. The theoretical indication is for the patient with a low turnover form of osteoporosis, where stimulation of bone formation is required.

The most effective dose is probably in the range of 60–75 mg of NaF daily, although side effects are more likely in this range. Beneficial effects may be seen with as little as 30 mg of NaF per day.

One of the major problems with fluoride therapy is that about 30% of patients do not respond, and so far it has not been possible to predict those who would not respond prior to initiating therapy.

Calcitriol and other vitamin D preparations

Description

Calcitriol (1,25-dihydroxyvitamin D_3) is the most active metabolite of vitamin D. Vitamin D and its analogs stimulate calcium absorption from the gut and are used in conditions associated with calcium malabsorption. They are also used for other diseases associated with impaired bone mineralization. The most widely used preparations include the parent compounds such as ergocholecalciferol or cholecalciferol, 25-hydroxyvitamin D_3, 1α-hydroxyvitamin D_3 and calcitriol (Table 5.3).

Mode of administration

As the most active metabolite of vitamin D, calcitriol is a fat-soluble vitamin that is well

Table 5.3 Vitamin D-like compounds in therapeutic use.

Nonproprietary name	Abbreviation	Commercial name	Effective daily dose	Time for reversal of toxic effects (days)
Cholecalciferol	Vitamin D_3	–	–	–
Ergocalciferol	Vitamin D_2	Calciferol	1–10 mg	17–60
Calcifediol	25(OH)D_3	Calderol	0.05–0.5 mg	7–30
Dihydrotachysterol		Dihydrotachysterol	0.1–1 mg	3–14
Alfacalcidol	1α(OH)D_3	One-alpha*	1–2 µg	5–10
Calcitriol	1,25(OH)$_2D_3$	Rocaltrol	0.5–1 µg	2–10

*Not available in the USA.

absorbed from the gastrointestinal tract in individuals with normal intestinal absorption. Because its biological half-life is so short, its toxicity is also very short-lived. Its toxic effects have disappeared after 48 hours.

Calcitriol (and other vitamin D preparations) increases the absorption of calcium from the gut and promotes the normal mineralization of bone. These are probably the major benefits it bestows in osteoporosis. It leads to a decrease in parathyroid hormone (PTH) secretion due to both direct and indirect effects. It also increases osteoclastic bone resorption and promotes the differentiation of cells of the osteoblast phenotype. It may also affect osteoclast function because of its effects on the production of osteotropic cytokines such as interleukin-1 and tumor necrosis factor (DeLuca 1982; Norman et al 1982; Bell 1985). The therapeutic significance of these latter effects is entirely unknown.

Efficacy

Calcitriol promotes calcium absorption from the gut. It is recommended for use in the treatment of patients with renal bone disease and secondary hyperparathyroidism, in postmenopausal osteoporosis and in rickets or osteomalacia associated with vitamin D deficiency, or with phosphate depletion due to oncogenic osteomalacia or sex-linked hypophosphatemic rickets. Its efficacy in these different conditions is variable. In renal bone disease it clearly decreases PTH secretion and promotes normal mineralization of bone. However, it will not correct mineralization defects associated with aluminum toxicity. Its efficacy in osteoporosis is fiercely debated. Vitamin D metabolites are widely believed by Japanese physicians to be a useful therapy for osteoporosis and are one of the most commonly prescribed drugs for postmenopausal osteoporosis in Japan. Calcitriol or other vitamin D metabolites are not as popular in other parts of the world. There are many conflicting reports on efficacy. Some studies have suggested therapy leads to an increase in bone mass and a decrease in vertebral fractures (Lindholm et al 1982; Orimo et al 1987). Others have shown decreased bone mass and increased fractures (Finn et al 1982; Ott and Chesnut 1989). What is clear is that elderly individuals are frequently vitamin D deficient, and that vitamin D supplementation of the diet can prevent hip fractures (Chapuy et al 1992).

Indications

Calcitriol (0.25 µg/day) is most likely to be effective in those osteoporotic patients who have impaired calcium absorption from the gut reflected by low urinary calcium excretion (< 100 mg/24 hours) and low serum calcitriol concentrations. This is relatively common in elderly patients with low turnover osteoporosis of the Type II variety. Parent vitamin D is a satisfactory and cheaper alternative in the elderly (Chapuy et al 1992).

Calcitriol is also used in rickets or osteomalacia associated with phosphate depletion due to oncogenic osteomalacia and sex-linked hypophosphatemia. It should be used in conjunction with oral phosphate therapy in these conditions. It is less effective in this type of osteomalacia than it is in osteomalacia due to vitamin D deficiency.

Adverse effects

Calcitriol may cause hypercalciuria and hypercalcemia especially in the elderly and should be used only with careful monitoring. In pharmacologic amounts it is also likely to increase osteoclastic bone resorption leading to actual bone loss. There is a very narrow window between therapeutic and toxic doses.

Plicamycin (mithramycin)

Description

Plicamycin therapy has been widely used for treatment of hypercalcemia of malignancy and less widely for Paget's disease of bone. At the present time, its place in both these conditions is limited following the advent of safer drugs that are at least equally efficacious. The introduction of gallium nitrate and powerful bisphosphonates, such as pamidronate, have made plicamycin almost obsolete.

Mechanism of action

Plicamycin inhibits DNA-dependent RNA synthesis (Yarbro et al 1966; Wollheim et al 1968; Northrop et al 1969). Its beneficial effects on serum calcium were found serendipitously. It was used as an anticancer agent in the 1960s and was found to cause a lowering of the serum calcium (Kofman et al 1964; Brown and Kennedy 1965). Its inhibitory effects on bone resorption have been shown in organ cultures (Cortes et al 1972; Minkin 1973). It is probably toxic to bone cells because its effects appear to be irreversible.

Mode of administration

Although plicamycin can be administered as an intravenous infusion or as a bolus infusion, the recommended mode of administration is by intravenous infusion. The dose should be 15–25 μg/kg body weight administered over 4 hours. Its clearance is reduced by impaired renal function. Plicamycin's effect on serum calcium lasts for variable periods. In some patients with hypercalcemia of malignancy, the serum calcium remains normal for 2 weeks following a single infusion. In others, the serum calcium may rise after 3 or 4 days (Mundy and Martin 1982; Mundy et al 1983).

Efficacy

Plicamycin works in approximately 80% of patients with the hypercalcemia of malignancy, causing a lowering of the serum calcium to the normal range (Mundy et al 1983). It is one of the most effective of antihypercalcemic therapies, although it is probably not as effective as the newer bisphosphonates (Figure 5.10). It is rather slow-acting, taking 24–48 hours to produce its maximal effects. It is also very effective in the treatment of Paget's disease of bone. Its use has not been as widespread in this situation because of its potential toxicity, but it has been effective in patients who have been refractory to other forms of therapy.

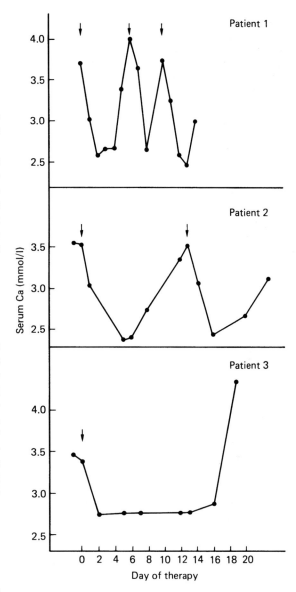

Figure 5.10

Effects of plicamycin (mithramycin) (25 μg/kg body weight per day) on serum calcium in three patients with the hypercalcemia of malignancy. Note the different patterns of response. Time of plicamycin infusion is indicated by the arrows. Note the rebound effect in Patient 3. (Reproduced from Mundy et al (1983).)

Adverse effects

Plicamycin has many toxicities, although it is used in lower doses in the treatment of hypercalcemia than when used as an anticancer agent. It may cause liver damage, with an increase in hepatocellular enzymes, and may also cause bone marrow suppression, nausea, vomiting and diarrhea. It has also been associated with a bleeding diathesis, which is not related to thrombocytopenia. It also may cause nephrotoxicity, and since it is cleared by the kidneys, its toxic effects are enhanced in patients with poor renal function.

Indications

Plicamycin can be used in several ways in the management of hypercalcemia of malignancy, either as one initial infusion followed by repeated infusions when the serum calcium increases, or infusions can be given on five successive days. There is no general agreement on which is the best approach.

Oral phosphate therapy

Description

Oral phosphate therapy is used in the treatment of hypercalcemia due to malignancy or primary hyperparathyroidism if the serum phosphorus is low. It is possibly most useful in the medical treatment of primary hyperparathyroidism.

Mechanism of action

Oral phosphate therapy probably has three separate modes of action on calcium homeostasis. It decreases calcium absorption from the gut because it binds calcium in the gut lumen, it causes soft tissue calcium deposition and it inhibits osteoclastic bone resorption (Raisz and Niemann 1969; Mundy and Martin 1982; Lorenzo et al 1984; Yates et al 1991). Its effects on osteoclastic bone resorption have been shown both in vitro and in vivo. Its effects on osteoclasts may be related to a physicochemical effect (Lorenzo et al 1984). Its effects to cause soft tissue calcium deposition depend on the speed of administration. When it is given rapidly, precipitation in soft tissues is more likely to occur, particularly in patients who are markedly hypercalcemic, who have poor renal function or who have high serum phosphate concentrations. This leads to serious toxicity (see below).

Mode of administration

Phosphate therapy should only be given orally. It should not be given intravenously since this frequently leads to soft tissue calcium deposition. It may be administered orally as tablets or as an elixir. Rectal suppositories have also been used. It is given in divided doses of 2–3 g/day of neutral sodium phosphate.

To avoid diarrhea associated with oral phosphate therapy, the dose can be reduced, or it can be given with antidiarrheal agents. It is frequently used successfully in conjunction with other agents, particularly in the treatment of hypercalcemia of malignancy.

Efficacy

Oral phosphate therapy is reasonably effective in lowering the serum calcium in patients who are hypophosphatemic (less than 4 mg/dl) and who have normal renal function (Figure 5.11). Since low serum phosphate enhances bone resorption, it is very effective in hypophosphatemic patients, even if other agents are also being used to lower the serum calcium. In my experience, it almost always works in patients with primary hyperparathyroidism, at least transiently (Mundy et al 1983). The major problem with its continued use is troublesome diarrhea.

Adverse effects

The most common side effect associated with continued oral phosphate therapy is diarrhea.

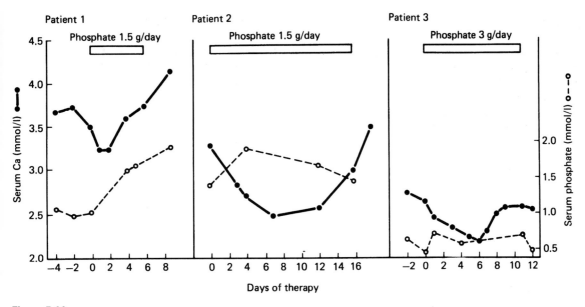

Figure 5.11

Effects of oral phosphate therapy on the serum calcium and serum phosphate in three patients with hypercalcemia of malignancy. (Reproduced from Mundy et al (1983).)

Although the mechanism responsible for diarrhea is not known, the effect is dose-related and diarrhea may be reduced by lowering the dose of oral phosphate. Phosphate therapy can also lead to renal stones, muscle cramps and pain and to soft tissue calcification (Carey et al 1968; Dudley and Blackburn 1970; Ayala et al 1975). In patients with impaired renal function, it can cause soft tissue calcification in the kidney, lungs, heart and other organs. This may lead to death from corresponding organ failure.

Gallium nitrate

Description

Gallium nitrate is an anticancer drug that was found serendipitously in early clinical studies to cause hypocalcemia and increased urinary excretion of calcium (Krakoff 1979; Warrell et al 1983; Warrell et al 1985). Later, it was found that gallium nitrate decreases bone resorption in vitro (Warrell et al 1984).

Indications

Gallium nitrate is not available for treatment of bone disease as yet, but is mentioned here because it has considerable future promise. It is currently being used in investigational studies for hypercalcemia of malignancy, osteolytic bone disease, Paget's disease of bone and osteoporosis.

Studies to date

Gallium nitrate was initially used in a series of 10 patients with hypercalcemia of malignancy. Gallium was administered as a continuous intravenous infusion at 200 mg/m^2/day for 5–7 days. In all patients there was a fall in the serum calcium to the normal range (Warrell et al 1984). In a later dose-ranging study, it was found that 200 mg/m^2/day was superior to 100 mg/m^2/day and caused a more prolonged response in patients with hypercalcemia of malignancy (Warrell et al 1986). In several later randomized double-blind studies, it was found that gallium nitrate was more effective than calcitonin and etidronate.

To date, studies in metastatic bone disease and Paget's disease of bone are still preliminary. However, gallium nitrate administered as a continuous intravenous infusion daily for 5–7 days to 22 patients with lytic bone metastases led to a marked fall in urine calcium excretion and urinary hydroxyproline excretion. In preliminary studies in patients with myeloma or Paget's disease, it also appears that gallium nitrate may produce beneficial effects. The true efficacy of gallium nitrate for prolonged therapy of patients with these conditions, as well as metastatic bone disease, will require different modes of administration. Currently, experiments are being performed using gallium nitrate administered as a subcutaneous injection. However, an oral form of therapy will eventually be necessary. Although no significant side effects have so far been found, it has not been studied extensively in patients with impaired renal function.

Gallium nitrate may never receive widespread acceptance. It may be as efficacious as the newer bisphosphonates, but is unlikely to be better. It has not been investigated as widely, and there is no oral formulation.

References

Adamson BB, Gallagher SJ, Byars J et al (1993) Mineralization defects with pamidronate therapy for Paget's disease, *Lancet* **342**: 1459–60.

Aitken JM, Hart DM, Anderson JB et al (1973) Osteoporosis after oophorectomy for non-malignant disease, *Br Med J* **1**: 325–8.

Ayala G, Chertow BS, Shah JH et al (1975) Acute hyperphosphatemia and acute persistent renal insufficiency induced by oral phosphate therapy, *Ann Intern Med* **83**: 520–1.

Bell NH (1985) Vitamin D—endocrine system, *J Clin Invest* **76**: 1–6.

Berenson JR, Lichtenstein A, Porter L et al (1998) Long-term pamidronate treatment of advanced multiple myeloma patients reduces skeletal events, *J Clin Onc* **16**: 593–602.

Bijvoet OLM, van der Sluys Veer J, Jansen AP (1968) Effects of calcitonin on patients with Paget's disease, thyrotoxicosis, or hypercalcemia, *Lancet* **i**: 876–81.

Bijvoet OLM, Frijlink WB, Jie K et al (1980) APD in Paget's disease of bone. Role of the mononuclear phagocyte system? *Arthritis Rheum* **23**: 1193–204.

Binstock ML, Mundy GR (1980) Effect of calcitonin and glucocorticoids in combination in malignant hypercalcemia, *Ann Intern Med* **93**: 269–72.

Black DM (1996) Screening and treatment in the elderly to reduce osteoporotic fracture risk, *Br J Obstet Gynaecol* **103**: 2–7.

Bounameaux HM, Schifferli J, Montani JP et al (1983) Renal failure associated with intravenous diphosphonate, *Lancet* **i**: 471.

Boyce BF, Smith L, Fogelman I et al (1984) Focal osteomalacia due to low-dose diphosphonate therapy in Paget's disease, *Lancet* **i**: 821–4.

Brown JH, Kennedy BJ (1965) Mithramycin in the treatment of disseminated testicular neoplasms, *N Engl J Med* **272**: 111–18.

Burgener D, Bonjour JP, Caverzasio J (1995) Fluoride increases tyrosine kinase activity in osteoblast-like cells: regulatory role for the stimulation of cell proliferation and Pi transport across the plasma membrane, *J Bone Miner Res* **10**: 164–71.

Carano A, Teitelbaum SL, Konsek JD et al (1990) Bisphosphonates directly inhibit the bone resorption activity of isolated avian osteoclasts in vitro, *J Clin Invest* **85**: 456–61.

Carey RW, Schmitt GW, Kopald HH (1968) Massive extraskeletal calcification during phosphate treatment of hypercalcemia, *Arch Intern Med* **122**: 150–5.

Cauley JA, Seeley DG, Ensrud K et al (1995) Estrogen replacement and fracture protection in older women, *Ann Intern Med* **122**: 9–16.

Caverzasio J, Imai T, Ammann P et al (1996) Aluminum potentiates the effect of fluoride on tyrosine phosphorylation and osteoblast replication in vitro and bone mass in vivo, *J Bone Miner Res* **11**: 46–55.

Chambers TJ, Magnus CJ (1982) Calcitonin alters the behavior of isolated osteoclasts, *J Pathol* **136**: 27–40.

Chapuy MC, Arlot ME, Duboeuf F et al (1992) Vitamin D_3 and calcium to prevent hip fractures in the elderly woman, *N Engl J Med* **327**: 1637–42.

Christiansen C, Lindsay R (1990) Estrogens, bone loss and preservation, *Osteoporos Int* **1**: 7–13.

Christiansen MS, Hagen C, Christiansen C et al (1982) Dose-response evaluation of cyclic estrogen–gestagen in postmenopausal women. Placebo-controlled trial of its gynecologic and metabolic actions, *Am J Obstet Gynecol* **144**: 873–9.

Civitelli R, Gonnelli S, Zacchei F et al (1988) Bone turnover in postmenopausal osteoporosis. Effect of calcitonin treatment, *J Clin Invest* **82**: 1268–74.

Colditz GA, Hankinson SE, Hunter DJ et al (1995) The use of estrogens and progestins and the risk of breast cancer in post menopausal women, *N Engl J Med* **332**: 1589–93.

Cortes EP, Holland JF, Moskowitz R et al (1972) Effects of mithramycin on bone resorption in vitro, *Cancer Res* **32**: 74–6.

Couzi RJ, Helzlsouer KJ, Fetting JH (1995) Prevalence of menopausal symptoms among women with a history of breast cancer and attitudes toward estrogen replacement therapy, *J Clin Oncol* **13**: 2737–44.

De Groen PC, Lubde DF, Hirsch JL et al (1996) Esophagitis associated with the use of alendronate, *N Engl J Med* **335**: 1016–21.

DeLuca HF (1982) Metabolism and mechanism of action of vitamin D. In: Peck WA, ed, *Bone and Mineral Research, Annual 1* (Elsevier: Amsterdam) 7–73.

Dudley FJ, Blackburn CRB (1970) Extraskeletal calcification complicating oral neurophosphate therapy, *Lancet* **ii**: 628–30.

Ellerington MC, Hillard TC, Whitecroft SIJ et al (1996) Intranasal salmon calcitonin for the prevention and treatment of postmenopausal osteoporosis, *Calcif Tissue Int* **59**: 6–11.

Eriksen EF, Colvard DS, Berg NJ (1988) Evidence of estrogen receptors in normal human osteoblast-like cells, *Science* **241**: 84–6.

Ettinger B, Genant HK, Cann CE (1985) Long-term estrogen replacement therapy prevents bone loss and fractures, *Ann Intern Med* **102**: 319–24.

Farley JR, Wergedal JE, Baylink DJ (1983) Fluoride directly stimulates proliferation and alkaline phosphatase activity of bone-forming cells, *Science* **222**: 330–2.

Farley SM, Wergedal JE, Farley JR et al (1990) Fluoride decreases spinal fracture rate: a study of over 500 patients. In: Christiansen C, Overgaard K, eds, *Osteoporosis 1990, Third International Symposium on Osteoporosis*, Copenhagen, Denmark, Vol 3, 1330–4.

Finn GF, Christiansen C, Transbol I (1982) Treatment of postmenopausal osteoporosis. A controlled therapeutic trial comparing oestrogen/gestagen, 1,25-dihydroxyvitamin D_3, and calcium, *Clin Endocrinol* **16**: 515–24.

Fleisch H (1995) *Bisphosphonates in bone disease*. 2nd edn (Parthenon: Carnforth, England).

Fleisch H, Russell RGG, Francis MD (1969) Diphosphonates inhibit hydroxyapatite dissolution in vitro and bone resorption in tissue culture and in vivo, *Science* **165**: 1262–4.

Francis MD, Russell RGG, Fleisch H (1969) Diphosphonates inhibit formation of calcium phosphate crystals in vitro and pathological calcification in vivo, *Science* **165**: 1264–6.

Friedman J, Au WYW, Raisz LG (1968) Responses of fetal rat bone to thyrocalcitonin in tissue culture, *Endocrinology* **82**: 149–56.

Frijlink WB, Bijvoet OLM, te Velde J et al (1979) Treatment of Paget's disease with (3'-amino-1-hydroxypropylidene)-1,1-bisphosphonate (APD), *Lancet* **i**: 799–803.

Gruber HE, Ivey JL, Baylink DJ et al (1984) Long-term calcitonin therapy in postmenopausal osteoporosis, *Metabolism* **33**: 295–303.

Harris ST, Gertz BJ, Genant HK et al (1993) The effect of short-term treatment with alendronate on vertebral density and biochemical markers of bone remodeling in early postmenopausal women, *J Clin Endocrinol Metab* **76**: 1399–406.

Heaney RP (1965) A unified concept of osteoporosis, *Am J Med* **39**: 377–80.

Heaney RP (1991) Lifelong calcium intake and prevention of bone fragility in the aged, *Calcif Tissue Int* **49**: S42–S45.

Heaney RP, Recker RR, Saville PD (1978) Menopausal changes in bone remodeling, *J Lab Clin Med* **92**: 964–70.

Heaney RP, Gallagher JC, Johnston CC et al (1982) Calcium nutrition and bone health in the elderly, *Am J Clin Nutr* **36**: 986–1013.

Heersche JNM, Marcus R, Aurbach GD (1974) Calcitonin and the formation of 3',5'-AMP in bone and kidney, *Endocrinology* **94**: 241–7.

Hortobagyi GN, Theriault RL, Porter L et al (1996) Efficacy of pamidronate in reducing skeletal complications in patients with breast cancer and lytic bone lesions, *N Engl J Med* **335**: 1785–91.

Hortobagyi GN, Theriault RL, Lipton A et al (1998) Long-term prevention of skeletal complications of metastatic breast cancer with pamidronate, *Lancet* (in press).

Hughes DE, Tiffee JC, Li HH et al (1996) Estrogen promotes apoptosis of murine osteoclasts—mediated by TGFβ, *Nat Med* **7**: 1132–6.

Jilka RL, Hangoc G, Girasole G et al (1992) Increased osteoclast development after estrogen loss—mediation by interleukin-6, *Science* **257**: 88–91.

Johnston CC Jr, Miller JZ, Slemenda CW et al (1992) Calcium supplementation and increases in bone mineral density in children, *N Engl J Med* **327**: 82–7.

Kanis JA, Johnell O, Gullberg B et al (1992) Evidence for efficacy of drugs affecting bone metabolism in preventing hip fracture, *Br Med J* **305**: 1124–28.

Kleerekoper M, Peterson EL, Nelson DA et al (1991) A randomized trial of sodium fluoride as a treatment for postmenopausal osteoporosis, *Osteoporos Int* **1**: 155–61.

Kofman S, Medrek TJ, Alexander RW (1964) Mithramycin in the treatment of embryonal cancer, *Cancer* **17**: 938–48.

Komm BS, Terpening CM, Benz DJ (1988) Estrogen binding, receptor mRNA, and biologic response in osteoblast-like osteosarcoma cells, *Science* **241**: 81–4.

Krakoff IH, Newman RA, Goldberg RS (1979) Clinical toxicologic and pharmacologic studies of gallium nitrate, *Cancer* **44**: 1722–7.

Krane SM (1982) Etidronate disodium in the treatment of Paget's disease of bone, *Ann Intern Med* **96**: 619–25.

Lau KH, Farley JR, Freeman TK et al (1989) A proposed mechanism of the mitogenic action of fluoride on bone cells: inhibition of the activity of an osteoblastic acid phosphatase, *Metabolism* **38**: 858–68.

Liberman UA, Weiss SR, Broll J (1995) Effect of oral alendronate on bone mineral density and the incidence of fractures in postmenopausal osteoporosis, *N Engl J Med* **333**: 1437–43.

Liberman U, Karpf DB, Capizzi T et al (1996) Reply to letter to the Editor, *N Engl J Med* **334**: 734–5.

Lindholm TS, Nilsson OS, Widhe T et al (1982) Preventive treatment of osteoporosis with 1-alpha-hydroxyvitamin D_3 and calcium. Evaluation of bone histomorphometry in osteoporotics and age matched controls, *Acta Vitaminol Enzymol* **4**: 179–84.

Lindsay R (1996) The menopause and osteoporosis, *Obstet Gynecol* **87**: 16S–19S.

Lindsay R, Hart CM, Clarke DM (1983) The minimum effective dose of estrogen for prevention of postmenopausal bone loss, *Obstet Gynecol* **63**: 759–63.

Lipton A, Theriault RL, Hortobagyi GN et al (1998) Long-term treatment with pamidronate reduces skeletal morbidity in women receiving endocrine treatment for advanced breast cancer and lytic bone lesions, *J Clin Onc* (in press).

Lorenzo JA, Holtrop ME, Raisz LG (1984) Effects of phosphate on calcium release, lysosomal enzyme activity in the medium, and osteoclast morphometry in cultured fetal rat bones, *Metab Bone Dis Relat Res* **5**:187–90.

Lowik CW, Boonekamp PM, van de Ploym G et al (1986) Bisphosphonates can reduce osteoclastic bone resorption by two different mechanisms, *Adv Exp Med Biol* **208**: 275–81.

Lufkin EG, Wahner HW, O'Fallon WM et al (1992) Treatment of postmenopausal osteoporosis with transdermal estrogen, *Ann Intern Med* **117**: 1–9.

Marcus R, Madvig P, Crim M et al (1984) Conjugated estrogens in the treatment of postmenopausal women with hyperparathyroidism, *Ann Intern Med* **100**: 633–40.

Matkovic V, Kostial K, Simonovic I et al (1979) Bone status and fracture rates in two regions of Yugoslavia, *Am J Clin Nutr* **32**: 540–9.

McPherson K (1995) Breast cancer and hormonal supplements in post menopausal women, *Br Med J* **311**: 699–700.

Meunier PJ, Chapuy MC, Alexandre C (1979) Effects of disodium dichloromethylene diphosphonate on Paget's disease of bone, *Lancet* **ii**: 489–92.

Minkin C (1973) Inhibition of parathyroid hormone stimulated bone resorption in vitro by the antibiotic mithramycin, *Calcif Tissue Res* **13**: 249–57.

Mundy GR, Martin TJ (1982) The hypercalcemia of malignancy: pathogenesis and management, *Metabolism* **31**: 1247–77.

Mundy GR, Wilkinson R, Heath DA (1983) Comparative study of available medical therapy for hypercalcemia of malignancy, *Am J Med* **74**: 421–32.

Nagant C, Devogelaer JP, Stein F (1990) Fluoride treatment for osteoporosis, *Lancet* **336**: 48–9.

Newcomb PA, Longnecker MP, Storer BE et al (1995) Longterm hormone replacement therapy and risk of breast cancer in post-menopausal women, *Am J Epidemiol* **142**: 788–95.

Norman AW, Roth J, Orci L (1982) The vitamin D endocrine system: steroid metabolism, hormone, receptors, and biological response (calcium binding proteins), *Endocrinol Rev* **3**: 331–66.

Northrop G, Taylor SG III, Northrup RL (1969) Biochemical effects of mithramycin on cultured cells, *Cancer Res* **29**: 1916–19.

Nussbaum SR, Younger J, Van de Pol CJ et al (1993) Single-dose intravenous therapy with pamidronate for the treatment of hypercalcemia of malignancy. Comparison of 30-, 60-, and 90 mg dosages, *Am J Med* **95**: 297–304.

Orimo H, Shiraki M, Hayashi T et al (1987) Reduced occurrence of vertebral crush fractures in senile osteoporosis treated with 1-alpha (OH)-vitamin D_3, *Bone Miner* **3**: 47–52.

Ott SM, Chesnut CH III (1989) Calcitriol treatment is not effective in postmenopausal osteoporosis, *Ann Intern Med* **110**: 267–74.

Oursler MJ (1994) Osteoclast synthesis and secretion and activation of latent transforming growth factor β, *J Bone Miner Res* **9**: 443–52.

Oursler MJ, Osdoby P, Pyfferoen J et al (1991) Avian osteoclasts as estrogen target cells, *Proc Natl Acad Sci U S A* **88**: 6613–17.

Overgaard K, Riis BJ, Christiansen C et al (1989) Nasal calcitonin for treatment of established osteoporosis, *Clin Endocrinol* **30**: 435–42.

Overgaard K, Hansen MA, Jensen SB et al (1992) Effect of calcitonin given intranasally on bone mass and fracture rates in established osteoporosis—a dose-response study, *Br Med J* **305**: 556–61.

Pacifici R (1996) Estrogen, cytokines, and pathogenesis of postmenopausal osteoporosis, *J Bone Miner Res* **11**: 1043–51.

Pacifici R, Rifas L, Teitelbaum S et al (1987) Spontaneous release of interleukin-1 from human blood monocytes reflects bone formation in idiopathic osteoporosis, *Proc Natl Acad Sci U S A* **84**: 4616–20.

Pacifici R, Rifas L, McCracken R et al (1989) Ovarian steroid treatment blocks a postmenopausal increase in blood monocyte interleukin-1 release, *Proc Natl Acad Sci U S A* **86**: 2398–402.

Pak C, Sakhaee K, Zerwekh JE et al (1989) Safe and effective treatment of osteoporosis with intermittent slow release sodium fluoride: augmentation of vertebral bone mass and inhibition of fractures, *J Clin Endocrinol Metab* **68**: 150–9.

Pak CYC, Sakhaee K, Bell NH et al (1996a) Comparison of nonrandomized trials with slow-release sodium fluoride with a randomized placebo-controlled trial in postmenopausal osteoporosis, *J Bone Miner Res* **11**: 160–8.

Pak CYC, Zerwekh JE, Antich PP et al (1996b) Slow-release sodium fluoride in osteoporosis, *J Bone Miner Res* **11**: 561–4.

Parfitt AM (1979) Quantum concept of bone remodeling and turnover: implications for the pathogenesis of osteoporosis, *Calcif Tissue Int* **28**: 1–5.

Raisz LG, Niemann I (1969) Effect of phosphate, calcium and magnesium on bone resorption and hormonal responses in tissue culture, *Endocrinology* **85**: 446–52.

Ralston SH, Gardner MD, Dryburgh FJ et al (1985) Comparison of aminohydroxypropylidene diphosphonate, mithramycin, and corticosteroids/calcitonin in treatment of cancer-associated hypercalcaemia, *Lancet* **ii**: 907–10.

Ralston SH, Alzaid AA, Gardner MD et al (1986) Treatment of cancer associated hypercalcemia with combined aminohydroxypropylidene diphosphonate and calcitonin, *Br Med J* **292**: 1549–50.

Ralston SH, Patel U, Fraser WD et al (1989) Comparison of three intravenous bisphosphonates in cancer-associated hypercalcaemia, *Lancet* **ii**: 1180–2.

Reginster JY, Denis D, Albert A et al (1987) One year controlled randomised trial of prevention of early postmenopausal bone loss by intranasal calcitonin, *Lancet* **ii**: 1481–3.

Rico H, Hernandez ER, Revilla M et al (1992) Salmon calcitonin reduces vertebral fracture rate in postmenopausal crush fracture syndrome, *Bone Min* **16**: 131–38.

Riggs BL, Jowsey J, Kelly PJ et al (1976) Effects of oral therapy with calcium and vitamin D in primary osteoporosis, *J Clin Endocrinol Metab* **42**: 1139–44.

Riggs BL, Hodgson SF, O'Fallon WM et al (1990) Effect of fluoride treatment on the fracture rate in postmenopausal women with osteoporosis, *N Engl J Med* **322**: 802–9.

Riis BJ, Thomsen K, Strom V et al (1987) The effect of percutaneous estradiol and natural progesterone on postmenopausal bone loss, *Am J Obstet Gynecol* **156**: 61–5.

Rizzato G, Schiraldi G, Tosi G et al (1989) Administration of salmon calcitonin nasal spray for long-term treatment of corticosteroid-induced osteoporosis: a preliminary report, *Current Therapeutic Research* **45**: 761–6.

Rodan GA, Fleisch HA (1996) Bisphosphonates: mechanisms of action, *J Clin Invest* **97**: 2692–6.

Rogers MJ, Watts DJ, Russell RG et al (1994) Inhibitory effects of bisphosphonates on growth of amoebae of the cellular slime mold *Dictyostelium discoideum*, *J Bone Miner Res* **9**: 1029–39.

Rogers MJ, Watts DJ, Russell RG (1997) Overview of bisphosphonates. *Cancer* **80(8)**: 1652–60.

Russell RGG, Muhlbauer RC, Bisaz S et al (1970) The influence of pyrophosphate, condensed phosphates, phosphonates, and other phosphate compounds on the dissolution of hydroxyapatite in vitro and on bone resorption induced by parathyroid hormone in tissue culture and in thyroparathyroidectomized rats, *Calcif Tissue Res* **6**: 183–96.

Sahni M, Guenther HL, Fleisch H et al (1993) Bisphosphonates act on rat resorption through the mediation of osteoblasts, *J Clin Invest* **91**: 2004–11.

Sasaki T, Wantanabe C (1995) Stimulation of osteoinduction in bone wound healing by high-molecular hyaluronic acid, *Bone* **16**: 9–15.

Sato M, Grasser W, Endo N et al (1991) Bisphosphonate action—alendronate localization in rat bone and effects on osteoclast ultrastructure, *J Clin Invest* **88**: 2095–105.

Schmidt A, Rutledge SJ, Endo N et al (1996) Protein-tyrosine phosphatase activity regulates osteoclast formation and function: inhibition by alendronate, *Proc Natl Acad Sci U S A* **93**: 3068–73.

Schneider HPG, Birkhauser M (1995) Does HRT modify risk of gynecological cancers? *Int J Fertil* **40**: 40–53.

Selby PL, Peacock M (1986) Ethinyl estradiol and norethindrone in the treatment of primary hyperparathyroidism in postmenopausal women, *N Engl J Med* **314**: 1481–5.

Shane E, Baquiran DC, Bilezikian JP (1981) Effects of dichloromethylene diphosphonate on serum and urinary calcium in primary hyperparathyroidism, *Ann Intern Med* **95**: 23–7.

Singer FR, Fernandez M (1987) Therapy of hypercalcemia of malignancy, *Am J Med* **82** (Supp 2A): 34–41.

Singer FR, Krane SM (1990) Paget's disease of bone. In: Avioli LV, Krane SM, eds, *Metabolic bone disease*, 2nd edn (WB Saunders: Philadelphia) 546–615.

Siris ES, Hyman GA, Canfield RE (1983) Effects of dichloromethylene diphosphonate in women with breast carcinoma metastatic to the skeleton, *Am J Med* **74**: 401–6.

Siris ES, Sherman WH, Baquiran DC et al (1980) Effect of dichloromethylene diphosphonate on skeletal mobilization of multiple myeloma, *N Engl J Med* **302**: 310–15.

Sleeboom HP, Bijvoet OLM, van Oosterom AT et al (1983) Comparison of intravenous (3'-amino-1-hydroxypropylidene)-1,1-bisphosphonate and volume repletion in tumour-induced hypercalcemia, *Lancet* **ii**: 239–43.

Speroff L (1996) Postmenopausal hormone therapy and breast cancer, *Obstet Gynecol* **87** (supp): 44S–54S.

Storm T, Thamsborg G, Steiniche T et al (1990) Effect of intermittent cyclical etidronate therapy on bone mass and fracture rate in women with postmenopausal osteoporosis, *N Engl J Med* **322**: 1265–71.

Takahashi S, Goldring S, Katz M et al (1995) Downregulation of calcitonin receptor mRNA expression by calcitonin during human osteoclast-like cell differentiation, *J Clin Invest* **95**: 167–71.

Van Breukelen FJM, Bijvoet OLM, Van Oosterom AT (1979) Inhibition of osteolytic bone lesions by (3'-amino-1-hydroxypropylidene)-1,1-bisphosphonate (APD), *Lancet* **i**: 803–5.

Warrell RP, Coonley CJ, Straus DJ et al (1983) Treatment of patients with advanced malignant lymphoma using gallium nitrate administered as a seven day continuous infusion, *Cancer* **51**: 1982–7.

Warrell RP, Bockman RS, Coonley CJ et al (1984) Gallium nitrate inhibits calcium resorption from bone and is effective treatment for cancer-related hypercalcemia, *J Clin Invest* **73**: 1487–90.

Warrell RP, Isaacs M, Coonley CJ et al (1985) Metabolic effects of gallium nitrate administered by prolonged infusion, *Cancer Treat Rep* **69**: 653–5.

Warrell RP, Skelos A, Alcock NW et al (1986) Gallium nitrate for acute treatment of cancer-related hypercalcemia: clinicopharmacological and dose response analysis, *Cancer Res* **46**: 4208–12.

Weiss NS, Ure CL, Ballard JH et al (1980) Decreased risk of fractures of the hip and lower forearm with postmenopausal use of estrogen, *N Engl J Med* **303**: 1195–8.

Wener JA, Gorton SJ, Raisz LG (1972) Escape from inhibition of resorption in cultures of fetal bone treated with calcitonin and parathyroid hormone, *Endocrinology* **90**: 752–9.

Wollheim MS, Yarbro JW, Kennedy BJ (1968) Effect of mithramycin on HeLa cells, *Cancer* **21**: 22–5.

Yang NN, Venugopalan M, Hardikar S et al (1996) Identification of an estrogen response element activated by metabolites of 17β-estradiol and raloxifene, *Science* **273**: 1222–5.

Yarbro JW, Kennedy BJ, Barnum CP (1966) Mithramycin inhibition of ribonucleic acid synthesis, *Cancer Res* **26**: 36–9.

Yates AJP, Oreffo ROC, Mayor K et al (1991) Inhibition of bone resorption by inorganic phosphate is mediated both by reduced osteoclast formation and by impaired activity of mature osteoclasts, *J Bone Miner Res* **6**: 473–8.

CHAPTER 6

Hypercalcemia

Hypercalcemia occurs when the normal compensatory mechanisms responsible for the maintenance of the extracellular fluid calcium are overwhelmed. It is usually due to a combination of increased entry of calcium into the extracellular fluid from bone or the gastrointestinal tract, often combined with impaired capacity of the kidney to excrete the calcium load. In this chapter, normal calcium homeostasis will be reviewed with respect to its control by regulation of fluxes of calcium between bone and the extracellular fluid, as well as regulation of fluxes across the gut and the kidney. Traditional concepts of calcium homeostasis will be discussed and emphasis will be given to gaps in our knowledge, and to key concepts for understanding the pathophysiology and rational medical treatment of hypercalcemia.

Causes of hypercalcemia

The causes of hypercalcemia and their relative frequency are shown in Tables 6.1 and 6.2. As can be seen from these tables, primary hyperparathyroidism and malignancy comprise approximately 90% of all patients.

Table 6.1 Causes of hypercalcemia.

Primary hyperparathyroidism
Malignant disease
Hyperthyroidism
Immobilization
Vitamin D intoxication
Vitamin A intoxication
Familial hypocalciuric hypercalcemia (FHH)
Diuretic phase of acute renal failure
Chronic renal failure ± aluminum toxicity
Thiazide diuretics
Sarcoidosis and other granulomatous diseases
Milk–alkali syndrome
Addison's disease
Paget's disease (with immobilization or co-existent primary hyperparathyroidism)
Postpartum with lactation

Table 6.2 Relative frequency of causes of hypercalcemia.

	Number of patients	Percentage of cases
Primary hyperparathyroidism	111	54
Malignant disease	72	25
Lung	25	35
Breast	18	25
Hematologic (myeloma 5, lymphoma 4)	10	14
Head and neck	4	8
Renal	2	3
Prostate	2	3
Unknown primary	5	7
Others (gastrointestinal 4)	8	8

From Mundy and Martin (1982).

Traditional concepts of calcium homeostasis

The traditional but almost certainly overly simplistic view of calcium homeostasis is that ECF ionized calcium concentration is tightly regulated by the actions of two major hormones (parathyroid hormone and 1,25-dihydroxyvitamin D_3) acting on fluxes of calcium across the gut, kidney and bone (Figure 6.1, Table 6.3). The major storehouse of calcium in the body is the skeleton (which contains approximately 1 kg or 99% of total body calcium). The kidney filters approximately 10 g/day, of which more than 90% is reabsorbed in the proximal convoluted tubules and distal convoluted tubules (the former influenced by sodium reabsorption, the latter by PTH). In normal adults in zero calcium balance, renal calcium excretion equals net gut absorption. In this view, extracellular fluid calcium is regulated in much the same way as a domestic thermostat ("reactive regulation") by negative feedback loops, which control PTH and 1,25-dihydroxyvitamin D_3 production (either directly or indirectly) (Figure 6.2). Calcitonin may also be involved in short-term regulation, although its physiologic

Figure 6.1

Calcium homeostasis for a normal adult in zero calcium balance. The numbers are estimates of the amount of calcium exchanged between the extracellular fluid and gut, kidney and bone each day. The exchange system between bone fluid and the extracellular fluid is not taken into account. (From Mundy (1990).)

Figure 6.2

The relationship between PTH secretion rate and plasma calcium. Note that small changes in plasma calcium produce relatively large changes in PTH secretion rate. Also note that since PTH is either maximally increased with plasma calcium below 7.5 mg/dl (1.8 mmol/l) and maximally suppressed with plasma calcium greater than 12.0 mg/dl (3.0 mmol/l), PTH exerts effects on plasma calcium over only a relatively small range about the normal. (From Mundy (1990).)

Table 6.3 Effects of systemic calcium-regulating hormones on target tissues, and their regulatory mechanisms.

Hormone	Origin	Major tissue target	Effects	Control
Parathyroid hormone	Parathyroid glands	Kidney, bone	Ca↑, Pi↓	Ca↓
1,25(OH)$_2$ vitamin D_3	Proximal tubules of kidney	Gut, bone	Ca↑, Pi↑	Pi↓, Ca↓, PTH↑
Calcitonin	Thyroid parafollicular cells	Bone, kidney	Ca↓, Pi↓	Ca↑, gastrin

role remains unclear even after 30 years. The whole system is seemingly overlapping and redundant, but this may be the explanation for control that is so tight.

Pathophysiology of hypercalcemia

Primary hyperparathyroidism

In primary hyperparathyroidism, there is increased calcium reabsorption in the renal tubules, increased calcium absorption from the gut (an indirect effect due to increased production of 1,25-dihydroxyvitamin D_3) and increased bone turnover (Figure 6.3).

Malignancy

Hypercalcemia occurs in most patients with malignancy due to markedly increased bone resorption not balanced by new bone formation, and impaired calcium excretion by the kidney (Figure 6.4). In some patients, the latter is due to decreased glomerular filtration, and in most there is also increased renal tubular reabsorption of calcium (Tuttle et al 1991).

Unresolved issues (Table 6.4)

Control of calcium homeostasis by reactive regulation has been likened to a domestic thermostat, which reacts to externally imposed changes by bringing the variable it controls back to the mean. Two important characteristics of the homeostatic mechanism are set-point and error correction. The set-point is the mean value about which the extracellular fluid calcium is controlled. This

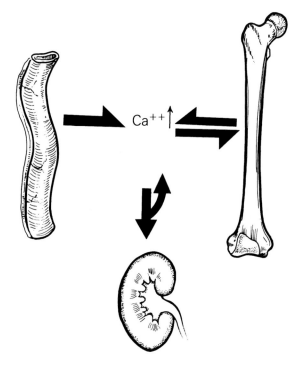

Figure 6.3
Abnormalities in calcium homeostasis in patients with primary hyperparathyroidism. These patients show increased bone turnover, increased renal tubular calcium reabsorption, and increased absorption of calcium from the gut. The increase in the absorption of calcium from the gut is mediated by 1,25-dihydroxyvitamin D_3, which is produced in the renal tubules in response to PTH. (From Mundy (1990).)

Table 6.4 Defenses against hypocalcemia and hypercalcemia—protection is better against hypocalcemia than against hypercalcemia.

Protection against decreased plasma calcium (for example, caused by dietary deficiency or hormonal deficiency)

- Glomerular filtration—filtered load of calcium decreases
- Calciotropic hormones (PTH, 1,25-dihydroxyvitamin D_3 and calcitonin)
    (a) Effects on bone and kidney—hypocalcemia stimulates PTH release, which increases plasma calcium by effects on renal tubules and osteoclasts
    (b) Effects on gut (adaptation)—increased fractional absorption of dietary calcium, mediated by 1,25-dihydroxyvitamin D_3

Protection against increases in plasma calcium (caused by bone destruction or large dietary calcium load)

- Glomerular filtration—filtered load of calcium increases
- Calciotropic hormones
    (a) PTH—but no further decrease in secretion if plasma calcium >11.5 mg/dl (2.9 mmol/l)
    (b) Calcitonin—but no long-term efficacy
    (c) 1,25-dihydroxyvitamin D_3—but gut effects are slow and limited
- Possible diuretic effect of chronic hypercalcemia eventually leading to sodium and volume depletion and to decreased calcium excretion (Harinck et al 1987)

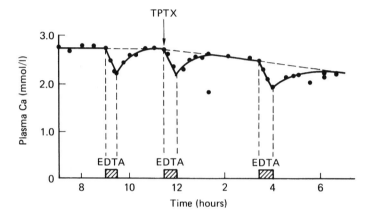

Figure 6.4

Effects of EDTA on plasma calcium in the hypoparathyroid dog. Note the relatively rapid correction of the plasma calcium and the maintenance of the plasma calcium at the predetermined set-point. TPTX = thyroparathyroidectomy. (Reproduced with permission from Parfitt AM, Equilibrium and disequilibrium hypercalcemia: new light on an old concept, *Metab Bone Dis Relat Res* **1**: 279–93. Copyright 1979 by Pergamon Press.)

mean concentration is exposed to insults such as dietary calcium loads, which cause deviations from the set-point. There are specific mechanisms for correction of these deviations (called error correction), which return the extracellular fluid calcium to the set-point. Although the calciotropic hormones can in part explain these characteristics, there must be important additional mechanisms since set-point and error correction occur in their absence (for example hypoparathyroidism (Figure 6.4)). Set-point and error correction are probably regulated by both hormonal (for example PTH) and nonhormonal (glomerular filtration, plasma–bone fluid exchange) mechanisms.

The domestic thermostat, automobile cruise control and automatic pilot have been used as analogies for the concepts of reactive regulation of physiological homeostatic mechanisms. However, these are not precise models for the "calciostat", in which the set-point is not imposed by an external influence separate from the system, nor do they have the component of "anticipatory" regulation seen in many homeostatic systems (Parfitt 1993).

Importance of pulsatile PTH secretion

It has been convincingly shown by a number of groups that PTH is secreted in a pulsatile manner, in bursts of about 7–8 pulses per hour (Harms et al 1989; Kitamura et al 1990; Samuels et al 1993). These pulses are unrelated to changes in extracellular fluid calcium concentrations (Figure 6.5). The molecular mechanism, presumably inherent to the parathyroid cell, rather than imposed from outside it, is unknown.

The physiological and pathological significance of pulsatile PTH secretion is also unknown. However, pulsatility of PTH secretion may be very

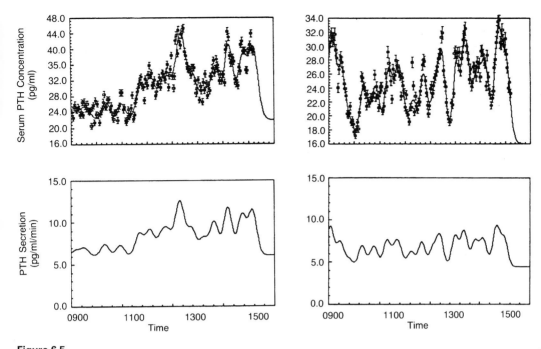

Figure 6.5

Demonstration of pulsatile pattern of secretion of PTH in normal individuals, a healthy young woman (left panel) and a healthy young man (right panel). The lower panels show a plot of PTH secretion rate over time. Note basal PTH secretion (about 30% of total) and the superimposed pulsatile pattern. (Reproduced from Samuels et al (1993).)

important for the following reasons.

- Pulsatile hormone secretion is important in other hormonal systems (for example, pituitary–hypothalamus);
- PTH has long been known to have effects on target bone cells that depend on whether they are exposed to PTH continuously or intermittently (Tam et al 1982).

In response to continuous exposure to PTH, there is an increase in bone turnover (increased bone resorption and bone formation). However, in response to low dose and intermittent PTH, the predominant effect is an increase in bone formation (the "anabolic" response to PTH).

It is not known if production of PTH-rP by tumor cells or normal cells is intermittent. Tumor cell production of PTH-rP may be regulated by external factors such as TGFβ in the bone microenvironment, but it seems likely that its production may be relatively constant. Differences in secretion patterns may be responsible for some of the differences in the syndromes of humoral hypercalcemia of malignancy and primary hyperparathyroidism (decreased rates of bone formation in the former, increased rates of bone formation in the latter).

Relative roles of the bone and kidney

The relative importance of the bone and kidney for the increase in extracellular fluid ionized calcium in hypercalcemia of malignancy has been frequently questioned. The kidney clearly plays an important role in many if not all patients with hypercalcemia of malignancy (Peacock et al 1969) (Figure 6.6). However, it is not clear what the

Figure 6.6
The relationship between urinary calcium excretion (CaE) and serum calcium in normal subjects during an acute calcium infusion, as first described by Peacock et al (1969). The shaded area represents the normal basal range. The solid line and the broken lines represent the mean values ± 2 SD, respectively.

relative contribution of increased renal tubular calcium reabsorption to the increase in extracellular fluid calcium in any particular patient is. In an attempt to distinguish the relative roles of bone and kidney, nomograms have been developed that can be used to make estimates in the individual patients (Percival et al 1985). This issue is very complex. PTH (and presumably PTH-rP) have differing effects on target cells depending on whether it is administered intermittently or continuously. There is still much to be learned of the effects of PTH on its target organs. Moreover, there is some evidence that prolonged hypercalcemia itself may have a direct and independent effect on influencing renal tubular calcium handling, as suggested by Bijvoet and colleagues (Harinck et al 1987).

Role of bone remodeling

- Changes in bone remodeling that are coupled and balanced probably have very little influence on normal calcium homeostasis. Marked increases in bone turnover (for example, Paget's disease and thyrotoxicosis) are rarely associated with severe hypercalcemia, as long as bone resorption and bone formation are balanced.

- Unbalanced bone remodeling is seen in most terminal cases of hypercalcemia of malignancy (although it is unclear if an increase in bone resorption alone without concomitant impairment in renal capacity to excrete the calcium load can cause hypercalcemia). Many patients with increased bone resorption do not have hypercalcemia.

Role of exchange of calcium between blood and the bone fluid–bone surface

This is the most poorly understood area of all.

- Neuman showed almost 40 years ago that a special bone fluid (analogous to the CSF) exists. This bone fluid is separated from the extracellular fluid by a "bone membrane", which is probably composed of the bone lining cells that cover bone surfaces in a continuum (Levinskas and Neuman 1955; Neuman 1982; Bushinsky et al 1989; Parfitt 1989).

- This bone membrane functions to keep calcium in the extracellular fluid and out of bone (the extracellular fluid is supersaturated with calcium compared with both the bone fluid and the crystalline surfaces of bone).

- There is no understanding of the hormonal mechanisms that might control calcium fluxes across the bone membrane, or whether these fluxes are influenced by disease states such as the hypercalcemia of malignancy or primary hyperparathyroidism. However, it is possible that these fluxes buffer fluctuations in extracellular fluid calcium caused by, for example, dietary calcium loads or calcium entry from bone destruction caused by malignancy. For example, these fluxes may be important in determining set-point. They could also be important in returning plasma calcium to the set-point (error correction) after a calcium load.

Humoral factors that have been implicated in the pathophysiology of hypercalcemia

The two commonest causes of hypercalcemia are primary hyperparathyroidism and malignancy. Together, these two conditions make up about 90% of all causes of hypercalcemia. (Tables 6.1 and 6.2 show a list of the causes of hypercalcemia with their relative frequencies.) Although primary hyperparathyroidism and malignancy are by far and away the most common causes, the pathogenetic mechanisms responsible for disruption of calcium homeostasis in these two disease states are different. In primary hyperparathyroidism, hypercalcemia occurs as a consequence of PTH production by the parathyroid glands (see Chapter 9). Hypercalcemia occurs because of the combined effects of PTH and 1,25-dihydroxyvitamin D_3 on renal tubular calcium reabsorption, gut absorption of calcium and bone resorption. The major effect is probably on the renal tubules. PTH (and PTH-rP) cause hypercalcemia acutely by effects that are not related to osteoclastic bone resorption, and probably not related to calcium absorption from the gut, since 1,25-dihydroxyvitamin D_3 formation in the kidneys is a relatively slow process requiring several different hydroxylation steps. Evidence that the acute effects of PTH and PTH-rP on calcium homeostasis are not mediated by osteoclastic bone resorption is demonstrated in osteopetrotic mice, which do not have osteoclasts capable of resorbing bone (Boyce et al 1992). In these mice, injections of PTH and PTH-rP cause similar elevations in serum calcium to normal littermates, indicating that functioning osteoclasts are not necessary for

Figure 6.7

Patterns of different abnormalities in calcium transport between the extracellular fluid and gut, kidney and bone in different types of hypercalcemia of malignancy. In myeloma (upper left), there is an increase in bone resorption and impaired glomerular filtration. In lung cancer (upper right), there is increased bone resorption and increased renal tubular calcium reabsorption, associated with increased nephrogenous cAMP. In breast cancer (lower right), there is increased bone resorption and increased renal tubular calcium reabsorption. In some lymphomas (lower left), there is increased bone resorption and increased gut absorption of calcium.

acute hypercalcemic responses to PTH or PTH-rP. Morphologic changes of increased bone turnover are prominent in only some patients with primary hyperparathyroidism.

In contrast, patients with hypercalcemia of malignancy develop hypercalcemia primarily because of an increase in osteoclastic bone resorption, although there is increasing evidence that a component of renal tubular calcium reabsorption is also important in most patients (Tuttle et al 1991) (Figure 6.7). The mediators implicated in myeloma are reviewed in Chapter 8. The other tumor-derived humoral factors that have been implicated are parathyroid hormone-related protein and parathyroid hormone, interleukin-1α and β, transforming growth factor α, tumor necrosis factor, lymphotoxin, interleukin-6, prostaglandins of the E series, and active vitamin D metabolites.

Figure 6.8

Effects of hPTH and hPTH-rP on bone resorption in organ culture. (Reproduced from Yates et al (1988).)

Parathyroid hormone-related protein (PTH-rP) and parathyroid hormone (PTH)

Parathyroid hormone-related protein (PTH-rP) was first discovered using in vitro bioassays for PTH in tumors derived from lung, breast and the kidney (Moseley et al 1987; Stewart et al 1987; Strewler et al 1987). This factor is now known to be expressed by many squamous cell carcinomas and has also been described in T-cell lymphomas that present with humoral hypercalcemia (Motokura et al 1989). It is a 141 amino acid peptide, which bears some homology to parathyroid hormone in the first 13 amino acids. It binds to and activates the PTH receptor, and this is presumably the reason it mimics the biological effects of PTH on bone, kidney and the gut (Figure 6.8; see also Chapter 4). It stimulates osteoclastic bone resorption and promotes renal tubular calcium reabsorption in similar concentrations to that of native PTH (Yates et al 1988). In some models of hypercalcemia associated with increased PTH-rP, hypercalcemia can be reversed by passive inoculation with neutralizing antibodies to PTH-rP (Kukreja et al 1988). It is now known that PTH-rP is produced by about 50% of primary breast cancers and its production may be enhanced at the bone site by bone-derived factors such as TGFβ (Powell et al 1991; Guise et al 1996). Radioimmunoassays have been developed for PTH-rP, although these assays have not shown a perfect relationship between the presence and severity of hypercalcemia and expression of the protein (Stewart et al 1987; Budayr et al 1989; Henderson and Pettipher 1989).

It is not surprising that there is a less than perfect correlation between circulating PTH-rP concentrations and hypercalcemia. The work of Guise et al (1996) shows that PTH-rP may be an important local mediator of bone resorption, particularly in breast cancer. Here it may cause local osteolysis with or without hypercalcemia (Figure 6.9). Thus, PTH-rP may cause two distinct tumor-related syndromes, HHM or localized osteolysis. The latter may or may not be associated with hypercalcemia, depending on the extent of the bone lesions.

Recently, we have created a model of PTH-rP-induced hypercalcemia in nude mice by transfecting Chinese hamster ovarian cells (CHO cells) with the human PTH-rP gene (Guise et al 1992). These cells are stably transfected with PTH-rP and express it in a constant manner. When these tumors are inoculated into nude mice, the tumor-bearing nude mice develop hypercalcemia, and increased plasma PTH-rP. In addition, they have other features that are identical to those seen with PTH excess, namely increased osteoclastic

Tumor syndromes associated
with PTH-rP production

Humoral hypercalcemia of malignancy (HHM)
- Hypercalcemia
- ↑Plasma [PTH-rP], [ncAMP]

Localized osteolysis
- ±Hypercalcemia
- No↑plasma [PTH-rP] or [ncAMP]

Figure 6.9
Recent data suggests that there are two distinct (although in some patients overlapping) tumor syndromes associated with PTH-rP. One is the well-known HHM syndrome, the other localized osteolysis where PTH-rP is overproduced locally in bone and does not necessarily cause increased plasma PTH-rP or hypercalcemia.

bone resorption associated with increased bone formation, and increased plasma 1,25-dihydroxyvitamin D_3 (Guise et al 1993). Since these features are not seen in the majority of patients dying with the syndrome of humoral hypercalcemia of malignancy, tumor increased production of PTH-rP alone cannot explain the syndrome. Our hypothesis is that other factors produced in conjunction with PTH-rP may modify the effects of PTH-rP on target tissues. Other data suggest that TGFα, IL-1α, IL-6 and TNFα may be synergistic with PTH-rP in vivo (Sato et al 1989; Guise et al 1993; De La Mata et al 1995; Uy et al 1996).

PTH-rP may have roles other than as a mediator of cancer hypercalcemia that have not yet been clearly determined. It has been found in lactating rat breast tissue as well as in human milk (Thiede and Rodan 1988; Budayr et al 1989). It has been suggested that it may be involved in placental calcium transport (Rodda et al 1988). PTH-rP has also been demonstrated in increased amounts in the amniotic fluid and is produced by amniotic cells (Bruns et al 1992). Its expression in amniotic cells decreases when the membranes rupture. It may have a role as a smooth muscle relaxant in this situation and be involved in labor and delivery. On the basis of these studies, it is possible that during embryonic life it may be an important hormone for calcium transport in the fetus.

Recently, in an attempt to study the normal physiological functions of PTH-rP, a null mutation was introduced into the PTH-rP gene by targeted disruption in embryonic stem cells followed by homologous recombination (Karaplis et al 1994). Resultant homozygous mice deficient in PTH-rP expression did not survive embryonic life. These mice showed marked abnormalities at the growth plate. Thus, PTH-rP expression may be important for normal endochondral bone formation.

This has been further emphasized in more recent studies. Point mutations in the PTH/PTH-rP receptor that are activating cause the condition Jansen's metaphyseal chondrodysplasia, a rare genetic disorder characterized by short-limbed dwarfism and severe, agonist-independent hypercalcemia (Schipani et al 1995). Moreover, the recent findings that PTH/PTH-rP receptor deficiency due to targeted gene disruption causes premature differentiation of chondrocytes, which leads to abnormalities in endochondral bone formation and can be reversed by adding PTH-rP, further emphasize this point (see Chapter 4) (Lanske et al 1996).

Recently, PTH itself has been implicated as a tumor mediator in several nonparathyroid tumors (Yoshimoto et al 1989; Nussbaum et al 1990; Strewler et al 1990). However, this is a rare occurrence (Simpson et al 1983). These tumors were a small cell lung cancer, a neuroectodermal tumor and an ovarian carcinoma. In one of these tumors, a DNA rearrangement in the region of the promoter was presumably responsible for overexpression of the PTH gene by the tumor. Most patients with nonparathyroid cancer who develop hypercalcemia and increased immunoreactive serum PTH have co-existent primary hyperparathyroidism.

Interleukin-1α and β

The interleukin-1s are powerful bone resorbing cytokines produced not only by activated monocytes, but also by many other cells. Interleukin-1α and interleukin-1β seem to have identical effects on bone resorption and bone forming cells (Sabatini et al 1988; Boyce et al 1989a,b). Interleukin-1α is expressed by many solid tumors as well as lymphomas (Fried et al 1989; Sato et al 1989; Nowak et al 1990). It may work in concert with PTH-rP to provoke hypercalcemia (Sato et al 1989). It has powerful effects on osteoclastic bone resorption in vivo (Sabatini et al 1988; Boyce et al 1989a,b). It inhibits differentiated function in osteoblasts in vitro but may promote their proliferation (Gowen et al 1985). Interleukin-1β has not been implicated in solid tumors associated with hypercalcemia, but several groups have recently shown that freshly isolated cells from the marrow of patients with myeloma produce interleukin-1β (Cozzolino et al 1989; Kawano et al 1989). Bone resorbing activity present in these cultured cell supernatants has been blocked by neutralizing antibodies to interleukin-1β.

Both interleukin-1α and interleukin-1β are powerful hypercalcemic agents (Chapter 4). This has been shown by infusions in normal intact mice as well as by repeated subcutaneous injections (Sabatini et al 1988; Boyce et al 1989a,b). The effects of interleukin-1 to cause hypercalcemia are clearly mediated by osteoclastic bone resorption. In osteopetrotic mice in whom osteoclasts are nonfunctional, hypercalcemia does not occur, in contrast to when PTH or PTH-rP are injected into osteopetrotic mice, where hypercalcemia occurs presumably due to the renal effects of the hormones (Boyce et al 1992).

Transforming growth factor α (TGFα)

Transforming growth factor α (TGFα) is produced by many solid tumors as well as breast carcinomas. TGFα is a powerful stimulator of osteoclast precursor proliferation and causes osteoclastic bone resorption and hypercalcemia in vivo (Ibbotson et al 1985; Tashjian et al 1985; Takahashi et al 1987). It has synergistic effects with PTH and more importantly with PTH-rP both on bone resorption and on hypercalcemia (Yates et al 1992; Guise et al 1993). Recent studies have suggested that TGFα is a cell membrane-associated protein and may exert biological effects while still incorporated into the cell membrane (Massague 1990). However, it is also clear that it can produce systemic effects on osteoclastic bone resorption and hypercalcemia, since Chinese hamster ovarian cells expressing and secreting TGFα cause hypercalcemia when inoculated into nude mice (Yates et al 1992).

The effects of TGFα on osteoclastic bone resorption may be exerted primarily on osteoclast progenitors (Takahashi et al 1986a,b). It stimulates progenitors to replicate, but not to differentiate. It exerts identical effects on osteoclasts as epidermal growth factor. In nude mice bearing CHO tumors expressing TGFα, hypercalcemia is associated with osteoclasts that are small in size and have fewer nuclei than the osteoclasts formed in response to PTH or PTH-rP (Yates et al 1992) (Figure 6.10). This suggests that these osteoclasts have been generated in response to a growth regulatory factor, and are consistent with the culture data indicating a primary proliferative effect of TGFα on osteoclast progenitor cells.

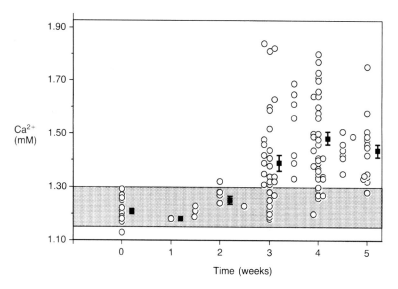

Figure 6.10

Effects of tumor production of TGFα in causing hypercalcemia in nude mice. Values shown are for mice bearing tumors transfected with TGFα. (Reproduced from Yates et al (1992).)

Tumor necrosis factor (TNF)

Tumor necrosis factor (TNF) has similar biological effects on osteoclasts to those of interleukin-1. It stimulates proliferation of precursors, enhances differentiation of committed precursors and activates the mature cell indirectly to stimulate the resorption of bone (Bertolini et al 1986; Johnson et al 1989; Uy et al 1995). It is not known to be produced by solid tumors. It is more likely that it may play a role in the bone destruction associated with solid tumors by being produced by normal host cells in excess amounts in response to the tumor. In this way, it may be associated with the paraneoplastic syndromes of cachexia, hypercalcemia and leukocytosis. There are several experimental examples in which this mechanism seems to be important. In the MH-85 tumor, a squamous cell carcinoma of the maxilla, both the original patient and nude mice carrying this tumor develop hypercalcemia, leukocytosis and cachexia (Yoneda et al 1991) (Figure 6.11). The tumor-bearing nude mice have increased circulating concentrations of tumor necrosis factor, although the tumor itself does not produce TNF, and when nude mice are treated with neutralizing antibodies to TNF, the hypercalcemia is markedly reduced. In these animals, it appears that tumor cells themselves are producing a circulating factor, which in turn is responsible for provoking TNF production. This mechanism has also been examined in two other models of hypercalcemia, the rat Leydig cell tumor and the A375 tumor. The rat Leydig cell tumor produces both PTH-rP and TGFα in large amounts. This is a tumor that causes profound hypercalcemia. However, the tumor-bearing rats also develop profound cachexia and hypertriglyceridemia, which is associated with increased circulating concentrations of TNF (Sabatini et al 1990a,b). Similarly, in the A375 human melanoma, nude mice bearing this tumor develop severe cachexia and hypercalcemia. These mice also have increased circulating concentrations of TNF. In this tumor, the factor responsible for provoking TNF production by the tumor cells has been purified and shown to be the colony-stimulating factor (CSF) for the granulocyte–macrophage series (GM-CSF) (Sabatini et al 1990a,b). The activity responsible for provoking TNF production in the MH-85 tumor cannot be ascribed to GM-CSF, but has still not been identified.

Lymphotoxin

Lymphotoxin has similar biological effects to those of tumor necrosis factor. It also is a powerful stimulator of osteoclastic bone resorption and causes hypercalcemia when infused or injected in vivo. It has been implicated in the hypercalcemia and bone destruction associated with myeloma (Garrett et al 1987). Long-term cultures of human myeloma cells express lymphotoxin messenger RNA. Moreover, there is lymphotoxin biological activity in conditioned media of cultured cells, and bone resorbing activity in the cell culture media of these cells can be blocked by neutralizing antibodies to lymphotoxin (Garrett et al 1987). Thus, possibly in association with other cytokines such as IL-1β and IL-6, lymphotoxin is likely to be important in the bone destruction associated with myeloma.

Interleukin-6 (IL-6)

Interleukin-6 (IL-6) is a more recently described cytokine that is a powerful B cell mitogen. It has a controversial role in myeloma. Some investigators believe it has an important paracrine or autocrine role in the pathophysiology of the dis-

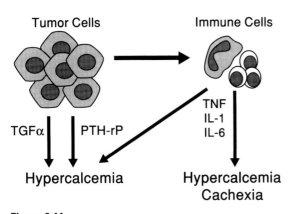

Figure 6.11

Hypothesis for production of bone resorbing cytokines by normal immune cells in hypercalcemia of malignancy.

ease (Bataille et al 1989). It also has controversial effects on bone resorption. It stimulates bone resorption in some systems but seems to be ineffective in other organ culture systems (Lowik et al 1989; Gowen et al 1990; Ishimi et al 1990). Its effects may depend on the presence of precursors for osteoclasts in the organ cultures. IL-6 clearly causes hypercalcemia in vivo. Chinese hamster ovarian cells that have been transfected with the IL-6 gene and which stably overexpress it cause hypercalcemia when inoculated into nude mice (Chapter 4). In addition, the nude mice develop leukocytosis, thrombocytosis and cachexia, which can be ascribed to IL-6 (Black et al 1991). It may be a stimulator of bone resorption acting early in the bone resorption process (Kukita et al 1990). IL-6 is produced by many solid tumors and must be a potential mediator of hypercalcemia and other paraneoplastic syndromes associated with malignancy.

However, the major role for IL-6 may not be as an independent factor but rather as a subsidiary factor enhancing the effects of other mediators. De La Mata et al (1995) showed that IL-6 markedly enhanced the effects of PTH-rP both on osteoclast formation and in generation of hypercalcemia in tumor-bearing mice. Since IL-6 is produced by bone cells in the presence of PTH and PTH-rP (Feyen et al 1989), this may be an important mechanism for hypercalcemia in some patients.

Recently, we have found that in a solid human tumor (a squamous cell carcinoma) that causes hypercalcemia in tumor-bearing nude mice, hypercalcemia may be reversed by treatment with neutralizing antibodies to IL-6 (Yoneda et al 1991). The source of the IL-6 is the tumor cells. Thus, IL-6 may be a contributory factor in hypercalcemia and other paraneoplastic syndromes associated not only with myeloma but with some solid tumors.

Prostaglandins of the E series

Prostaglandins of the E series have long been known to be relatively powerful bone resorbing factors (Klein and Raisz 1970). Their role in the bone destruction associated with malignancy remains unclear (Mundy 1990). However, it is known that at least part of the effects of some of the cytokines on osteoclastic bone resorption in vivo as well as in vitro are mediated through prostaglandin synthesis. Boyce et al (1989a,b) showed this by intermittent subcutaneous injections of IL-1 over the calvariae of mice, some of which were treated with indomethacin, which inhibits prostaglandin synthesis. They found that part of the effects of IL-1 on bone in vivo as assessed by histomorphometry could be blocked by indomethacin. However, it is also possible that prostaglandins of the E series may exert more direct effects on osteoclastic bone resorption. They are produced by cultured tumor cells in vitro. Whether a similar phenomenon will happen in vivo or not is unknown. One possibility is that prostaglandins, like cytokines such as TNF, could be produced by host immune cells in response to the tumor.

1,25-Dihydroxyvitamin D_3

Serum 1,25-dihydroxyvitamin D_3 is suppressed in most patients with bone destruction associated with hypercalcemia. However, in a small subset of patients with T-cell lymphomas, 1,25-dihydroxyvitamin D_3 production by the tumor tissue is increased and this is associated with increased calcium absorption from the gut (Breslau et al 1984). This mechanism is important in the pathophysiology of the hypercalcemia in these cases. This mechanism probably represents a small minority of all patients with T-cell lymphomas. An atypical metabolite of 1,25-dihydroxyvitamin D_3 has also been invoked in the hypercalcemia associated with one solid tumor associated with hypercalcemia (Shigeno et al 1985). This also appears to be an uncommon mechanism responsible for hypercalcemia of malignancy.

Implications for the medical treatment of hypercalcemia associated with increased bone resorption

Pharmacologic agents used in management of hypercalcemia of malignancy are discussed in more detail in Chapter 5. Here, some principles of treatment based on pathophysiological characteristics of the syndrome will be discussed briefly. Increased osteoclastic bone resorption is present in almost all patients with hypercalcemia of malignancy, and in most with primary hyperparathyroidism. In most patients with terminal malignancy, the increase in bone resorption is not accompanied by new bone formation (McDonnell et al 1982; Stewart et al 1982). Therapies that inhibit osteoclastic bone resorption effectively (for example, new generation bisphosphonates, gallium nitrate and plicamycin) are almost universally effective in the treatment of hypercalcemia of malignancy. Decreased renal calcium excretion is common to patients with hypercalcemia of malignancy and primary hyperparathyroidism. In malignancy, it has a number of causes:

- effects of factors (for example, PTH-rP) to enhance renal tubular calcium reabsorption;
- other mechanisms (still unclear at present) that also enhance renal tubular calcium reabsorption—seen in patients without PTH-rP production (for example, myeloma), and may be related to hypercalcemia per se;
- impaired glomerular filtration—associated with dehydration (reversible) or renal damage as in myeloma (irreversible). This causes increased renal tubular sodium reabsorption and associated increased renal tubular calcium reabsorption.

There are three current methods to promote renal calcium excretion: normal saline infusions; loop diuretics; and WR-2721. Of these, only normal saline is recommended. It is possible that part of the effect of calcitonin is to promote renal calcium excretion.

Since increased bone resorption is common to most patients, and patients with hypercalcemia of malignancy have progressive hypercalcemia due to increasing tumor burden, agents that transiently lower the serum calcium by promoting calcium diuresis are not sufficient therapy alone. All patients with malignancy-associated hypercalcemia should be treated with inhibitors of bone resorption, even when an initial episode of hypercalcemia has been brought under control, unless the primary tumor can be successfully treated. The most useful agents currently available for the treatment of hypercalcemia are the new generation bisphosphonates such as pamidronate. These are considered in detail in Chapter 5.

References

Bataille R, Jourdan M, Zhang XG et al (1989) Serum levels of interleukin-6, a potent myeloma cell growth factor, as a reflect of disease severity in plasma cell dyscrasias, *J Clin Invest* **84**: 2008–11.

Bertolini DR, Nedwin GE, Bringman TS et al (1986) Stimulation of bone resorption and inhibition of bone formation in vitro by human tumour necrosis factors, *Nature* **319**: 516–8.

Black K, Garrett IR, Mundy GR (1991) Chinese hamster ovarian cells transfected with the murine interleukin-6 gene cause hypercalcemia as well as cachexia, leukocytosis and thrombocytosis in tumour-bearing nude mice, *Endocrinology* **128**: 2657–9.

Boyce BF, Aufdemorte TB, Garrett IR et al (1989a) Effects of interleukin-1 on bone turnover in normal mice, *Endocrinology* **125**: 1142–50.

Boyce BF, Yates AJP, Mundy GR (1989b) Bolus injections of recombinant human interleukin-1 cause transient hypocalcemia in normal mice, *Endocrinology* **125**: 2780–83.

Boyce BF, Yoneda T, Lowe C et al (1992) Requirement of pp60$^{c\text{-}src}$ expression of osteoclasts to form ruffled borders and resorb bone, *J Clin Invest* **90**: 1622–7.

Breslau NA, McGuire JL, Zerwekh JE et al (1984) Hypercalcemia associated with increased serum calcitriol levels in three patients with lymphoma, *Ann Intern Med* **100**: 1–6.

Bruns DE, Ferguson JE, Weir EC et al (1992) Parathyroid hormone-related protein (PTH-rP): a novel hormone in human pregnancy, *J Bone Miner Res* **7** (Suppl 1): no 6.

Budayr AA, Halloran BP, King JC et al (1989) High levels of a parathyroid hormone-like protein in milk, *Proc Natl Acad Sci USA* **86**: 7183–5.

Bushinsky DA, Chabala JM, Levi-Setti R (1989) Ion microprobe analysis of mouse calvariae in vitro: evidence for a "bone membrane", *Am J Physiol* **256**: E152–E158.

Cozzolino F, Torcia M, Aldinucci D et al (1989) Production of interleukin-1 by bone marrow myeloma cells, *Blood* **74**: 380–7.

De La Mata J, Uy H, Guise TA et al (1995) IL-6 enhances hypercalcemia and bone resorption mediated by PTH-rP in vivo, *J Clin Invest* **95**: 2846–52.

Feyen JHM, Elford P, Dipadova FE et al (1989) Interleukin-6 is produced by bone and modulated by parathyroid hormone, *J Bone Miner Res* **4**: 633–8.

Fried RM, Voelkel EF, Rice RH et al (1989) Two squamous cell carcinomas not associated with humoral hypercalcemia produce a potent bone resorption-stimulating factor which is interleukin-1 alpha, *Endocrinology* **125**: 742–51.

Garrett IR, Durie BGM, Nedwin GE et al (1987) Production of the bone resorbing cytokine lymphotoxin by cultured human myeloma cells, *N Engl J Med* **317**: 526–32.

Gowen M, Wood DD, Russell RGG (1985) Stimulation of the proliferation of human bone cells in vitro by human monocyte products with interleukin-1 activity, *J Clin Invest* **75**: 1223–9.

Gowen M, Chapman K, Littlewood A et al (1990) Production of tumor necrosis factor by human osteoblasts is modulated by other cytokines but not by osteotropic hormones, *Endocrinology* **126**: 1250–5.

Guise TA, Chirgwin JM, Favarato G et al (1992) Chinese hamster ovarian cells transfected with human parathyroid hormone-related protein cDNA cause hypercalcemia in nude mice, *Lab Invest* **67**: 477–85.

Guise TA, Yoneda T, Yates AJ et al (1993) The combined effect of tumor-produced parathyroid hormone-related protein and transforming growth factor alpha enhance hypercalcemia in vivo and bone resorption in vitro, *J Clin Endocrinol Metab* **77**: 40–5.

Guise TA, Yin JJ, Taylor SD et al (1996) Evidence for a causal role of parathyroid hormone-related protein in the pathogenesis of human breast cancer-mediated osteolysis, *J Clin Invest* **98**: 1544–9.

Harinck HIJ, Bijvoet OLM, Plantingh AST (1987) Role of bone and kidney in tumor-induced hypercalcemia and its treatment with bisphosphonate and sodium chloride, *Am J Med* **82**: 1133–42.

Harms HM, Captaina U, Kulpmann WR et al (1989) Pulse amplitude and frequency modulation of parathyroid hormone in plasma, *J Clin Endocrinol Metab* **69**: 843–51.

Henderson B, Pettipher ER (1989) Arthritogenic actions of recombinant IL-1 and tumour necrosis factor alpha in the rabbit: evidence for synergistic interactions between cytokines in vivo, *Clin Exp Immunol* **75**: 306–10.

Ibbotson KJ, Twardzik DR, D'Souza SM et al (1985) Stimulation of bone resorption in vitro by synthetic transforming growth factor-alpha, *Science* **228**: 1007–9.

Ishimi Y, Miyaura C, Jin CH et al (1990) IL-6 is produced by osteoblasts and induces bone resorption, *J Immunol* **145**: 3297–303.

Johnson RA, Boyce BF, Mundy GR et al (1989) Tumors producing human TNF induce hypercalcemia and osteoclastic bone resorption in nude mice, *Endocrinology* **124**: 1424–7.

Karaplis AC, Luz A, Glowacki J et al (1994) Lethal skeletal dysplaces from targeted disruption of the parathyroid-related peptide gene, *Genes Dev* **8**: 277–89.

Kawano M, Tanaka H, Ishikawa H et al (1989) Interleukin-1 accelerates autocrine growth of myeloma cells through interleukin-6 in human myeloma, *Blood* **73**: 2145–8.

Kitamura N, Shigeno C, Shiomi K et al (1990) Episodic fluctuation in serum intact parathyroid hormone concentration in men, *J Clin Endocrinol Metab* **70**: 252–63.

Klein DC, Raisz LG (1970) Prostaglandins: stimulation of bone resorption in tissue culture, *Endocrinology* **86**: 1436–40.

Kukita A, Bonewald L, Rosen D et al (1990) Osteoinductive factor inhibits formation of human osteoclast-like cells, *Proc Natl Acad Sci USA* **87**: 3023–6.

Kukreja SC, Shevrin DH, Wimbiscus SA et al (1988) Antibodies to parathyroid hormone-related protein lower serum calcium in athymic mouse models of malignancy-associated hypercalcemia due to human tumors, *J Clin Invest* **82**: 1798–802.

Lanske B, Karaplis AC, Lee K et al (1996) PTH/PTHrP receptor in early development and Indian hedgehog-related bone growth, *Science* **273**: 653–66.

Levinskas GJ, Neuman WF (1955) The solubility of bone mineral. I. Solubility studies of synthetic hydroxyapatite, *J Physiol Chem* **59**: 164–8.

Lowik CWGM, Vanderpluijm G, Bloys H et al (1989) Parathyroid hormone (PTH) and PTH-like protein (Plp) stimulate interleukin-6 production by osteogenic cells—a possible role of interleukin-6 in osteoclastogenesis, *Biochem Biophys Res Commun* **162**: 1546–52.

Massague J (1990) Transforming growth factor alpha. A model for membrane-anchored growth factors, *J Biol Chem* **265**: 21 393–6.

McDonnell GD, Dunstan CR, Evans RA et al (1982) Quantitative bone histology in the hypercalcemia of malignant disease, *J Clin Endocrinol Metab* **55**: 1066–72.

Moseley JM, Kubota M, Diefenbach-Jagger H et al (1987) Parathyroid hormone-related protein purified from a human lung cancer cell line, *Proc Natl Acad Sci USA* **84**: 5048–52.

Motokura T, Fukumoto S, Matsumoto T et al (1989) Parathyroid hormone related protein in adult T-cell leukemia-lymphoma, *Ann Intern Med* **111**: 484–8.

Mundy GR (1990) *Calcium homeostasis: hypercalcemia and hypocalcemia*, 2nd edn (Martin Dunitz: London).

Mundy GR, Martin TJ (1982) The hypercalcemia of malignancy: pathogenesis and management, *Metabolism* **31**: 1247–77.

Neuman NW (1982) Blood:bone equilibrium, *Calcif Tissue Int* **34**: 117–20.

Nowak RA, Morrison NE, Goad DL et al (1990) Squamous cell carcinomas often produce more than a single bone resorption-stimulating factor—role of interleukin-1-alpha, *Endocrinology* **127**: 3061–9.

Nussbaum SR, Gaz RD, Arnold A (1990) Hypercalcemia and ectopic secretion of parathyroid hormone by an ovarian carcinoma with rearrangement of the gene for parathyroid hormone, *N Engl J Med* **323**: 1324–8.

Parfitt AM (1989) Plasma calcium control at quiescent bone surfaces, a new approach to the homeostatic function of bone lining cells, *Bone* **10**: 87–8.

Parfitt AM (1993) Calcium homeostasis. In: Mundy GR, Martin TJ, eds, *Physiology and pharmacology of bone. Handbook of experimental pharmacology* (Springer Verlag: Berlin) 1–65.

Peacock M, Robertson WG, Nordin BEC (1969) Relation between serum and urine calcium with particular reference to parathyroid activity, *Lancet* **i**: 384–6.

Percival RC, Yates AJP, Gray RES et al (1985) Mechanisms of malignant hypercalcemia in carcinoma of the breast, *Br Med J* **291**: 776–9.

Powell GJ, Southby J, Danks JA et al (1991) Localization of parathyroid hormone-related protein in breast cancer metastases: increased incidence in bone compared with other sites, *Cancer Res* **51**: 3059–61.

Rodda CP, Kubota M, Heath JA et al (1988) Evidence for a novel parathyroid hormone-related protein in fetal lamb parathyroid glands and sheep placenta: comparisons with a similar protein implicated in humoral hypercalcemia of malignancy, *J Endocrinol* **117**: 261–71.

Sabatini M, Boyce B, Aufdemorte T et al (1988) Infusions of recombinant human interleukin-1α and β cause hypercalcemia in normal mice, *Proc Natl Acad Sci USA* **85**: 5235–9.

Sabatini M, Yates AJ, Garrett R et al (1990a) Increased production of tumor necrosis factor by normal immune cells in a model of the humoral hypercalcemia of malignancy, *Lab Invest* **63**: 676–82.

Sabatini M, Chavez J, Mundy GR et al (1990b) Stimulation of tumor necrosis factor release from monocytic cells by the A375 human melanoma via granulocyte–macrophage colony stimulating factor, *Cancer Res* **50**: 2673–8.

Samuels MH, Veldhuis J, Cawley C et al (1993) Pulsatile secretion of parathyroid hormone in normal young subjects: assessment by deconvolution analysis, *J Clin Endocrinol Metab* **77**: 399–403.

Sato K, Fujii Y, Kasono K (1989) Parathyroid hormone-related protein and interleukin-1α synergistically stimulate bone resorption in vitro and increase the serum calcium concentration in mice in vivo, *Endocrinology* **124**: 2172–8.

Schipani E, Kruso K, Joppner H (1995) A combitatively active mutane PTH-PTHrP receptor in Jansen-type metaphyseal chondrodysplasia, *Science* **268**: 98–100.

Shigeno C, Yamamoto I, Dokoh S et al (1985) Identification of 1,24(R)-dihydroxyvitamin D_3-like bone-resorbing lipid in a patient with cancer-associated hypercalcemia, *J Clin Endocrinol Metab* **61**: 761–8.

Simpson EL, Mundy GR, D'Souza SM et al (1983) Absence of parathyroid hormone messenger RNA in non-parathyroid tumors associated with hypercalcemia, *N Engl J Med* **309**: 325–30.

Stewart AF, Vignery A, Silvergate A et al (1982) Quantitative bone histomorphometry in humoral hypercalcemia of malignancy—uncoupling of bone cell activity, *J Clin Endocrinol Metab* **55**: 219–27.

Stewart AF, Wu T, Goumas D et al (1987) N-terminal amino acid sequence of two novel tumor-derived adenylate cyclase-stimulating proteins: identification of parathyroid hormone-like and parathyroid hormone-unlike domains, *Biochem Biophys Res Commun* **146**: 672–8.

Strewler GJ, Budayr AA, Bruce RJ (1990) Secretion of authentic parathyroid hormone by a malignant tumor, *Clin Res* **38**: 462A.

Strewler GJ, Stern PH, Jacobs et al (1987) Parathyroid hormone-like protein from human renal carcinoma cells: structural and functional homology with parathyroid hormone, *J Clin Invest* **80**: 1803–7.

Takahashi N, MacDonald BR, Hon J et al (1986a) Recombinant human transforming growth factor alpha stimulates the formation of osteoclast-like cells in long term human marrow cultures, *J Clin Invest* **78**: 894–8.

Takahashi N, Mundy GR, Roodman GD (1986b) Recombinant human interferon-γ inhibits formation of human osteoclast-like cells, *J Immunol* **137**: 3544–9.

Takahashi N, Mundy GR, Kuehl TJ et al (1987) Osteoclast like formation in fetal and newborn long term baboon marrow cultures is more sensitive to 1,25-dihydroxyvitamin D_3 than adult long term marrow cultures, *J Bone Miner Res* **2**: 311–17.

Tam CS, Heersche JNM, Murray TM et al (1982) Parathyroid hormone stimulates the bone apposition rate independently of its resorptive action: differential effects of intermittent and continuous administration, *Endocrinology* **110**: 506–12.

Tashjian AH, Voelkel EF, Lazzaro M et al (1985) Alpha and beta transforming growth factors stimulate prostaglandin production and bone resorption in cultured mouse calvaria, *Proc Natl Acad Sci USA* **82**: 4535–8.

Thiede MA, Rodan GA (1988) Expression of a calcium-mobilizing parathyroid hormone-like peptide in lactating mammary tissue, *Science* **242**: 278–80.

Tuttle KR, Kunau RT, Loveridge N et al (1991) Altered renal calcium handling in hypercalcemia of malignancy, *J Am Soc Nephrol* **2**: 191–9.

Uy HL, Dallas M, Calland JW et al (1995) Use of an in vivo model to determine the effects of interleukin-1 on cells at different stages in the osteoclast lineage, *J Bone Miner Res* **10**: 295–301.

Uy HL, Mundy GR, Boyce BF et al (1996) Tumor necrosis factor enhances parathyroid hormone related protein (PTH-rP)—induced hypercalcemia in vivo, *J Bone Miner Res* **11** (Suppl 1): S447.

Yates AJP, Gutierrez GE, Smolens P et al (1988) Effects of a synthetic peptide of a parathyroid hormone-related protein on calcium homeostasis, renal tubular calcium reabsorption and bone metabolism, *J Clin Invest* **81**: 932–8.

Yates AJP, Favarato G, Aufdemorte TB et al (1992) Expression of human transforming growth factor α by Chinese hamster ovarian tumors in nude mice causes hypercalcemia and increases osteoclastic bone resorption, *J Bone Miner Res* **7**: 847–53.

Yoneda T, Alsina MM, Chavez JB et al (1991) Evidence that splenic cytokines play a pathogenetic role in the paraneoplastic syndromes of cachexia, hypercalcemia and leukocytosis in a human tumor in nude mice, *J Clin Invest* **87**: 977–85.

Yoshimoto K, Yamasaki R, Sakai H et al (1989) Ectopic production of parathyroid hormone by small cell lung cancer in a patient with hypercalcemia, *J Clin Endocrinol Metab* **68**: 976–81.

CHAPTER 7

Metastatic bone disease

The skeleton is the third most favored site for metastasis of solid tumors. Bone metastasis is a catastrophic complication for most patients, although in the early stages it may be inapparent and unexpected. It usually means that the malignant process is incurable, and it causes not only intractable pain, but other local complications such as fracture after trivial injury and nerve compression. Extensive bone destruction can lead to hypercalcemia, the most rapidly fatal complication. In this chapter, some special aspects of the process of bone metastasis will be reviewed, including what is known of why it occurs, why some tumors favor the skeleton as a metastatic site, and what the future holds for prevention or treatment of established metastases.

Classification of bone metastases

Tumors cause two distinct types of skeletal lesions when they spread to bone (Figure 7.1). The most common is the destructive or osteolytic lesion. In this type of metastatic bone lesion, tumor products distort the normal remodeling sequence so that there is an increase primarily in osteoclast activity. The secondary osteoblast response seen in normal bone remodeling is almost always impaired to a varying degree, so that the lesion is predominantly lytic. Less common is the osteoblastic response, which occurs without previous resorption. The mechanisms which are responsible for distinctive and discrete effects on osteoblasts and osteoclasts involved in normal bone remodeling remain obscure. Table 7.1 is a simple outline of a classification for bone metastases.

Frequency of bone metastases

The commonest malignant tumors that affect humankind involve the skeleton. Approximately 700 000 people die of cancer in the United States each year (Wingo et al 1995), and at least two-thirds of these have bone metastases. Over 220 000 people die with lung and breast cancer, and the frequency of bone metastases in these patients is even greater. Although bone metastasis occurs frequently with nearly all tumors, there are special types of cancers that have a special predilection for the skeleton. In particular, breast cancer and prostate cancer almost always metastasize to the skeleton and other common solid tumors such as lung cancer frequently do. Bone metastases also occur commonly in thyroid and renal cancers. This special pattern of types of solid tumors that are associated with metastatic bone lesions is exemplified by Tables 7.2–7.4 and Figures 7.2 and 7.3.

Please note that these estimates of the frequency of metastasis depend on the sensitivity of the diagnostic technique. The techniques that have been mostly used are bone scans, X-rays

Malignant disease and the skeleton

Figure 7.1
Tumors have two effects on the skeleton—either to cause osteolytic lesions and in some patients hypercalcemia, or osteoblastic lesions. Osteolytic lesions are far more common than osteoblastic lesions.

Table 7.1 Spectrum of bone lesions seen in malignancy.

	Myeloma	Breast cancer	Prostate cancer
X-rays	Osteolytic	Mixed	Osteosclerotic
Histology	Osteoclasts increased	Mixed osteoclastic and osteoblastic	Osteoblastic bone formation
Serum alkaline phosphatase	Normal	Increased	Markedly increased
Bone scans	Normal	Increased activity	Markedly increased activity

and histologic examination of autopsy specimens. Both radiologic and histologic assessments are limited by the extent of the sample evaluated. Bone scans survey the whole body, but because isotope accumulation depends on osteoblast activity, those lesions with very little osteoblastic component cannot be detected.

Skeletal involvement is also common in hematologic malignancies. Myeloma almost always causes osteolytic lesions, which are present in at least 95% of cases (Mundy and Bertolini 1986). In some patients with myeloma there may be a mixture of discrete osteolytic and diffuse osteopenic lesions. For example, it is common to find patients who have multiple discrete osteolytic lesions in the skull and diffuse osteoporosis in the vertebral column. Hypercalcemia occurs late in the disease in approximately 30% of patients with myeloma (Mundy 1990). Both osteolytic and osteoblastic lesions can occur in patients with lymphomas, particularly Hodgkin's disease, but these are not as common as they are in patients with myeloma. In a small percentage of patients with myeloma, osteosclerosis occurs due to a generalized stimulation of osteoblast activity.

Table 7.2 Frequency of skeletal metastases at autopsy.[a]

Tumor	Frequency of skeletal metastasis (%)
Breast	50–85
Prostate	60–85
Thyroid	28–60
Kidney	33–60
Lung	32–64
Esophagus	6
Gastrointestinal tract	3–10
Rectum	8–60
Bladder	42
Uterine cervix	50
Ovaries	9
Liver	16
Melanoma	7

[a]Modified from Galasko (1986b).

Table 7.3 Frequency of skeletal metastases, as detected by scintigraphy.[a]

Primary site	Percent with metastases
Breast	84
Prostate	70
Thyroid	43
Kidney	60
Bronchus	64
Rectum	61
Uterine cervix	56

[a]Modified from Galasko (1986b).

Table 7.4 Destruction of bone metastases detected by scintigraphy.[a]

Primary tumour	Distribution of skeletal metastases (%)				
	Skull	Spine	Rib cage	Pelvis	Appendicular skeleton
Breast	28	60	59	38	32
Lung	16	43	65	25	27
Prostate	14	60	50	57	38
Cervix	26	26	22	43	43
Bladder	13	47	53	47	7
Rectum	21	36	29	43	43

[a]From Tofe et al (1975).

Favored sites of skeletal involvement by malignant disease

Tumor cells most frequently affect those parts of the skeleton that are the most heavily vascularized, and in particular the red bone marrow of the axial skeleton and the proximal ends of the long bones, the ribs and the vertebral column. This is true in both hematologic malignancies and for all solid tumors. Although metastases to the appendicular skeleton occur less frequently, they may be seen particularly in patients with melanoma and renal cancer. Breast cancer cells sometimes metastasize to the posterior clinoid processes. The precise reasons for these unusual distributions of bone lesions are not clear. Galasko (1986a,b) has reviewed in detail the distribution of

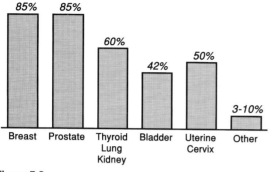

Figure 7.2

Frequency of bone metastases associated with common malignancies. These represent patients with advanced disease.

skeletal metastases from various solid tumors. The major, but not the sole, determinant of the site of metastasis is blood flow from the primary site. Since prostate cancer frequently metastasizes to the vertebral column, it was suggested 50 years ago that access through the vertebral venous plexus (Batson's plexus) is key. Batson's plexus is a low pressure, high volume system of vertebral veins that can communicate with the intercostal veins and runs up the spine. Batson's vertebral plexus has been suggested as being responsible for the distribution of prostate tumor cell metastasis to the spine. This plexus has extensive intercommunications, which apparently function independently of other major venous systems such as the pulmonary, caval and portal

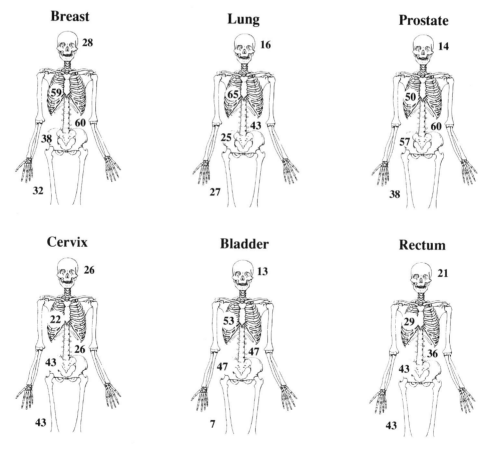

Figure 7.3

Distribution of bone metastases throughout the skeleton in common malignancies that metastasize to bone. (Modified from Tofe et al (1975).)

systems (Batson 1940). It has been studied by the injection of dye into the dorsal vein of the penis in cadavers and experimental animals (Batson 1940). A number of workers have suggested that this system may be important for the spread of tumor cells to the axial skeleton (Coman and DeLong 1951; Van den Brenk et al 1975; Galasko 1986a,b). However, Dodds et al (1981) have questioned whether prostate cancer cells do in fact spread preferentially through this paravertebral plexus to the spine.

Clinical consequences of skeletal involvement by cancer

Bone pain

Frequent bone pain is common in patients with either osteolytic or osteoblastic lesions. The mechanisms responsible for bone pain are unclear, and bone may undergo remissions and exacerbations without apparent change in nature or behavior of the underlying metastasis. Bone pain is a major symptomatic problem in patients with bone metastases.

Pathologic fractures

Pathologic fractures following trivial injury are frequent in patients with metastatic bone disease, and particularly in those with osteolytic lesions. These fractures occur most frequently in the vertebral bodies and the proximal ends of long bones, at the common sites of metastasis.

Nerve compression syndromes

Nerve compression syndromes may occur because of tumors that impinge directly on the spinal cord, but occur more frequently because severe destructive osteolytic lesions lead to nerve fracture and fragility of the vertebral body and compression of the cord as a result of the subsequent deformity. Nerve compression syndromes also occur occasionally in patients with osteoblastic lesions because of bony overgrowth impinging directly on nerves or narrow foramina or canals. Prostate cancer that metastasizes to the vertebral spine may cause spinal cord compression, cauda equina syndromes and paraparesis, and metastases to the base of the skull can impinge on cranial nerve foramena.

Hypercalcemia

Hypercalcemia occurs commonly in patients with metastatic bone disease, and particularly in patients with osteolytic lesions. It is very uncommon in patients with prostate cancer. Approximately 30% of patients with breast cancer will develop hypercalcemia at some time during the course of the disease, and usually late in the disease (Galasko and Burn 1971). Myeloma also causes hypercalcemia in at least one-third of patients during the disease process, and usually later in the disease as the tumor burden increases (Mundy 1990). Hypercalcemia is almost always due primarily to an increase in bone resorption, which is caused in turn by the production of bone-active agents by the tumor cells that stimulate osteoclastic bone resorption. However, in almost all these patients, there is an impairment of the kidney's capacity to compensate for this increased calcium load.

Although hypercalcemia usually occurs in association with osteolytic bone lesions, it also occurs without evidence of localized osteolysis. In most situations, hypercalcemia is due to one (or more) systemic factor produced by the tumor cells, which stimulates osteoclastic bone resorption and usually increases renal tubular calcium reabsorption. This latter situation has frequently been referred to as the humoral hypercalcemia of malignancy. It is not particularly helpful to distinguish hypercalcemia due to localized bone destruction from hypercalcemia associated with metastasis. In some patients with osteolytic lesions, it is clear that systemic mediators are produced by the tumor cells and they are likely to play a major role in the pathophysiology of hypercalcemia. These factors may be particularly important if they are produced in large amounts locally at the metastatic sites and the concentrations of these factors that bathe osteoclasts are high. These factors are described in more detail in

Chapter 6. In the past, a distinction between humoral hypercalcemia and osteolytic hypercalcemia has been made by some groups. These distinctions have been determined by measurements of nephrogenous cyclic AMP (Stewart et al 1980), a parameter of PTH-rP production. However, PTH-rP is not the only factor associated with the hypercalcemia of malignancy, and some patients with humoral hypercalcemia do not have increased nephrogenous cyclic AMP. Moreover, PTH-rP is often secreted by metastatic tumor cells associated with osteolytic lesions.

Studies by Tuttle et al (1991) have shown that renal tubular calcium reabsorption is increased not only in patients with humoral hypercalcemia, but almost universally in patients with the hypercalcemia of malignancy, and even in patients with hypercalcemia due to myeloma. It had previously been recognized that renal tubular calcium reabsorption was frequently increased in patients with solid tumors associated with hypercalcemia (Peacock et al 1969), but widely thought that hypercalcemia associated with osteolytic lesions or with myeloma was not usually associated with increased renal tubular calcium reabsorption. The studies of Tuttle et al (1991) and the earlier studies of Percival et al (1985) have refuted that conclusion. Gallacher et al (1990) also showed that in patients with breast cancer there was frequently an increase in reabsorption of calcium in the renal tubules that could not be accounted for by PTH-rP. In the studies of Tuttle et al (1991), glomerular filtration rate was carefully measured as well as hydration status, and renal tubular calcium reabsorption was compared with control patients who were matched for impairment of renal function. The mechanisms responsible for the increase in renal tubular calcium reabsorption are not entirely clear, although obviously there is an increase in production of PTH-rP in some patients. In those patients who do not produce PTH-rP, the mechanism is likely to be related to other factors that have not yet been explained. Harinck et al (1987) suggested that calcium reabsorption may be due to changes in volume status caused by chronic hypercalcemia, so that subsequent volume depletion increased sodium reabsorption in the proximal tubules and this is associated with increased calcium reabsorption. However, Tuttle et al (1991) showed that increased renal tubular calcium reabsorption was essentially universal in patients with the hypercalcemia of malignancy independent of PTH-rP status and the increase in renal tubular calcium reabsorption also occurred independent of hydration status.

Pathophysiology of the metastatic process

The metastasis of tumor cells to specific sites in the skeleton is clearly not a simple random event determined solely by blood flow, but rather a directed and multistep process that is dependent on specific properties of the tumor cells as well as factors in the bone microenvironment that favor metastasis. Liotta and colleagues have suggested that although the distribution of metastases in distant organs can be predicted by the anatomic distribution of blood flow from the primary site in 30% of cases, in the majority there are specific properties at the metastatic site that determine whether the metastasis can become established (Liotta and Kohn 1990). Over 100 years ago, this nonrandom concept for tumor metastasis was recognized by Paget (1889) who described the "seed and soil" hypothesis of tumor spread.

The recognition that tumor metastasis is a multistep process involving separate discrete steps, raises the possibility that interruption of one or more of these steps can inhibit the metastatic process (Figure 7.4). Each of these discrete steps is due to specific determinants of both the tumor and the tissue (Liotta and Kohn 1990; Zetter et al 1990). The steps involved in the shedding of tumor cells from the primary site involve detachment of tumor cells from adjacent cells, followed by invasion of adjacent tissue in the primary organs. The cells then enter tumor capillaries (stimulated by specific angiogenesis factors produced by the tumor) and via these capillaries reach the general circulation (Weiss et al 1989). The steps involved in entering the tumor blood vessels at the primary site are similar to those involved in exit from the vasculature in the bone marrow cavity. These steps include the attachment of the tumor cells to basement membrane, the secretion of proteolytic enzymes that enable tumor cells to disrupt the basement membrane and then migration of the tumor cells through the basement membrane (Liotta et al 1980, 1986;

Figure 7.4

The multistep progression of events involved in the pathophysiology of bone metastasis. See text for details.

Figure 7.5

Metastatic cascade in bone as described by Liotta et al (1986), involving (A) attachment to basement membranes; (B) proteolysis and disruption of basement membranes; and (C) chemotaxis or unilateral migration of tumor cells out of blood vessels into the tissue stroma. See text for details.

Liotta and Steeg 1990) (Figure 7.5).

Attachment of tumor cells to other cells and to extracellular structures is critical for the metastatic process. Cell adhesion molecules (CAMs) such as laminin and E-cadherin are particularly likely to play a key role in several important events involved in cancer cell invasion and metastasis. CAMs mediate cell-to-cell and cell-to-substratum communications. Cancer cell adhesion to normal host cells and to extracellular matrix through CAMs has been shown to regulate tumor cell invasiveness and proliferation (Albelda and Buck 1990).

At the primary site, loss of CAMs causes disruption of the interconnections between cancer cells and promotes the detachment of cancer cells from the primary tumor, which results in initiation of local invasion and eventually in the development of metastasis. In contrast, at the metastatic site, elevated expression of CAMs might be a prerequisite for cancer cells to arrest through the attachment to extracellular matrix. Subsequently, expression of CAMs might be diminished to free cancer cells from direct contact-mediated regulation by host immune cells. Recent studies have demonstrated that metastatic breast and ovarian cancers show heterogeneous expression of E-cadherin (Oka et al 1993), and E-cadherin expression in these cancer cells may be reversibly modulated according to culture conditions in vitro (Hashimoto et al 1989) and environmental factors in vivo (Mareel et al 1991). Therefore, cancer cells may express either decreased or increased levels of CAMs depending on the stage of metastasis development and sites of metastasis. We think it likely that the CAMs E-cadherin and laminin are involved in bone metastasis (see below).

Integrins are the most abundant CAMs and are responsible for a variety of cell–cell and cell–matrix interactions (Haynes 1992), and have been implicated in hematogenous dissemination (Nip et al 1992). In cancer metastasis, integrins have been shown to mediate cancer cell attachment to vascular endothelial cells and to matrix proteins such as laminin and fibronectin that underlie endothelium, an initial step in tumor colonization (Albelda and Buck 1990). For example, it has recently been demonstrated that A375 human melanoma cells express high levels of the $\alpha_v\beta_3$ integrin (vitronectin receptor) on the cell surface when they bind to and invade the basement membrane matrix matrigel (Seftor et al 1992).

Because of their complex structural and functional diversity, it seems unlikely at the present time that multiple integrins could potentially be involved in bone metastasis.

Laminin

We have found that synthetic antagonists to laminin inhibit osteolytic bone metastasis formation by A375 cells in nude mice (Nakai et al 1992). To perform these studies, we developed a model for bone metastasis based on the technique first described by Arguello et al (1988) to study metastasis to bone of human tumor cells (Figure 7.6). We inoculated human melanoma cells into the left ventricle of nude mice and examined the formation of osteolytic metastases by radiographs and histology. This process was prevented by a synthetic antagonist to laminin (Figures 7.7–7.9).

We are aware that our bone metastasis model does not allow us to study the roles of CAMs in the steps *before* cancer cell entry into the circulation since we inject cells into the left ventricle of the heart. However, we will be able to examine

Figure 7.6

Technique for studying bone metastasis as described by Arguello et al (1988) and modified by Yoneda and colleagues (Nakai et al 1992) to study the capacity of human tumors to metastasize to bone.

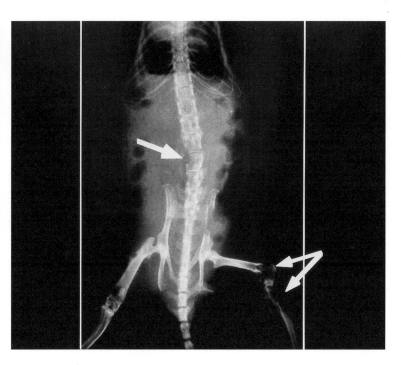

Figure 7.7

Osteolytic lesions formed by human melanoma cells after injection into the left ventricle of the heart of nude mice after 3 weeks. (Reproduced from Nakai et al (1992).)

Figure 7.8

The laminin molecule, indicating specific sites in the glycoprotein to which antagonists and the control peptides used by Nakai et al (1992) were derived. The domain designated YIGSR is critical for bone metastasis.

CAMs for their importance in the events involved specifically after intravasation of cancer cells. In these steps, increased expression of integrins may be required for cancer cells to arrest and form microfoci at metastatic sites.

E-cadherin

E-cadherin (uvomorulin) is a 120 kilodalton cell surface glycoprotein involved in calcium-dependent epithelial cell-specific cell adhesion. E-cadherin has homophilic properties in cell–cell adhesion and thus causes homotypic cell aggregation, which may be important in controlling embryogenesis and morphogenesis (Takeichi 1991). Recent evidence has shown that E-cadherin also plays a role in cancer invasion and metastasis. Treatment of epithelial noninvasive Madin–Darby canine kidney (MDCK) cells with monoclonal antibodies to E-cadherin rendered these cells more invasive (Behrens et al 1989). Overexpression of the E-cadherin gene in highly invasive cancer cells dramatically suppressed their invasiveness and conversely the introduction of E-cadherin-specific antisense RNA rendered noninvasive epithelial cells invasive (Vleminckx et al 1991). E-cadherin expression was increased in populations of MCF-7 breast cancer cells with reduced invasiveness, whereas relatively low levels of E-cadherin were detected in the highly invasive human breast cancer cells MDA-231 (Sommers et al 1991).

Anti–laminin Peptide on Bone Metastasis

Control　　Laminin　　YIGSR　　YOSH

Figure 7.9

Effects of laminin antagonists on bone resorption. Note that control mice, mice treated with laminin, and mice treated with control peptide (YOSH) all have multiple osteolytic lesions—most pronounced with laminin. However, in the mice treated with the synthetic laminin antagonist (YIGSR), there was reduction in the number of metastases. (Reproduced from Nakai et al (1992).)

We have examined the capacity of the human breast cancer cell lines MCF-7 (high E-cadherin expression) and MDA-231 cells (low E-cadherin expression) to form bone metastases (Mbalaviele et al 1996). We have found that MDA-231 cells are much more effective at forming osteolytic bone lesions in vivo. This experiment has been performed multiple times on a total of 50 mice for MDA-231 cells and 40 mice for MCF-7 cells. Whereas MDA-231 cells form obvious osteolytic lesions by 4 weeks after inoculation into the left ventricle, MCF-7 cells take more than 8 weeks to form similar lesions. At 4 weeks, no lesions are apparent in mice inoculated with MCF-7 cells. However, when MDA-231 cells were transfected with E-cadherin cDNA, their capacity to form osteolytic bone lesions was markedly reduced (Mbalaviele et al 1996).

Secretion of proteolytic enzymes by the tumor cells or by host cells may be responsible for disruption of the basement membranes of blood vessels and the tissue stroma, processes that are required for tumor cell egress from the circulation. These enzymes may include Type IV collagenase as well as other proteolytic enzymes. Tumor cells may cross the basement membrane by a process of directed migrational chemotaxis, but increased random movement (or chemokinesis) may also be responsible. Tumor cells produce motility factors that can increase their locomotive capacity and result in increased migration through defects in the basement membrane (Liotta et al 1986). Tumor cells have varying capacity for metastasis. Primary tumors comprise heterogeneous populations of cells, which have been shown in many studies to have differing invasive properties and different metastatic potentials (Fidler 1978; Carr and Orr 1983; Heppner 1984; Fidler and Post 1985; Poste 1986). Tumor cells are unstable phenotypically for reasons that are not completely understood, although this has been the subject of many studies (Nowell 1976; Miller 1983). As tumors grow, they undergo rapid clonal diversification (Reedy and Fialkow 1980). Some of the possibilities for this variability in individual tumor behavior include a host selection process, which may be due to some cells having the capability of surviving naturally occurring immune defense mechanisms, or the effects of treatment with anticancer drugs or radiation therapy, which may lead to acquired genetic variability. It is now well recognized that the genetic component of tumor cells can greatly influence their metastatic potentials as well as their invasive capabilities and tumorigenicity (Garbisa et al 1987; Liotta and Kohn 1990). In breast cancers, expression of the Her-2/Neu oncogene occurs in parallel with aggressive behavior of the cells (Slamon et al 1987). In some tumors, particularly melanoma, expression of the NM23 oncogene appears to inhibit the capability of the tumor to metastasize (Steeg et al 1988; Liotta and Steeg 1990). As already noted, the expression of laminin receptors on tumor cells may cause enhanced metastatic capabilities. Deletions of chromosomal material on chromosome 11p have been noted in aggressive breast cancers (Ali et al 1987) and deletions of chromosomes 17 and 18 may be found in colon carcinomas that arise from colonic polyps (Vogelstein et al 1988; Baker et al 1989).

There are multiple mechanisms that protect against tumor metastasis. Current evidence suggests that less than 1% of tumor cells survive in the circulation (Liotta and Kohn 1990). Tumors probably survive best in the circulation as aggregates, which may prevent the loss of individual cells in the circulation from mechanical shear forces or from anoxia.

The blood coagulation mechanism appears to be important in promoting tumor cell metastasis (Winterbauer et al 1968; Warren and Vales 1972; Hilgard and Gordon-Smith 1974). Anticoagulants of the coumadin class have been tested over many years for their capacity to inhibit metastasis and promote survival, although the data remain inconclusive and controversial. Once within the bone marrow cavity, tumor cells pass through wide-channelled marrow sinusoids. The cellular and molecular events involved in their passage from the marrow sinusoid to the bone surface are similar to the events involved in their escape from the primary site. Again, the tumors must attach to basement membranes of blood vessels, disrupt these basement membranes by the production of proteolytic enzymes and then migrate through the basement membrane to invade the tissue stroma. A fourth step is involved in the pathophysiology of the bone metastasis, and this involves the destruction of bone. There is some controversy over the mechanisms by which this may occur (see below). Recently, we have studied several human tumors (A375 melanoma cells and cultured breast cancer cells) to determine their capability of growing metastases in bone using a modification of the technique described by Arguello et al (1988). We have used inhibitors of specific cell adhesion molecules to determine their effects on the metastatic process. Tumor cells bind to basement membranes on endothelial cells at the metastatic site (Auerbach et al 1987) through specific cell adhesion molecules such as fibronectin and laminin. We have used synthetic antagonists of laminin, which interfere with the binding of laminin to laminin receptors on the tumor cells, to determine the effects on the formation of the bone metastasis. We have found that a synthetic antagonist YIGSR totally inhibits this process in bone. A similar result was found when this antagonist was used in a lung metastasis model (McCarthy et al 1988). There may be a 50-fold increase in laminin receptors on the surface of high invasive and metastatic tumor cells compared with other tumor cells that do not have the capability of metastasis or invasion (Wewer et al 1987).

Secretion of proteolytic enzymes

Tumor cells produce proteolytic enzymes to degrade basement membranes and traverse the vessels to enter the tissue stroma. This process can involve direct production of proteolytic enzymes by tumor cells such as Type IV collagenase, or even production of proteolytic enzymes by host cells. Garbisa et al (1987) have pointed out the potential role of the production of Type IV collagenase by tumor cells and its potential for degradation of the capillary basement membrane. Basset et al (1990) have shown that host cells associated with some invasive breast carcinomas expressed a gene that encodes a metalloproteinase. This gene was expressed by fibroblasts and stromal cells that were present adjacent to the breast cancer cells. Expression of this metalloproteinase was stimulated by growth factors produced by the breast cancer cells such as platelet-derived growth factor (PDGF), TGFα and basic fibroblast growth factor (bFGF).

Cell motility

Tumor cells may be attracted from the vasculature towards bone surfaces by a number of chemotactic factors. Bone itself contains multiple factors with chemotactic potential for tumor cells. These include fragments of Type I collagen, which have been shown to cause unidirectional migration of tumor cells (Mundy et al 1981), and fragments of the bone protein osteocalcin, which may cause chemotaxis of tumor cells and monocytes (Mundy and Poser 1983). The conditioned media harvested from resorbing or remodeling bones contain chemotactic activity, which stimulates the unidirectional migration of rat and human tumor cells (Orr et al 1979, 1980). The nature of the factor responsible has not been identified, but may be TGFβ, which is present in abundant amounts in bone (Hauschka et al 1986).

Tumor cell mediation of bone destruction at the metastatic site

The cellular mechanism responsible for local destruction of bone by tumor cells has been a controversial issue for some years (Figure 7.10). Although definitive proof is still not available, it is likely that the predominant mechanism for bone destruction is an increase in osteoclast activity. In other words, tumors produce local factors that stimulate osteoclasts, which then in turn are responsible for the resorption of bone. The alternative possibility is that tumor cells may destroy bone directly without the addition of osteoclasts. The evidence in favor of osteoclastic bone resorption being the predominant mechanism is twofold. First, when looked for carefully using techniques such as scanning electron microscopy, osteoclasts are invariably found to be present adjacent to tumor deposits (Boyde et al 1986) (Figure 7.11). Moreover, distinctive osteoclast resorption lacunae are universally present. Such studies show no evidence of smaller resorption lacunae corresponding to the size of the tumor cells. Secondly, drugs that effectively inhibit osteoclast activity such as the bisphosphonates, plicamycin and gallium nitrate work very effectively in the hypercalcemia of malignancy, which is due predominantly to increased bone

Figure 7.11

Demonstration that osteoclasts are the major mechanism by which solid tumors cause bone destruction. Multiple Howship's lacunae are seen in this scanning electron micrograph of the cancellous bone surface of a vertebral body in this patient with metastatic pancreatic cancer. This figure shows successively higher powers of the same site on the cancellous bone surface. (From Boyde et al (1986).)

Figure 7.10

X-ray showing characteristic lytic lesions seen in a patient with metastatic breast cancer.

resorption caused by tumors. These data suggest that since these drugs work through the inhibition of osteoclast function, osteoclasts are major (possibly sole) mediators of the bone destruction. Nevertheless, there is in vitro evidence suggesting that breast cancer cells have the capacity to cause bone resorption in vitro. When breast cancer cells have been added to devitalized bone, they cause both mineral release and matrix degradation (Eilon and Mundy 1978).

Mechanisms of osteoclast stimulation at the metastatic site

As indicated above, the major cellular mechanism for bone destruction in osteolytic bone disease is osteoclastic. Consequently, there is interest in determining the mediator responsible for this increase in osteoclast activity. Recent studies suggest that the factor responsible in at least some of these patients is PTH-rP, the tumor peptide that has been associated with humoral hypercalcemia of malignancy. This is so even though many of these patients do not have increased plasma PTH-rP or increased nephrogenous cyclic AMP. Indicating the absence of these latter parameters does not mean that PTH-rP is unimportant. Recently, it has been shown by immunohistochemistry that there is increased expression of PTH-rP in bone sites compared with either soft tissue metastases or primary tumors in patients with carcinoma of the breast (Powell et al 1991).

One example we have studied, in which the human breast cancer cell line MDA-MB-231 has been inoculated into the left cardiac ventricle of nude mice and the development of osteolytic lesions followed over the following 4–6 weeks, found that there is an increase in PTH-rP expression in the tumor cells that metastasize to bone. This is associated with the development of typical osteolytic bone lesions seen in patients with the disease. When tumor-bearing nude mice are treated with neutralizing antibodies to PTH-rP, not only is there a decrease in the development of the osteolytic bone lesions, but there is also a decrease in the tumor burden in bone (Guise et al 1996) (Figures 7.12–7.14). The most likely explanation for the increase in PTH-rP production in

No treatment   IgG   PTH-rP-Ab

Figure 7.12

Effects of neutralizing antibodies to PTH-rP on the capacity of human MDA-MB-231 breast cancer cells to cause osteolytic bone lesions following intracardiac injection in nude mice. The neutralizing antibodies to PTH-rP prevent the development of osteolytic lesions (Guise et al 1996).

Figure 7.13

Quantitation of lesion area from the experiment described in Figure 7.12 (Guise et al 1996). Impairment of the development of osteolytic lesions is caused by neutralizing antibodies to PTH-rP.

Figure 7.14

Histomorphometric analysis of data shown in Figures 7.12 and 7.13. Neutralizing antibodies to PTH-rP not only reduce the number of osteoclasts adjacent to metastatic human breast cancer cells, but also markedly reduces tumor burden in bone.

the bone microenvironment is that bone provides a fertile environment for the growth of tumor cells and also enhances the production of PTH-rP. More recent studies have shown that a likely mechanism responsible for this effect is production of transforming growth factor β (TGFβ), which is released from bone in active form when bone resorbs (Pfeilschifter and Mundy 1987). Studies by Yin et al (1996) have shown that when MDA-MB-231 cells are transfected with a dominant-negative type II TGFβ receptor, which makes the cells unresponsive to TGFβ, PTH-rP production is not enhanced in the bone microenvironment and the development and progression of osteolytic bone lesions are significantly less compared with this metastasis caused by parental MDA-MB-231. It is also likely that there are other mechanisms for bone destruction associated with tumor cells that metastasize to bone. These may involve production by the tumor cells or by host immune cells in the bone microenvironment of mediators such as TGFα, interleukin 1α, tumor necrosis factor and interleukin 6, each of which acting alone or in combination with PTH-rP represents a strong stimulus to increase bone resorption (De La Mata et al 1995).

Bone-derived tumor growth factors at the metastatic site

Bone provides a very favorable niche for tumor cells and it is clear that in this microenvironment many tumors grow very well. In part, the reason may be that bone is a large repository or storehouse for growth regulatory factors (Hauschka et al 1986) (Figure 7.15). In particular, bone is rich in TGFβ, but also stores other growth regulatory factors that may act as tumor growth factors including bone morphogenetic proteins, heparin binding fibroblast growth factors, platelet-derived growth factors, and insulin-like growth factors I and II. These factors are presumably the reason that bone is resorbed so avidly in metastases. They may be made available locally through bone resorption. This has been shown particularly in the case of TGFβ. TGFβ may alter the behavior of many tumor cells, and in particular breast cancer cells, to enhance the production of parathyroid hormone-related protein (Zakalik et al 1992). The mouse metastasis model, which has been described above, provides a very useful approach for studying osteolytic bone metastasis (Sasaki and Watanabe 1995). The bone lesions are typical of patients with the disease. The tumor cells can be modified by transfection with genes that are likely to be involved in the metastatic process, or by determining whether or not a specific mechanism is responsible by transfecting the cells with genes that interfere with this function, such as TIMP or dominant-negative type II TGFβ receptors (Yin et al 1996). These approaches can provide considerable insights into the molecular mechanisms responsible for osteolytic bone metastasis.

Another factor that may be important in tumor cell behavior in the bone microenvironment is calcium. Calcium released by resorbing bone may

TYPE	CONCENTRATION (ng/g)
Insulin-Like Growth factor II	1500
Transforming Growth Factor β	450
Insulin-Like Growth Factor I	100
Platlet-Derived Growth Factor	60
Basic Fibroblast Growth Factor	50
Acidic Fibroblast Growth Factor	10
Bone Morphogenic Protein	1-2

Figure 7.15

Growth factors stored in the bone matrix are released during the process of resorption in an active form, and are then potentially available to modulate tumor growth and activity (Hauschka et al 1986).

- CAMs
- MMPs

- CAMs
- MMPs

- PTH-rP
- Cytokines
- src

Figure 7.16

Molecular mechanisms involved in breast cancer cell metastasis to bone. Some of these steps are general steps and some are steps that are specific for bone. These molecular mechanisms have been clarified by the recent studies of Sasaki and Guise (Sasaki et al 1995; Guise et al 1996).

alter tumor cell proliferation (Rizzoli and Bonjour 1989). Unfortunately, there is still little information on this topic.

One of the major difficulties that has limited the study of bone metastasis has been the lack of suitable animal models. Although this has retarded the accumulation of knowledge in the pathophysiology of bone metastasis, it has not been a problem in investigating other types of metastases, and in particular lung metastases (Fidler and Post 1985). Arguello et al (1988) devised a technique where tumor cells are injected directly into the left ventricle of mice. This leads to the colonization of bone in regions containing hematopoietic bone marrow by appropriate tumor cells with potential to metastasize to bone. This leads to multiple lytic lesions resembling those seen in patients with cancer. In these models, bone metastasis occurs when tumor cells have ready access to the arterial circulation. We have modified this model by the use of human tumor cells in nude mice (Nakai et al 1992). By inoculating human breast cancer cells into the left ventricle of nude mice, we have been able to characterize a number of steps involved in osteolytic bone metastasis. By treating the animals with antagonists or antibodies to specific molecules involved in the process (for example, E-cadherin and PTH-rP), by transfecting the tumor cells with specific genes (for example, E-cadherin,

Figure 7.17

Effects of increasing local bone turnover on the development of osteolytic bone lesions in nude mice. In this experiment, interleukin-1 (IL-1) was administered for 3 days over the calvaria of a nude mouse to increase bone turnover. Following IL-1 injections, the mice were inoculated with MDA-MB-231 cells into the left cardiac ventricle. Note the obvious development of osteolytic lesions in the calvarium in which bone turnover was stimulated by IL-1, compared with a calvarium where bone turnover was not increased. This effect of IL-1 was inhibited by simultaneous treatment with the bisphosphonate ibandronate, which inhibits bone resorption.

TIMP-2, src, and PTH-rP) and showing their roles in this process, and by treating the animals with agents (for example, bisphosphonates and growth factors), which regulate normal bone cell function, the interaction between bone cells and tumor cells in the bone microenvironment can be determined. Some of the molecular mechanisms likely to be involved in the process of breast cancer metastasis to bone that have been identified using this technique are shown diagrammatically in Figure 7.16. With a special modification of this technique, Yoneda et al (1995) have developed a method for specifically examining metastasis to the calvarium to give a better picture of the progressive development of bone metastasis (Figure 7.17).

Shevrin et al (1988) used prostate cancer cells to induce bone metastases following intravenous injection and occlusion of the inferior vena cava. Pollard and Luckert (1975) and Pollard et al (1988) used rat prostate adenocarcinoma cells in Lobund–Wistar rats to show that these tumors cause a profound local change in bone formation. When this tumor is injected adjacent to a bone surface where the periosteum is often mildly damaged by scratching with a needle tip, the tumor stimulates adjacent new woven bone formation (Figure 7.20).

Specific treatments for metastatic osteolytic bone disease

The best form of treatment for metastatic bone disease is ablative therapy for the tumor. Unfortunately, as already indicated, in the vast majority of patients this is not feasible. Most attention at the present time is being focused on drugs that inhibit osteoclast activity such as the bisphosphonates. Over the last 20 years there have been many studies examining the effects of bisphosphonates in patients with osteolytic bone metastases, and there is accumulating evidence that several bisphosphonates (pamidronate and clodronate have been most extensively studied) are extremely effective at inhibiting skeletal-related events (for example, pathological fractures, need for radiation or surgery for osteolytic bone disease, prevention of spinal cord compression due to vertebral collapse, and prevention of episodes of hypercalcemia). The more recent of these studies have been double-blind, randomized and controlled. Most of them have been performed with pamidronate used intravenously by infusion every month. Pamidronate clearly reduces the number of skeletal-related events and also delays the onset of the first skeletal-related event in breast cancer patients with osteolytic bone metastases (Hortobagyi et al 1996). There are varying reports of the effects of pamidronate on tumor mass in soft tissue or bone. Our findings in the model described above in which MDA-MB-231 cells are inoculated into the left ventricle of nude mice suggest that bisphosphonates not only reduce osteolytic bone lesions, but also markedly reduce tumor burden in bone (Sasaki et al 1995). This is likely due to the decreased production of growth factors in the bone microenvironment by inhibition of bone remodeling. It remains unclear whether this is also associated with effects of bisphosphonates to increase or alter tumor burden in other metastatic sites, although this seems unlikely from recent studies (Yoneda and Michigami, unpublished observations, 1997). Bisphosphonates do not have any direct effect on tumor mass as has been shown in a number of studies (Wingen and Schmahl 1985; Krempien et al 1988). It is hoped that new generation bisphosphonates that are orally active may be useful not only in the treatment of patients with established metastases, but also in the prevention of the development of new metastases. Although information is not currently available in this regard, it seems likely that inhibitors of osteoclastic bone resorption may be even more effective in the prevention of new metastases than in the treatment of established metastases. Theoretically, inhibition of continued resorption would leave the patient with a residual lytic lesion in bone (although occasional patients may show some sclerosis of the healing lesion). On the other hand, in those patients who have malignancies with a predilection for the skeleton, such as breast cancer, preventative treatment with an inhibitor of osteoclastic bone resorption may prevent the initial development of an osteolytic metastasis.

As indicated earlier, attention should not be focused solely on the osteoclasts. Drugs such as laminin antagonists, which prevent binding of tumor cells to basement membranes, inhibitors of proteolytic enzyme disruption of the basement membrane or tumor cell chemotaxis, may also turn out to be useful in the prevention or treatment of established metastases. Laminin antagonists prevent tumor metastasis in an experimental model. Recently, we have used neutralizing antibodies of PTH-rP to prevent progression of osteolytic bone lesions in animal models of human metastatic breast cancer (Guise et al 1996) and also transfected the human tumor cells with inhibitors of the matrix metalloproteinases, namely tissue inhibitor of matrix metalloproteinase-2 (TIMP-2), and shown a decrease in osteolytic bone lesions (Williams et al 1995).

Models such as these may have predictive value prior to the initiation of clinical trials with experimental therapies such as laminin antagonists and inhibitors of proteolytic enzyme digestion.

Osteoblastic metastases

Tumors affect the skeleton not only by causing osteolytic metastases, but also occasionally by causing metastases characterized by the formation of new bone around the tumor cell deposits (Figures 7.18 and 7.19). This occurs without prior

Figure 7.18

Characteristic X-ray of a patient with an osteoblastic metastasis, showing vertebral body sclerosis.

Figure 7.19

Osteoblastic metastases in a vertebral body caused by solid tumor deposits in the marrow cavity tumor deposits.

osteoclastic resorption, and the newly formed bone is laid down directly on trabecular bone surfaces without a preceding resorptive episode (Charhon et al 1983). Prostate cancer is the commonest tumor that causes this response. Essentially, all patients with prostate cancer will develop osteoblastic bone metastases if they live long enough (Galasko 1986a,b; Mundy 1993).

The mechanisms responsible for the osteoblastic metastasis are unknown, but are attracting great interest. From the histomorphometric studies of Charhon et al (1983), osteoblastic metastases are likely due to soluble factors produced by the metastasizing cancer cells and which stimulate bone formation. Many investigators have attempted to identify factors produced by prostate cancer cells that have proliferative effects on cells with the osteoblast phenotype in vitro. Jacobs and Lawson (1980) found that extracts of a well differentiated prostatic carcinoma stimulated [^{3}H]thymidine incorporation into fibroblasts. Similar effects were seen with extracts of benign prostatic hyperplasia. Preliminary characterization of this activity showed it to have an apparent molecular weight of greater than 67 kilodaltons. In retrospect, this activity may have represented a combination of growth factors now known to be produced by prostate cancer cells, and may not have had any relationship to bone growth stimulatory effects.

Others, including Simpson et al (1985) and Koutsilieris et al (1987), have described osteoblast stimulating activity produced by prostatic cancer tissue. Simpson et al (1985) took extracts from the human prostate cancer cell line PC3, injected total RNA into Xenopus oocytes and then examined the conditioned media for bone stimulatory activity. These extracts stimulated both mitogenesis and alkaline phosphatase activity in osteosarcoma cells with the osteoblast phenotype. Koutsilieris et al (1987) took extracts of prostate cancer tissue as well as extracts of normal prostatic tissue and also found growth proliferative activity for bone cells.

As noted above, most studies to date that have attempted to identify bone growth regulatory factors produced by prostate cancer cells have utilized well established human prostate cancer cell lines. However, these have not turned out to be satisfactory models. These human cancer cells when inoculated into nude mice cause bone resorption rather than bone formation. This occurs whether the cells are implanted in the peritoneum, intramuscularly, subcutaneously or adjacent to the calvarium. The reasons these cells do not produce osteoblastic lesions in vivo are not clear. However, human prostate carcinoma cells are notoriously difficult to grow in vitro, and the established cell lines that are available have changed some of their characteristics while in culture. For example, PC3 is no longer a hormone-responsive tumor. A better model may be the PA-III model of rat prostate adenocarcinoma. Pollard developed a strain of rats, Lobund–Wistar, which give a high frequency (10%) of spontaneous prostate adenocarcinoma (Pollard and Luckert 1975; Pollard et al 1988). Several cell lines have been derived from these tumors, and one of these, PA-III, has been studied extensively and stimulates new bone formation in Lobund–Wistar rats (Pollard et al 1988). We confirmed that when PA-III cells were injected in nude mice near a bone site associated with local damage to the periosteum, the prostate tumors induced a strong local osteoblastic response with extensive new woven bone (Figure 7.20). This increase in bone formation could not be accounted for by previous bone resorption, and as such, resembles the osteoblastic response to prostate cancer in humans. We have found these PA-III tumor cells to express a variety of BMPs, and that transfection of the tumor cells with antisense constructs of the BMP-3 gene reduces their capacity to stimulate an osteoblastic response in vivo (Harris et al 1992).

Figure 7.20

The Pollard model of rat prostate adenocarcinoma (PA-III) causing increased bone formation. The tumor has been inoculated into nude mice adjacent to the scapula. New woven bone is seen radiating out from the scapula. The tumor has been in situ for approximately 3 weeks.

A number of other models of prostate cancer have been utilized. The Mat Ly/Lu variant of the rat Dunning prostate cancer causes bone metastases in vivo, which are more pronounced when the cells overexpress rat urokinase-type plasminogen activator (uPA) (Achbarou et al 1994). Recently, Gingrich et al (1996) have used transgenic mice in which the transgene is a regulatory element to the rat probasin gene linked to SV40 T antigen and showed the spontaneous development of bone metastases. This TRAMP (transgenic adenocarcinoma mouse prostate) model is currently being evaluated for the insights it may provide into osteoblastic metastasis. It was first described by Greenberg et al (1995).

A number of factors have been suggested as potential mediators of osteoblastic metastasis associated with prostate cancer:

- *Transforming growth factor β2.* TGFβ2 is abundant in PC3 human prostatic cancer cells, and was purified from the human prostate cancer cell line PC3 (Marquardt et al 1987). TGFβ2 stimulates proliferation of osteoblasts in vitro, as well as bone formation in vivo.
- *Fibroblast growth factor.* Prostatic cancer cells express large amounts of both acidic and basic fibroblast growth factors (FGFs) (Matuo et al 1987; Mansson et al 1989) and these are potential mediators of osteoblast proliferation in patients with this disease (Canalis et al 1987, 1988). Both acidic and basic FGFs (also called FGF-1 and -2) cause profound stimulation of bone formation in vivo (Mayahara et al 1993; Dunstan et al 1995). Izbicka et al (1996) have shown that a human tumor cell line causes bone formation in vivo and produces a mitogenic factor for osteoblastic cells, which was identified as an extended form of FGF-2.
- *Plasminogen activator sequence.* There have been several reports of purification of mitogenic activity for rat calvarial osteoblastic cells present in the conditioned media of the human prostatic cancer cell line PC3 (Rabbani et al 1990a,b). The first 10 amino acids were sequenced and shown to be identical to the serine protease urokinase (uPA). Overexpression of uPA in rat prostate cancer cells leads to bone metastases in vivo (Achbarou et al 1994). An amino terminal fragment of uPA that contains EGF-like repeats has been shown to have mitogenic activity for osteoblasts (Rabbani et al 1992). The carboxy-terminal proteolytic domain may be responsible for tumor invasiveness or growth factor activation. The expression of proteases in the microenvironment of growth factors such as TGFβ may be very important for their activator in bone (Dallas et al 1994, 1995). Plasmin-sensitive cleavage sites are present in the latent TGFβ binding protein that masks TGFβ activity.
- *Bone morphogenetic proteins.* We have found that both normal and neoplastic prostate tissue express a variety of BMPs. We have examined human and rat neoplastin prostate tissue, and found evidence of BMP-2, 3, 4, and 6 mRNA (Harris et al 1994). In one of these tumors, the bone formation response seems to depend on the amount of BMP-3 expressed (see below).
- *PTH-rP.* Cultured prostatic cancer cells frequently express PTH-rP, which in appropriate doses has an anabolic effect on bone (Stewart 1996). It is possible that this tumor peptide may be related to the anabolic effect of prostate cancers (L McCauley, personal communication, 1996). There is no direct data as yet to support this notion.
- *Prostate specific antigen (PSA).* This serine protease that is expressed by prostate cancer cells can cleave PTH-rP at the amino-terminus

(Cramer et al 1996) and could also potentially activate other growth factors produced by prostate carcinomas. PSA is a serine protease produced in excessive amounts by prostate carcinoma cells, and is used as a marker of tumor burden. Whether it has harmful effects is unknown, but one possibility is that its enzymatic action could be responsible for activating anabolic agents such as IGF-I and TGFβ, by cleaving them from their binding proteins, or by cleaving PTH-rP to an anabolic fragment. It has been shown to cleave PTH-rP (Cramer et al 1996).

- *Endothelin-1*. Endothelin-1 has recently been implicated as an osteoblast stimulant in metastatic prostate cancer (Nelson et al 1995). It is a powerful mitogenic factor for osteoblasts (Takuwa et al 1989, 1990) and is produced in large amounts by the prostatic epithelium (Langenstroer et al 1993). Circulating concentrations are increased in patients with metastatic prostate cancer (Nelson et al 1995). However, whether it has more pathophysiologic significance than the numerous other growth regulatory factors for bone cells produced by prostate carcinomas remains unknown.

References

Achbarou A, Kaiser S, Tremblay G et al (1994) Urokinase overproduction results in increased skeletal metastasis by prostate cancer cells in vivo, *Cancer Res* **54**: 2372–7.

Albelda SM, Buck CA (1990) Integrins and other cell adhesion molecules, *FASEB J* **4**: 2868–80.

Ali IU, Lidereau R, Theillet C et al (1987) Reduction to homozygosity of genes on chromosome 11 in human breast neoplasia, *Science* **238**: 185–8.

Arguello F, Baggs RB, Frantz CN (1988) A murine model of experimental metastasis to bone and bone marrow, *Cancer Res* **48**: 6876–81.

Auerbach R, Lu WC, Pardon E et al (1987) Specificity of adhesion between murine tumor cells and capillary endothelium: an in vitro correlate of preferential metastasis in vivo, *Cancer Res* **47**: 1492–6.

Baker SJ, Fearon ER, Nigro JM et al (1989) Chromosome 17 deletions and p53 gene mutations in colorectal carcinomas, *Science* **244**: 217–21.

Basset P, Bellocq JP, Wolf C et al (1990) A novel metalloproteinase gene specifically expressed in stromal cells of breast carcinomas, *Nature* **348**: 699–704.

Batson OV (1940) The function of the vertebral veins and their role in the spread of metastases, *Ann Surg* **112**: 138–49.

Behrens J, Mareel MM, Van Roy FM et al (1989) Dissecting tumor cell invasion: epithelial cells acquire invasive properties after the loss of uvomorulin-mediated cell–cell adhesion, *J Cell Biol* **108**: 2435–47.

Boyde A, Maconnachie E, Reid SA et al (1986) Scanning electron microscopy in bone pathology: review of methods. Potential and applications, *Scanning Electron Microsc* **4**: 1537–54.

Canalis E, Centrella M, McCarthy T (1988) Effects of basic fibroblast growth factor on bone formation in vitro, *J Clin Invest* **81**: 1572–7.

Canalis E, Lorenzo J, Burgess WH et al (1987) Effects of endothelial cell growth factor on bone remodeling in vitro, *J Clin Invest* **79**: 52–8.

Carr I, Orr FW (1983) Current reviews: invasion and metastasis, *Can Med Assoc J* **128**: 1164–7.

Charhon SA, Chapuy MC, Delving EE et al (1983) Histomorphometric analysis of sclerotic bone metastases from prostatic carcinoma with special reference to osteomalacia, *Cancer* **51**: 918–24.

Coman DR, De Long RP (1951) The role of the vertebral venous system in the metastasis of cancer to the spinal column; experiments with tumour cell suspension in rats and rabbits, *Cancer* **4**: 610–18.

Cramer SD, Chen Z, Peehl DM (1996) Prostate specific antigen cleaves parathyroid hormone-related protein in the PTH-like domain: inactivation of PTH-rP stimulated cAMP accumulation in mouse osteoblasts, *J Urology* **156**: 526–31.

Dallas SL, Park-Snyder S, Miyazono K et al (1994) Characterization and autoregulation of latent TGFβ complexes in osteoblast-like cell lines: production of a latent complex lacking the latent TGFβ-binding protein (LTBP), *J Biol Chem* **269**: 6815–22.

Dallas SL, Miyazono K, Skerry TM et al (1995) Dual role for the latent transforming growth factor-beta binding protein in storage of latent TGF-beta in the extracellular matrix and as a structural matrix protein, *J Cell Biol* **131**: 539–49.

De La Mata J, Uy HL, Guise TA et al (1995) Interleukin-6 enhances hypercalcemia and bone resorption mediated by parathyroid hormone-related protein in vivo, *J Clin Invest* **95**: 2846–52.

Dodds PR, Caride VJ, Lytton B (1981) The role of vertebral veins in the dissemination of prostatic carcinoma, *J Urol* **126**: 753–5.

Dunstan CR, Garrett IR, Adams R et al (1995) Systemic fibroblast growth factor (FGF-1) prevents bone loss, increases new bone formation, and restores trabecular microarchitecture in ovariectomized rats, *J Bone Miner Res* **10** (Suppl 1): P279.

Eilon G, Mundy GR (1978) Direct resorption of bone by human breast cancer cells in vitro, *Nature* **276**: 726–8.

Fidler IJ (1978) Tumor heterogeneity and the biology of cancer invasion and metastasis, *Cancer Res* **38**: 2651–60.

Fidler IJ, Poste G (1985) The cellular heterogeneity of malignant neoplasms: implications for adjuvant chemotherapy, *Semin Oncol* **12**: 207–21.

Galasko CSB (1986a) Skeletal metastases, *Clin Orthop* (September): 18–30.

Galasko CSB (1986b) *Skeletal metastases* (Butterworth: London).

Galasko CSB, Burn JI (1971) Hypercalcemia in patients with advanced mammary cancer, *Br Med J* **3**: 573–7.

Gallacher SJ, Fraser WD, Patel U et al (1990) Breast cancer-associated hypercalcaemia: a reassessment of renal calcium and phosphate handling, *Ann Clin Biochem* **27**: 551–6.

Garbisa S, Pozzatti R, Muschel RJ et al (1987) Secretion of type IV collagenolytic protease and metastatic phenotype: induction by transfection with c-Ha-ras but not c-Ha-ras plus AD2-Ela, *Cancer Res* **47**: 1523–8.

Gingrich JR, Barrios RJ, Morton RA et al (1996) Metastatic prostate cancer in a transgenic mouse, *Cancer Res* **56**: 4096–102.

Greenberg NM, DeMayo F, Finegold MJ et al (1995) Prostate cancer in a transgenic mouse, *Proc Natl Acad Sci USA* **92**: 3439–43.

Guise TA, Mundy GR (1996) Physiological and pathological roles of parathyroid hormone-related protein, *Curr Opin Nephrol* **5**: 307–15.

Guise TA, Yin JJ, Taylor SD et al (1996) Evidence for a casual role of parathyroid hormone-related protein in the pathogenesis of human breast cancer-mediated osteolysis, *J Clin Invest* **98**: 1544–9.

Harinck HI, Bijvoet OL, Plantingh AS et al (1987) Role of bone and kidney in tumor-induced hypercalcemia and its treatment with bisphosphonate and sodium chloride, *Am J Med* **82**: 1133–42.

Harris SE, Boyce B, Feng JQ et al (1992) Antisense bone morphogenetic protein 3 (BMP 3) constructions decrease new bone formation in a prostate cancer model, *J Bone Miner Res* **7** (suppl 1): no. 92.

Harris SE, Bonewald LF, Harris MA et al (1994) Effects of transforming growth factor beta on bone nodule formation and expression of bone morphogenic protein 2, osteocalcin, osteopontin, alkaline phosphatase, and type 1 collagen mRNA in long-term cultures of fetal rat calvarial osteoblasts, *J Bone Miner Res* **9**: 855–63.

Hashimoto M, Niwa O, Nitta Y (1989) Unstable expression of E-cadherin adhesion molecules in metastatic ovarian tumor cells, *Jpn J Cancer Res* **80**: 459–63.

Hauschka PV, Mavrakos AE, Iafrati MD et al (1986) Growth factors in bone matrix, *J Biol Chem* **261**: 12 665–74.

Haynes RO (1992) Integrins: versatility, modulation, and signaling in cell adhesion, *Cell* **69**: 11–25.

Heppner G (1984) Tumor heterogeneity, *Cancer Res* **214**: 2259–65.

Hilgard P, Gordon-Smith EL (1974) Microangiopathic hemolytic anemia and experimental tumor-cell emboli, *Br J Haematol* **26**: 651–9.

Hortobagyi GN, Theriault RL, Porter L et al (1996) Efficacy of pamidronate in reducing skeletal complications in patients with breast cancer and lytic bone metastases, *N Eng J Med* **335**: 1785–91.

Izbicka E, Dunstan C, Esparza J et al (1996) Human amniotic tumor which induces new bone formation in vivo produces a growth regulatory activity in vitro for osteoblasts identified as an extended form of basic fibroblast growth factor (bFGF), *Cancer Res* **56**: 633–6.

Jacobs SC, Lawson R (1980) Mitogenic factors in human prostate extracts, *Urology* **16**: 488–91.

Koutsilieris M, Rabbani SA, Bennett HP et al (1987) Characteristics of prostate-derived growth factors for cells of the osteoblast phenotype, *J Clin Invest* **80**: 941–6.

Krempien B, Wingen F, Eichmann T et al (1988) Protective effects of a prophylactic treatment with the bisphosphonate 3-amino-1-hydroxypropane-1, 1-bisphosphonic acid on the development of tumor osteopathies in the rat: experimental studies with the Walker carcinosarcoma 256, *Oncology* **45**: 41–6.

Langenstroer P, Tang R, Shapiro E et al (1993) Endothelin-1 in the human prostate: tissue levels, source of production and isometric tension studies, *J Urol* **150**: 495–9.

Liotta LA, Kohn E (1990) Cancer invasion and metastases, *JAMA* **263**: 1123–6.

Liotta LA, Steeg PS (1990) Clues to the function of Nm23 and Awd proteins in development, signal transduction, and tumor metastasis provided by studies of dictyostelium discoideum, *J Natl Cancer Inst* **82**: 1170–2.

Liotta LA, Tryggvason K, Garbisa S et al (1980) Metastatic potential correlates with enzymatic degradation of basement membrane collagen, *Nature* **284**: 67–8.

Liotta LA, Mandler R, Murano G et al (1986) Tumor cell autocrine motility factor, *Proc Natl Acad Sci USA* **83**: 3302–6.

Mansson PE, Adams P, Kan M et al (1989) HBGF1 gene expression in normal rat prostate and two transplantable rat prostate tumors, *Cancer Res* **49**: 2485–94.

Mareel MM, Behrens J, Birchmeier W et al (1991) Down-regulation of E-cadherin expression in Madin–Darby canine kidney (MDCK) cells inside tumors of nude mice, *Int J Cancer* **47**: 922–8.

Marquardt H, Lioubin MN, Ikeda T (1987) Complete amino acid sequence of human transforming growth factor type beta 2, *J Biol Chem* **262**: 12 127–30.

Matuo Y, Nishi N, Matsui S et al (1987) Heparin binding affinity of rat prostate growth factor in normal and cancerous prostate: partial purification and characterization of rat prostate growth factor in the Dunning tumor, *Cancer Res* **47**: 188–92.

Mayahara H, Ito T, Nagai H et al (1993) In vivo stimulation of endosteal bone formation by basic fibroblast growth factor in rats, *Growth Factors* **9**: 73–80.

Mbalaviele G, Dunstan CR, Sasaki A et al (1996) E-cadherin expression in human breast cancer cells suppress the development of osteolytic bone metastases in experimental metastasis model, *Cancer Res* **56**: 4063–70.

McCarthy JB, Skubitz APN, Palm SL et al (1988) Metastasis inhibition of different tumor types by purified laminin fragments and a heparin-binding fragment of fibronectin, *J Natl Cancer Inst* **80**: 108–16.

Miller FR (1983) Tumor subpopulation interactions in metastasis, *Invasion Metastasis* **3**: 234–42.

Mundy GR (1990) *Calcium homeostasis: hypercalcemia and hypocalcemia*, 2nd edn (Martin Dunitz: London).

Mundy GR (1993) Pathophysiology of skeletal complications of cancer. In: Mundy GR, Martin TJ, eds, *Physiology and pharmacology of bone. Handbook of experimental pharmacology* (Springer-Verlag: Berlin) 641–71.

Mundy GR, Poser JW (1983) Chemotactic activity of the gamma-carboxyglutamic acid containing protein in bone, *Calcif Tissue Int* **35**: 164–8.

Mundy GR, Bertolini DR (1986) Bone destruction and hypercalcemia in plasma cell myeloma, *Semin Oncol* **13**: 291–9.

Mundy GR, DeMartino S, Rowe DW (1981) Collagen and collagen-derived fragments are chemotactic for tumor cells, *J Clin Invest* **68**: 1102–5.

Nakai M, Mundy GR, Williams PJ et al (1992) A synthetic antagonist to laminin inhibits the formation of osteolytic metastases by human melanoma cells in nude mice, *Cancer Res* **52**: 5395–9.

Nelson JB, Hedican SP, George DJ et al (1995) Identification of endothelin-1 in the pathophysiology of metastatic adenocarcinoma of the prostate, *Nature Med* **1**: 944.

Nip J, Shibata H, Loskutoff DJ et al (1992) Human melanoma cells derived from lymphatic mestastases use integrins $\alpha_v\beta_3$ to adhere to lymph node vitronectin, *J Clin Invest* **90**: 1406–13.

Nowell PS (1976) The clonal evolution of tumor cell subpopulations, *Science* **194**: 23–38.

Oka H, Shiozaki H, Kobayashi K et al (1993) Expression of E-cadherin cells adhesion molecules in human breast cancer tissues and its relationship to metastasis, *Cancer Res* **53**: 1696–701.

Orr W, Varani J, Gondek MD et al (1979) Chemotactic responses of tumor cells to products of resorbing bone, *Science* **203**: 176–9.

Orr FW, Varani J, Gondek MD et al (1980) Partial characterization of a bone derived chemotactic factor for tumor cells, *Am J Pathol* **99**: 43–52.

Paget S (1889) The distribution of secondary growths in cancer of the breast, *Lancet* **i**: 571–3.

Peacock M, Robertson WG, Nordin BEC (1969) Relation between serum and urine calcium with particular reference to parathyroid activity, *Lancet* **i**: 384–6.

Percival RC, Yates AJP, Gray RES et al (1985) Mechanisms of malignant hypercalcaemia in carcinoma of the breast, *Br Med J* **291**: 776–9.

Pfeilschifter J, Mundy GR (1987) Modulation of transforming growth factor beta activity in bone cultures by osteotropic hormones, *Proc Natl Acad Sci USA* **84**: 2024–8.

Pollard M, Luckert PH (1975) Transplantable metastasizing prostate adenocarcinoma in rats, *J Natl Cancer Inst* **54**: 643–59.

Pollard M, Luckert MS, Scheu J (1988) Effects of diphosphonate and X-rays on bone lesions induced in rats by prostate cancer cells, *Cancer* **61**: 2027–32.

Poste G (1986) Pathogenesis of metastatic disease: implications for current therapy and for the development of new therapeutic strategies, *Cancer Treat Rev* **70**: 183–99.

Powell GJ, Southby J, Danks JA et al (1991) Localization of parathyroid hormone-related protein in breast cancer metastases—increased incidence in bone compared with other sites, *Cancer Res* **51**: 3059–61.

Rabbani SA, Desjardins J, Bell AW et al (1990a) An amino-terminal fragment of urokinase isolated from a prostate cancer cell line (PC-3) is mitogenic for osteoblast-like cells, *Biochem Biophys Res Commun* **173**: 1058–64.

Rabbani SA, Desjardins J, Bell AW et al (1990b) Identification of a new osteoblast mitogen from a human prostate cancer cell line, PC-3, *J Bone Miner Res* **5**: no 549.

Rabbani SA, Mazar AP, Bernier SM et al (1992) Structural requirements for the growth factor activity of the amino-terminal domain of urokinase, *J Biol Chem* **267**: 14 151–6.

Reedy AL, Fialkow PJ (1980) Multicellular origin of fibrosarcomas in mice induced by the chemical carcinogen 3-methylcholanthrene, *J Exp Med* **150**: 878–86.

Rizzoli R, Bonjour JP (1989) High extracellular calcium increases the production of a parathyroid hormone-like activity by cultured Leydig tumor cells associated with humoral hypercalcemia, *J Bone Miner Res* **4**: 839–44.

Sasaki A, Boyce BF, Story B et al (1995) Bisphosphonate risedronate reduces metastatic human breast cancer burden in bone in nude mice, *Cancer Res* **55**: 3551–7.

Seftor REB, Seftor EA, Gehlsen KR et al (1992) Role of the $\alpha_v\beta_3$ integrin in human melanoma cell invasion, *Proc Natl Acad Sci U S A* **89**: 1557–61.

Shevrin D, Kukreja SC, Ghosh L et al (1988) Development of skeletal metastasis by human prostate cancer in athymic nude mice, *Clin Exp Metastasis* **6**: 401–9.

Simpson EL, Harrod J, Eilon G et al (1985) Identification of a mRNA fraction in human prostatic cancer cells coding for a novel osteoblast stimulating factor, *Endocrinology* **117**: 1615–20.

Slamon DJ, Clark GM, Wong SG et al (1987) Human breast cancer: correlation of relapse and survival with amplification of the HER-2/neu oncogene, *Science* **235**: 177–32.

Sommers CL, Thompson EW, Torri JA et al (1991) Cell adhesion molecule uvomorulin expression in human breast cancer cell lines: relationship to morphology and invasive capacities, *Cell Growth Diff* **2**: 365–71.

Steeg PS, Bevilacqua G, Kopper L et al (1988) Evidence for a novel gene associated with low tumor metastatic potential, *J Natl Cancer Instit* **80**: 200–4.

Stewart AF (1996) PTHrP (1–36) as a skeletal anabolic agent for the treatment of osteoporosis, *Bone* **19**: 303–6.

Stewart AF, Horst R, Deftos LJ et al (1980) Biochemical evaluation of patients with cancer-associated hypercalcemia: evidence for humoral and nonhumoral groups, *N Engl J Med* **303**: 1377–83.

Takeichi M (1991) Cadherin cell adhesion receptors as a morphogenetic regulator, *Science* **251**: 1451–4.

Takuwa Y, Masaki T, Yamashita K (1990) The effects of the endothelin family peptides on cultured osteoblastic cells from rat calvariae, *Biochem Biophys Res Commun* **170**: 998–1005.

Takuwa Y, Ohue Y, Takuwa N et al (1989) Endothelin-1 activates phopholipase C and mobilizes Ca^{2+} from extra- and intracellular pools in osteoblastic cells, *Am J Physiol* **257**: E797–803.

Tofe AJ, Francis MD, Harvey WJ (1975) Correlation of neoplasms with incidence and localization of skeletal metastases. An analysis of 1355 diphosphonate bone scans, *J Nucl Med* **16**: 986–9.

Tuttle KR, Kunau RT, Loveridge N et al (1991) Altered renal calcium handling in hypercalcemia of malignancy, *J Am Soc Nephrol* **2**: 191–9.

Van den Brenk HAS, Burch WM, Kelley H et al (1975) Venous diversion trapping and growth of blood-borne cancer cells en route to the lungs, *Br J Cancer* **31**: 46–61.

Vleminckx K, Vakaet L, Mareel M et al (1991) Genetic manipulation of E-cadherin expression by epithelial tumor cells reveals an invasion suppressor role, *Cell* **66**: 107–19.

Vogelstein B, Fearon ER, Hamilton SR et al (1988) Genetic alterations during colorectal tumor development, *N Engl J Med* **319**: 525–32.

Warren BA, Vales O (1972) The adhesion of thromboplastic tumor emboli to vessel walls in vivo, *Br J Exp Pathol* **53**: 301–13.

Weiss L, Orr FW, Honn KV (1989) Interactions between cancer cells and the microvasculature: a rate-regulator for metastasis, *Clin Exp Metastasis* **7**: 127–67.

Wewer UM, Taraboletti G, Sobel ME et al (1987) Laminin receptor: role in tumor cell migration, *Cancer Res* **47**: 5691–8.

Williams P, Mbalaviele G, Sasaki A et al (1995) Multi-step inhibition of breast cancer metastasis to bone, *J Bone Miner Res* **10** (suppl 1): no 121.

Wingen F, Schmahl D (1985) Distribution of 3-amino-1-hydroxypropane-1, 1-diphosphonic acid in rats and effects on rat osteosarcoma, *Drug Res* **35**: 1565–71.

Wingo PA, Tong T, Bolden S (1995) Cancer statistics, *CA Cancer J Clin* **45**: 8–30.

Winterbauer RH, Elfenbein IB, Ball WC (1968) Incidence and clinical significance of tumor embolization to the lungs, *Am J Med* **45**: 271–90.

Yin JJ, Chirgwin JM, Taylor SD et al (1996) Dominant negative blockade of the transforming growth factor β (TGFβ) type II receptor decreases breast cancer-mediated osteolysis, *J Bone Miner Res* **11** (suppl 1): no 180.

Yoneda T, Williams P, Dunstan C et al (1995) Growth of metastatic cancer cells in bone is enhanced by bone derived insulin-like growth factors (IGFs), *J Bone Miner Res* **10** (Suppl 1): P269.

Zakalik D, Diep D, Hooks MA et al (1992) Transforming growth factor beta increases stability of parathyroid hormone related protein messenger RNA, *J Bone Miner Res* **7** (Suppl 1): no 104.

Zetter BR (1990) The cellular basis of site-specific tumor metastasis, *N Engl J Med* **322**: 605–12.

CHAPTER 8

Myeloma bone disease

Introduction

Bone remodeling is profoundly disturbed in almost all patients with myeloma. Although patients with other malignancies may have skeletal manifestations, they are rarely as severe and certainly not as common as in myeloma. Understanding the mechanisms responsible in myeloma may not only lead to better treatments for this disease, but also should improve our understanding of normal mechanisms for bone remodeling.

Bone destruction in myeloma is responsible for the most prominent and distressing clinical features of this disease, namely intractable bone pain, fractures occurring either spontaneously or following trivial injury, and hypercalcemia with its attendant symptoms and signs. Although myeloma is not a common malignancy, there are probably about 30 000 patients in the United States with this condition at any one point in time, and essentially all of them have the bone disease. The annual incidence rate is 5–10 new cases per 100 000 population per year, and the median survival is about 3 years. Occasional patients live for 15 years. The extent of the bone lesions is an important factor in the prognosis. Eighty percent of patients present with bone pain as a predominant symptom (Snapper and Kahn 1971). The bone lesions occur in several patterns (Figure 8.1). Occasionally, patients develop single osteolytic lesions that are associated with solitary

Figure 8.1

Clinical picture of clinical manifestations of myeloma, showing destructive lesion in the skeleton, accumulation of myeloma cells in the marrow cavity, monoclonal protein production in the serum and/or urine, and characteristic vertebral collapse in osteopenia.

Osteolytic (5T2)   Osteosclerotic (5T14)

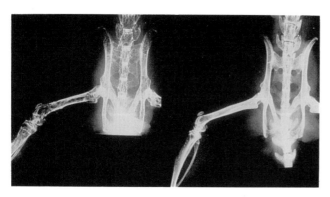

Figure 8.2
5T murine model of myeloma studied by Dr Jiri Radl and colleagues (Radl et al 1988). The bone disease in this model is very similar to the bone disease seen in patients with myeloma. Note the characteristic lytic lesions found in the mice with the osteolytic variant, and sclerosis found in the mice with the osteosclerotic variant.

plasmacytomas. Some patients have diffuse osteopenia, which mimics the appearance of osteoporosis, and is due to the myeloma cells being spread diffusely throughout the axial skeleton. In most patients there are multiple discrete lytic lesions occurring at the site of deposits or nests of myeloma cells. Hypercalcemia occurs as a consequence of bone destruction in about one-third of patients with advanced disease. Rarely, patients with myeloma do not have lytic lesions or bone loss, but rather have an increase in the formation of new bone around myeloma cells. This rare situation is known as osteosclerotic myeloma.

A number of rodent models of myeloma have been described, although the only one that mimics the bone lesions of human myeloma is the 5T murine model described by Radl (Radl et al 1988) (Figure 8.2). Recently, a model of human myeloma bone disease has been described in which human myeloma cells are inoculated into SCID mice (Alsina et al 1996).

Pathophysiology of the bone lesions

Osteolytic bone lesions are by far the most common bone lesions in patients with myeloma. Although the precise molecular mechanisms remain unclear, observations over 25 years have shown a number of facts:

- The mechanism by which bone is destroyed in myeloma is via the osteoclast, the normal bone resorbing cell.

- Osteoclasts accumulate on bone resorbing surfaces in myeloma adjacent to collections of myeloma cells. Thus, it appears that the mechanism by which osteoclasts are stimulated in myeloma is a local one.

- It has been known now for many years that cultures of human myeloma cells in vitro produce several osteoclast activating factors.

- Various mediators have been implicated in the stimulation of osteoclast activity including lymphotoxin (tumor necrosis factor β), interleukin-1β and interleukin-6.

- Hypercalcemia occurs in approximately one-third of patients with myeloma sometime during the course of the disease. Hypercalcemia is always associated with markedly increased bone resorption and frequently with impairment in glomerular filtration.

- The increase in osteoclastic bone resorption in myeloma is usually associated with a marked impairment in osteoblast function. Alkaline phosphatase activity in the serum is decreased or in the normal range, unlike patients with other types of osteolytic bone disease, and radionuclide scans do not show evidence of increased uptake, indicating an impaired osteoblast response to the increase in bone resorption.

- Occasional patients with myeloma show predominantly an increase in new bone formation with subsequent osteosclerosis. This is often associated with the POEMS syndrome (see below).

Most available evidence suggests that the cellular mechanism of bone destruction in myeloma is due to an increase in osteoclast activity (Figure 8.3). This was first studied systematically on autopsy and biopsy samples of bone from a series of 37 patients with myeloma (Mundy et al 1974a,b). Active osteoclastic bone resorption was correlated with the presence of infiltrations of more than 20% myeloma cells in the adjacent marrow cell population. In biopsy specimens of bone from myeloma patients that contained few or no myeloma cells, little osteoclast activity or evidence of active bone resorption was observed. This suggested that the myeloma cells caused an increase in local osteoclast activity that led to increased bone resorption. There have been some recent suggestions that osteoclasts in patients with myeloma may not be as large as the osteoclasts in patients with primary hyperparathyroidism or even solid tumors associated with bone destruction. The association between increased osteoclasts on bone resorbing surfaces and areas of heavy myeloma cell infiltration was confirmed in a later study using quantitative bone histomorphometry on transiliac bone biopsies from 118 patients (Valentin-Opran et al 1982). Abnormalities in bone formation were also confirmed. Bone forming surfaces were increased away from the areas of heavy myeloma cell infiltration, but the osteoid seams were reduced in thickness and had a lowered calcification rate. The authors concluded that the activity of individual osteoblasts was reduced in many patients with myeloma. More detailed studies on bone formation rates in early and overt myeloma were reported by Bataille et al (1991). These workers suggested that bone formation rates were markedly suppressed in patients with advanced disease, but surprisingly were increased earlier in the disease course.

Further evidence that the mechanism of bone resorption in myeloma is primarily osteoclastic is provided by data showing drugs that are relatively specific inhibitors of osteoclast activity, for example, the bisphosphonates, plicamycin, and calcitonin are usually very effective in lowering the serum calcium in patients with myeloma (Binstock and Mundy 1980; Mundy and Martin 1982; Mundy et al 1983).

Bone scans in myeloma often show no abnormality. Isotopic bone scans are performed with labeled bisphosphonates that are taken up at sites of mineral deposition and reflect increased activity of bone forming cells. Myeloma is characterized by discrete lytic lesions with little increase in formation and this is probably the explanation for the difference in appearance between the bone scans in myeloma and the bone scans in breast cancer, where osteoblast activity is frequently increased. Similarly, serum alkaline phosphatase, which also reflects osteoblast activity, is usually not increased in patients with myeloma, unless they have coexistent pathological fractures.

In occasional patients with myeloma (probably less than 1% in the experience of most clinicians), osteosclerosis, rather than osteolytic bone destruction, is the major radiologic finding (Bardwick et al 1980). Valentin-Opran et al (1982) reported morphologic bone biopsy data from 118 patients, three of whom had increased trabecular bone volume, suggesting that these biopsies represented the osteosclerotic variant. The molecular mechanism responsible for the increase in osteoblast activity is unknown. These patients frequently have peripheral neuropathy and they may or may not have other multisystem features that

Figure 8.3

The cellular mechanism of bone resorption in myeloma. In this histologic section of bone from a patient with myeloma, myeloma cells can be seen in the marrow cavity adjacent to active bone-resorbing osteoclasts. (Reproduced from Mundy et al (1974b).)

have been referred to as the polyneuropathy, organomegaly, endocrinopathy, M protein, and skin changes (with the acronym, POEMS) syndrome (Farhangi and Merlini 1986). Hypercalcemia has not been described in this condition.

Pathogenetic factors

The increase in osteoclast activity in myeloma is likely to be due to production of local factors or cytokines by the myeloma cells (or host cells) that increases osteoclast activity. The supporting evidence for factors produced by myeloma cells comes from in vitro studies in which it has been shown that lymphoid cell lines derived from patients with myeloma (Mundy et al 1974a,b), marrow myeloma cells (Mundy et al 1974a,b; Josse et al 1981), and explants of bone containing myeloma cells (Gailani et al 1976), produce a factor or factors that stimulate osteoclast activity in organ cultures of fetal rat bones. This bone resorbing activity had similar chemical and biological characteristics to the bone resorbing activity present in phytohemagglutinin-stimulated peripheral blood leukocyte cultures, which was then known as osteoclast activating factor or OAF (Horton et al 1972). One of these lymphoid cell lines, 8226, produced gamma light chains with the same antigenic determinants as the Bence Jones protein in the urine of the patient from whom this cell line was derived, suggesting that this lymphoid cell line was in fact derived from the myeloma cells. Short-term cultures of marrow cells aspirated from patients with myeloma contained similar activity (Mundy et al 1974a,b). Similar bone resorbing activity was not present in cells taken from a series of patients with other types of hematologic disorders not usually associated with bone lesions or hypercalcemia. These findings were confirmed by Josse et al (1981) who also showed that the bone resorbing factor produced by marrow myeloma cell cultures had no effect on cyclic AMP accumulation in bone, and the production of the factor was inhibited by indomethacin, suggesting that it was dependent on prostaglandin synthesis. These workers showed that the effects of the factor on bone were independent of inhibition of prostaglandin synthesis. Similar results had been shown previously for the OAF produced by activated peripheral blood leukocytes (Raisz et al 1975; Yoneda and Mundy 1979a,b).

Similar bone resorbing activity has been found in other hematologic neoplasms. In patients with various forms of lymphomas, macromolecular bone resorbing activity similar to that present in lymphoid cell lines derived from patients with lymphoma, normal activated peripheral blood leukocytes, and myeloma cell cultures has been identified. In one patient with lymphosarcoma cell leukemia, the bone resorbing activity was characterized in some detail (Mundy et al 1978). In this patient, the cultured tumor cells produced a bone resorbing factor that was chromatographically and pharmacologically similar to the osteoclast activating factor produced by normal peripheral blood leukocytes. Many of these patients have a T-cell lymphoma that is associated with the HTLV type I virus (Bunn et al 1983). HTLV type I infected cells produce PTH-rP and a range of lymphokines including macromolecular bone resorbing activity (Bertolini et al 1984; Motokura et al 1989). Some of these patients have increased circulating concentrations of 1,25-dihydroxyvitamin D_3 (Breslau et al 1984; Davies et al 1985; Rosenthal et al 1985; Zaloga et al 1985), and these tumor cells also have the capacity to metabolize 25-hydroxyvitamin D_3 to its most biologically active metabolite, 1,25-dihydroxyvitamin D_3, which may play a part in the pathogenesis of hypercalcemia by increasing calcium absorption from the gut as well as increasing bone resorption (Fetchick et al 1986). The circulating concentrations of 1,25-dihydroxyvitamin D_3 are usually low or low–normal in patients with myeloma.

Potential factors involved in the bone destruction in myeloma

The pathogenesis of the bone lesions is related to increased production of a local bone resorbing factor in the bone marrow of patients with myeloma. This bone resorbing factor has similar characteristics to the bone resorbing activity produced by activated peripheral blood leukocytes that was formerly called osteoclast activating factor or OAF. OAF represents a family of bone resorbing factors that are produced by lymphocytes and monocytes following exposure to an antigen to which they have previously been exposed or a nonspecific mitogen such as phytohemagglutinin (Horton et al 1972). The OAFs that have been implicated in myeloma are lymphotoxin, interleukin-1β and interleukin-6.

Lymphotoxin

Lymphotoxin is a normal activated lymphocyte product, which is also produced by lymphoid cell lines in culture. In particular, B-lymphoblastoid cell lines express and secrete lymphotoxin. It has now been shown that in a number of cell culture lines isolated from patients with myeloma, the tumor cells express lymphotoxin messenger RNA and contain cytotoxic activity in the conditioned media (Garrett et al 1987) (Figure 8.4). This cytotoxic activity can be ascribed to lymphotoxin. The conditioned media also contains bone resorbing activity that can be partially neutralized by lymphotoxin neutralizing antibodies.

Lymphotoxin increases bone resorption (Bertolini et al 1986), and stimulates the formation of osteoclasts from precursors in marrow cell cultures (Pfeilschifter et al 1989). In addition, lymphotoxin can activate mature osteoclasts to form resorption pits (Thomson et al 1987). Lymphotoxin has identical effects to those of tumor necrosis factor on bone resorption, and overlapping effects with those of interleukin-1α and β. Repeated injections of recombinant human lymphotoxin cause hypercalcemia in normal mice (Garrett et al 1987).

Interleukin-1β (IL-1β)

Interleukin-1α and β are powerful stimulators of osteoclastic bone resorption (Gowen et al 1983a,b, 1986). In addition, IL-1 can cause hypercalcemia (Sabatini et al 1988) and markedly increased osteoclastic bone resorption in vivo (Sabatini et al 1988; Boyce et al 1989). Freshly isolated marrow cells from patients with myeloma, which contain myeloma cells plus stromal cells, have been shown to produce IL-1β in the conditioned media (Cozzolino et al 1989; Kawano et al 1989). Bone resorbing activity produced by these cultures can be neutralized by antibodies to IL-1β. In contrast, established cell lines from patients with myeloma do not express IL-1β (Garrett et al 1987). The reason for these discrepancies probably relates to the nature of the cells that are studied. Artifacts could occur in both models. Established cell lines could have changed in culture to produce factors that the parent cells in situ did not. Alternatively, the freshly isolated cells (which contain dead and dying elements) are

Figure 8.4

Expression of lymphotoxin mRNA in human myeloma cells (lanes a,b,c) shown by Northern blot analysis (left). These tumors also express tumor necrosis factor mRNA (right), but tumor necrosis factor does not appear to be secreted into the cell culture media. Lanes d and e represent rat myelomas. (Reproduced from Garrett et al (1987).)

likely to release factors that they did not release in situ (as has been shown previously for prostaglandins).

IL-1 stimulates the formation of osteoclasts from progenitor cells (Pfeilschifter et al 1989). IL-1 also activates mature osteoclasts to resorb bone (McSheehy and Chambers 1986). This is possibly the most powerful peptide bone resorbing factor known.

Interleukin-6 (IL-6)

Interleukin-6 is a recently described multifunctional cytokine, which may play an important role in the pathophysiology of myeloma. There is considerable evidence to suggest it may be an important growth factor in myeloma, and recently it has been suggested that neutralizing antibodies to IL-6 may have important effects on the course of the disease (Bataille et al 1989). We have tested IL-6 for its effects on bone resorption and calcium homeostasis in vitro and in vivo (Black et al 1991). IL-6 has effects that are different from those of IL-1 and tumor necrosis factor. IL-6 does not stimulate osteoclastic bone resorption in organ cultures of fetal rat long bones. Its effects in neonatal mouse calvariae are also minor or possibly nonexistent. However, in other types of organ culture it has been shown to stimulate osteoclastic bone resorption (Lowik et al 1989; Ishimi et al 1990). IL-6 causes hypercalcemia in vivo. When IL-6 is stably transfected into Chinese hamster ovarian (CHO) cells, these cells from tumors in nude mice express IL-6. Mice carrying tumors with CHO cells expressing IL-6 develop increasing levels of IL-6 in the serum as the tumor grows. These mice become progressively hypercalcemic, and in addition develop leukocytosis, thrombocytosis and cachexia (Black et al 1991). This increase in serum calcium is due to an increase in osteoclastic bone resorption in vivo.

IL-6 may also have effects in the bone microenvironment that are different from those of the other cytokines. Although bone cells isolated from trabecular bone surfaces (bone lining cells) express cytokines such as IL-1, tumor necrosis factor, colony-stimulating factors and IL-6, it is only in the case of IL-6 that these bone cells produce more of a cytokine when exposed to osteotropic factors such as parathyroid hormone, IL-1 and tumor necrosis factor (Feyen et al 1989). In the case of the other cytokines, production by bone cells may be enhanced by nonphysiologic stimuli such as lipopolysaccharide. In addition, it has been shown recently that bone cell expression of IL-6 can be decreased by exposure of the bone cells to estrogen (Girasole et al 1992; Jilka et al 1992).

Which of these cytokines is the most important in bone lesions associated with myeloma is at present unknown. It is possible in myeloma that a combination of these cytokines works in concert to enhance bone resorption. It is also possible that other factors may be involved. For example, in some patients, PTH-rP has been implicated (Budayr et al 1989; Suzuki et al 1994; Firkin et al 1996).

Models of myeloma bone disease

One of the difficulties in studying the mechanisms involved in myeloma bone disease has been the lack of suitable animal models for this aspect of the disease. This has been unlike the situation in hypercalcemia of malignancy due to solid tumors, where solid human tumors readily grow in nude mice and findings that are made in vitro can readily be confirmed in vivo. However, there have been until recently no suitable animal models of myeloma bone disease, and it has not been possible to grow human myeloma cells in nude mice. Two recent animal models have been described that may overcome these problems. In the murine model of myeloma described by Radl et al (1988), typical lesions of myeloma bone disease occur in tumor-bearing mice. This form of myeloma occurs spontaneously in aging C57BL/KaLwRij mice at the rate of about one in every 200 mice. Osteolytic lesions are typical of myeloma bone disease that occurs in humans. Some of these tumors have now been established in permanent cell culture (Manning et al 1992). A second animal model is that described recently by Alsina et al (1996). In this model, human myeloma cells grow in irradiated mice with severe combined immunodeficiency (SCID) and also cause typical myeloma bone lesions and hypercalcemia. Either or both of these models may provide the background for more detailed study of molecular mechanisms responsible for human myeloma bone disease.

Effects of bone and bone cell products on myeloma cells

Since the observation that myeloma cells cause bone destruction by producing factors that stimulate osteoclasts to resorb bone, the attention of the field has been focused on the identification of the responsible mediators. However, the interactions between myeloma cells and bone cells may be much more complicated than simple excess production of a factor by myeloma cells that stimulates osteoclasts. Recent data have suggested the hypothesis that the avidity with which myeloma cells grow in bone compared with other hematologic malignancies is likely to be influenced by products produced as a consequence of osteoclastic bone resorption, and in particular the cytokine IL-6, which is a major growth regulatory factor for myeloma cells. Thus, bone may not be simply a passive bystander in this disease, but rather act to amplify the growth of myeloma cells in bone. If this concept is correct, then a vicious cycle may exist between myeloma cells and osteoclastic bone resorption, whereby myeloma cells stimulate osteoclasts to resorb bone by the production of osteotropic cytokines such as TNFβ, IL-1β and IL-6, but that during the process of osteoclastic bone resorption the cytokine IL-6 is generated in prodigious amounts by cells

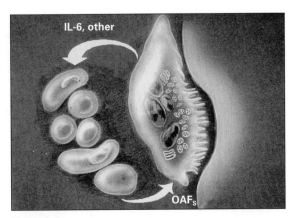

Figure 8.5

Potential interactions between interleukin-6 and myeloma cells in patients with myeloma bone disease. Note that interleukin-6 is produced in large amounts by osteoclasts, and that myeloma cells enhance the capacity of osteoclasts to produce more interleukin-6.

involved in the resorption process, and this enhances the growth of myeloma cells in bone (Figure 8.5). This vicious cycle could mean that the greater the bone destruction, the more aggressive the behavior of myeloma cells, which then may cause even greater bone destruction.

This concept is based on the recent information that osteoclasts produce considerably more IL-6 than any other cell, and certainly more than other types of bone cells (Table 8.1). The only cells that produce comparable amounts of IL-6 are endometrial cells. However, it should be recognized that these data do not indicate which cell in bone is the most abundant source, since osteo-

Table 8.1 Amounts of interleukin-6 (IL-6) produced by various cells during 24–48 hours of culture.

Cell source	Production of IL-6	Reference
Osteoclasts from human giant cell tumor	55 pg/cell/h	Gilles et al (1993)
Osteoclasts from human giant cell tumor	38 pg/cell/h	Ohsaki et al (1992)
Osteoclast-like cells in human marrow cultures from Paget's and normal	2–20 fg/cell/h	Roodman et al (1992)
SaOS ± PTH	2.5–25 fg/cell/h	Feyen et al (1989)
Human osteoblastic cells ±PTH	6–60 fg/cell/h	Linkhart et al (1991)
Peripheral blood mononuclear cells	2–20 fg/cell/h	Schindler et al (1990)
Endometrial cells	1–10 pg/cell/h	Tabibzadeh et al (1989)

Figure 8.6

Interleukin-6 (IL-6) has a complicated role in myeloma, and possibly in myeloma bone disease. It is produced in large amounts by osteoclasts and by stromal cells in the bone marrow microenvironment. In both these types of cells, its production is likely to be regulated by osteoclast activating factors (OAFs) secreted by myeloma cells. Since IL-6 is (1) the most important growth regulatory factor for myeloma cells; and (2) an important subsidiary factor in osteoclast formation, it very likely plays an important role in myeloma bone disease. We know that its production by myeloma cells may require direct cell–cell contact between myeloma cells and stromal cells.

clasts are much fewer in number than are other cells. Nevertheless, IL-6 production by bone organ cultures and by osteoclasts is reduced by treatment with calcitonin, suggesting that osteoclast production of IL-6 is clearly regulated by factors that control osteoclast function.

It is certainly possible that production of IL-6 in the bone microenvironment could result from direct cellular interactions between myeloma cells and other cells such as stromal cells, osteoblasts or even osteoclasts (Figure 8.6) (Lokhorst et al 1994).

Recent studies have shown that cell-cell attachment molecules may be important in the production of bone resorbing activity in the bone microenvironment. Michigami et al (1997) found that myeloma cells attach to stromal cells in the marrow microenvironment by mechanisms which involve the integrin $\alpha_4\beta_1$ expressed on myeloma cells and VCAM-1 bone marrow stromal cells.

Pathogenesis of the hypercalcemia

Hypercalcemia in myeloma is due primarily to increased bone resorption. However, the pathogenesis is more complex than just a simple increase in bone resorption. First, only about 20–40% of patients with myeloma develop hypercalcemia (Snapper and Kahn 1971). Moreover, although hypercalcemia occurs in those patients who have the largest tumor volume, not all patients with the largest tumor burdens develop hypercalcemia. In addition, we have found that measurements of total body myeloma cell number and production of bone resorbing activity by bone marrow myeloma cells in vitro do not correlate closely with the production of hypercalcemia (Durie et al 1981). However, there is a highly significant correlation ($P<0.001$) between the amounts of bone resorbing activity produced by cultured marrow myeloma cells and the extent of bone destruction as determined by radiologic lesions in the patient. Thus, other factors in addition to production of bone resorbing activity must be involved in the pathogenesis of the hypercalcemia. Impaired renal function is common in myeloma for a number of reasons. These include, in addition to hypercalcemia, uric acid nephropathy, amyloid nephropathy, myeloma kidney due to Bence Jones protein excretion, and chronic infections. Because hypercalcemia occurs almost always in patients with impairment of renal function, we suggest that this is an important contributing factor in the pathophysiology of hypercalcemia. Increased bone resorption in myeloma leads to increased entry of calcium into the extracellular fluid, but many patients with normal homeostatic control mechanisms (particularly patients with normal renal function) are able to compensate for this increase in extracellular fluid calcium and maintain the serum calcium in the normal range by increasing urine calcium excretion. However, in patients with impaired renal function, this increase in bone resorption overwhelms the kidney's capacity to compensate and these patients develop hypercalcemia. This is more likely to occur in patients who produce Bence Jones protein or are predisposed to impaired renal function for other reasons (Snapper and Kahn 1971). In many cases, impairment of renal function may also be due to the direct effects of hypercalcemia on the kidney.

Since the mechanisms responsible for hypercalcemia in patients with myeloma are different from those in patients with other types of malignancy, there are subtle differences in laboratory test findings at the time of diagnosis. Because of renal impairment in many patients with myeloma, a large number of them have increased serum phosphorus rather than decreased serum phosphorus, which is common with other types of malignancy. In addition, serum alkaline phosphatase, a marker of osteoblast activity, is usually not increased in patients with myeloma since there is little active new bone formation. For similar reasons, as noted earlier, bone scans may also be negative.

Treatment of bone destruction and hypercalcemia in myeloma will be considered under two categories, first, the treatment of osteolytic bone lesions and second, the treatment of hypercalcemia.

Indications for treatment

We consider that all patients with hypercalcemia require specific treatment to inhibit bone resorption. As in other malignant diseases, hypercalcemia due to increased bone resorption is likely to worsen very rapidly. This is particularly true for myeloma, where renal function is so tenuous because of a number of complicating factors deleterious to the kidney such as Bence Jones proteinuria, hyperuricemia, urinary tract infection and, in a few patients, amyloid.

Principles of treatment

Underlying disease

Hypercalcemia and increased bone resorption are improved in many patients with myeloma by treatment with cytotoxic drugs. This often leads to a decrease in bone pain and a lowering of the serum calcium. This is particularly likely to occur if corticosteroids, which also inhibit bone resorption in myeloma, are part of the treatment regimen. Even in patients with myeloma who respond to cytotoxic drug therapy, bone lesions are unlikely to recalcify (Snapper and Kahn 1971), possibly because there is usually only about a one log reduction in myeloma cell mass.

Inhibition of the bone resorption

The primary goal of therapy for the hypercalcemia of myeloma should be the inhibition of osteoclastic bone resorption. A number of therapeutic agents that inhibit osteoclastic bone resorption are available. These include lowering serum calcium by drugs such as corticosteroids, calcitonin, plicamycin, and the bisphosphonates. In patients with myeloma bone disease, the most effective of these are the new generation bisphosphonates, one of which (pamidronate) has now been approved by the FDA in the treatment of myeloma bone disease.

Bisphosphonates

The bisphosphonates are very effective inhibitors of osteoclastic bone resorption. These drugs are pyrophosphate analogues that suppress bone resorption by mechanisms that are still not clearly defined, but probably involve binding of the drug to the bone surface as well as direct inhibition of osteoclast activity (Mundy and Martin 1982). The agent 3-amino-1-hydroxypropane-1,1-diphosphonate (pamidronate) has been shown to be particularly effective in patients with secondary osteolytic lesions due to breast cancer and myeloma, and has also been extremely effective in lowering the serum calcium (Van Breukelen et al 1979; Mundy et al 1983). Unfortunately, pamidronate and other amino bisphosphonates may cause upper gastrointestinal mucosal ulcers when used in oral form (Mundy et al 1983), which limits its usefulness when taken over prolonged periods, but it is extremely effective over short periods when used parenterally. Other bisphosphonates, such as clodronate, are also very effective in lowering the serum calcium, relieving bone pain, and reducing bone turnover in patients with myeloma (Siris et al 1980). The older bisphosphonate, ethane-1-hydroxy-1,1-diphosphonate (EHDP), or etidronate, has been used intravenously in the treatment of hypercalcemia (Ryzen et al 1983). Its effects are possibly slower and less reliable than the newer bisphosphonates, and its current use is not recommended. Clodronate was withdrawn from testing in the United States because of unfounded fears of its potential toxicity. The use of bisphosphonates to treat myeloma bone disease without hypercalcemia will be considered below.

Unfortunately, as noted above, most patients with myeloma and hypercalcemia also have some impairment of renal function. There is limited experience in the use of bisphosphonates (or any other hypercalcemic agent for that matter) in this circumstance, and bisphosphonates probably should be used with caution in any patient with a serum creatinine greater than 3 mg/dl.

Corticosteroids

Corticosteroids are frequently effective in controlling osteoclastic bone resorption in myeloma (Lazor and Rosenberg 1964). As already indicated, they are usually part of the initial cytotoxic regimen. The inhibitory effects of corticosteroids on bone resorption are dependent on the stimulus. They are much less effective against PTH than they are against other factors. Corticosteroids inhibit the bone resorbing activity produced by activated peripheral blood leukocytes in low concentrations (Mundy et al 1978; Strumpf et al 1978), and this is possibly why they are very effective in lowering the serum calcium in many patients with myeloma and related diseases. The mechanism by which they exert this effect may be due to impairment of formation of new osteoclasts, as has been shown in a feline marrow cell culture system for generation of cells with osteoclast characteristics (Suda et al 1983). Although most patients with myeloma and hypercalcemia respond to corticosteroid therapy, some do not (Binstock and Mundy 1980), particularly those late in the course of their disease.

Plicamycin (mithramycin)

Plicamycin is an agent that is a powerful inhibitor of bone resorption, possibly by exerting a cytotoxic effect on bone resorbing cells (Minkin 1973). It is frequently used as a form of treatment of hypercalcemia and is usually effective (Stamp et al 1975; Mundy et al 1983). However, we do not advocate its use as a primary agent in myeloma (or any other situation) because it is directly nephrotoxic and its side effects are more frequent in patients with impaired renal function (Mundy and Martin 1982). Because many patients with myeloma and hypercalcemia have impaired renal function before treatment, we think it should be used as a third-line drug for therapy.

Calcitonin and corticosteroids

Calcitonin and corticosteroids used in conjunction are almost always effective in patients with hypercalcemia due to myeloma (Binstock and Mundy 1980). These patients may be extremely difficult to treat because they frequently do have impaired renal function, which makes the use of other agents that lower the serum calcium, such as oral phosphate or plicamycin, undesirable. Combined corticosteroid/calcitonin therapy is not harmful when used for short periods in patients with impaired renal function. Although the effects may be relatively short-lived, we find that withdrawal of calcitonin for several days followed by its reintroduction almost always results in return of the serum calcium into the normal range or into a range that is not associated with symptoms due to hypercalcemia. We have treated several patients for a number of months with this form of therapy in situations where no other agent was suitable (Mundy and Martin 1982). Moreover, the effects of combined therapy are very rapid, with lowering of serum calcium usually occurring within 12 hours. The combination is more effective than either agent used alone and seems to be more effective in myeloma than in patients with solid tumors and hypercalcemia (Binstock and Mundy 1980).

Calcitonin and glucocorticoids are also very effective inhibitors of bone resorption in vitro. Calcitonin treatment alone leads to the escape phenomenon, characterized by loss of effectiveness despite the continued presence of calcitonin (Wener et al 1972). Glucocorticoids prevent the escape phenomenon both in vitro and in vivo (Au 1975; Binstock and Mundy 1980; Mundy and Martin 1982). Whether the effects of the combination on bone, as suggested by these data, or on the kidney, as proposed by Ralston et al (1985), are more important will require further study.

Other agents

Recently, other cytotoxic drugs such as gallium nitrate (Warrell et al 1984) and cisplatinum (Kukla et al 1984) have been used in the therapy of hypercalcemia associated with malignant disease. Gallium nitrate is a very effective inhibitor of osteoclastic bone resorption, which is apparently useful both in the treatment of hypercalcemia of malignancy as well as in patients with myeloma. It seems to have a similar spectrum of activity to the new generation bisphosphonates and to mithramycin. It is discussed in more detail in Chapter 5.

Promotion of renal calcium excretion

As in other forms of hypercalcemia, promotion of a saline diuresis in myeloma may transiently lower the serum calcium and improve renal function because sodium and calcium handling by the renal tubules are linked. This can be achieved with the use of saline infusions. Some workers also use furosemide, although that produces marginal additional benefits to saline infusion (Suki et al 1970; Mundy and Martin 1982). Great care must be exercised in the use of large volumes of intravenous fluids in myeloma, since frequently the impairment of renal function is fixed and large volumes of fluids will lead to the rapid onset of congestive cardiac failure. For this reason, administration of large volumes of fluids to patients with myeloma should be accompanied by central venous pressure monitoring.

Practical guide to treatment

Our own approach to the treatment of hypercalcemia in myeloma is as follows:

- Institution of cytotoxic drugs for treatment of myeloma.

- The cautious use of intravenous saline to promote a saline diuresis, with careful observation for the development of cardiac failure.

- The administration of pamidronate 60–90 mg by intravenous infusion, which is almost always effective in patients with serum creatinine less than 3 mg/dl.

- The institution of calcitonin and corticosteroids, which can be used safely and effectively in those patients with hypercalcemia and renal failure. Calcitonin and glucocorticoids are reserved for those patients with renal failure, or when a rapid (less than 24 hours) response is required. We use salmon calcitonin in doses of 200–400 IU intramuscularly or subcutaneously each 12 hours, and prednisone 40–60 mg daily or equivalent doses of hydrocortisone parenterally.

Bone markers

Bone markers are very important for monitoring the progress of osteolytic bone disease. The current most useful marker for bone resorption is the measurement of deoxypyridinoline crosslinks of collagen (Delmas 1992). These can be readily measured in the urine either by chemical assay or by ELISA. Hopefully this marker may eventually be measurable in the serum. This measurement provides a very accurate and precise parameter of osteoclastic bone resorption, which is much improved over previous markers such as urinary hydroxyproline or fasting urine calcium. New markers such as this should improve our ability to monitor the progress of patients treated with agents that inhibit bone resorption much more precisely. In myeloma, serum osteocalcin (bone Gla protein) concentrations are decreased in patients with advanced disease and extensive lesions, but either normal or even increased in patients early in the disease (Bataille et al 1990).

Figure 8.7

Bisphosphonates cause a marked reduction in bone lesions in the 5T murine model of myeloma bone disease, but no effect on markers of tumor burden such as monoclonal proteins. Data are not yet available to determine whether bisphosphonates exert a beneficial effect on tumor burden in patients with myeloma bone disease.

Treatment of painful bone lesions without hypercalcemia

For a number of years, clinicians have attempted to devise therapeutic approaches in myeloma that would relieve disabling symptoms due to skeletal destruction. This was first attempted with the use of fluoride and later calcium and fluoride, although this combination was ineffective and, in fact, detrimental because of the associated side effects. More recently, several groups have shown that the newer generation bisphosphonates will relieve bone pain, and produce a rapid, sustained, and significant decrease in the urinary excretion of calcium and hydroxyproline indicating decreased bone turnover (Van Breukelen et al 1979; Siris et al 1980). This was shown first with pamidronate (Van Breukelen et al 1979) and then with clodronate (Siris et al 1980).

The FDA approved the use of pamidronate for myeloma bone disease in 1995. Pamidronate has been shown to reduce skeletal events, to reduce the need for radiation therapy, and to reduce episodes of hypercalcemia and pathologic fracture when given in doses of 90 mg over 4 hours by intravenous infusion monthly for 9 months (Berenson et al 1996). More recent studies have shown that pamidronate continued in this regimen for 21 months is safe and well tolerated (Berenson et al 1998). The number of skeletal events was almost halved in patients taking pamidronate. Moreover, an objective assessment of the quality of life showed a beneficial effect of bisphosphonates. Similar studies in Finland and Great Britain involving hundreds of patients have also suggested that potent bisphosphonates such as clodronate are effective in improving performance status, reducing vertebral fractures, reducing the progress of osteolytic bone lesions, and preventing hypercalcemic episodes. The bisphosphonates seem to be more effective in patients with minimal disease, but they are appropriate for essentially all patients. Early data suggest that survival may be improved (Berenson et al 1996). The results are comparable with either parenteral or oral agents. A reasonable conclusion from the current data is that all patients should be treated, and the real issues are cost, which bisphosphonate and which route of administration. It is not clear as yet whether the use of bisphosphonates to inhibit bone resorption will also reduce the tumor burden in bone, but that is possible (Figure 8.7). For example, by reducing the production of cytokines such as IL-6, which promote myeloma cell growth and are produced during states of increased bone resorption, it could be expected that this may lead to a decrease in total myeloma cell burden (Berenson et al 1996).

References

Alsina M, Boyce B, Devlin RD et al (1996) Development of an in vivo model of human multiple myeloma bone disease, *Blood* **87**: 1495–501.

Au WYW (1975) Calcitonin treatment of hypercalcemia due to parathyroid carcinoma–synergistic effect of prednisone on long-term treatment of hypercalcemia, *Arch Intern Med* **135**: 1594–7.

Bardwick PA, Zvaifler NJ, Gill GN et al (1980) Plasma cell dyscrasia with polyneuropathy, organomegaly, endocrinopathy, M protein, and skin changes: the POEMS syndrome, *Medicine* **59**: 311–22.

Bataille R, Jourdan M, Zhang XG et al (1989) Serum levels of interleukin-6, a potent myeloma cell growth factor, as a reflect of dyscrasias, *J Clin Invest* **84**: 2008–11.

Bataille R, Delmas PD, Chappard D et al (1990) Abnormal serum bone Gla protein levels in multiple myeloma, *Cancer* **66**: 167–72.

Bataille R, Chappard D, Marcelli C et al (1991) Recruitment of new osteoblasts and osteoclasts is the earliest critical event in the pathogenesis of human multiple myeloma, *J Clin Invest* **88**: 62–6.

Berenson JR, Lichtenstein A, Porter L et al (1996) Efficacy of pamidronate in reducing skeletal events in patients with advanced multiple myeloma, *N Engl J Med* **334**: 488–93.

Berenson JR, Lichtenstein A, Porter L et al (1998) Long-term pamidronate treatment of advanced multiple myeloma patients reduces skeletal events, *J Clin Oncol* **16**: 593–602.

Bertolini DR, Sarin P, Mundy GR (1984) Production of macromolecular bone resorbing activity by human T-cell leukemia virus (HTLV) transformed cell lines, *Calcif Tissue Int* **36**: 284A.

Bertolini DR, Nedwin GE, Bringman TS et al (1986) Stimulation of bone resorption and inhibition of bone formation in vitro by human tumour necrosis factors, *Nature* **319**: 516–18.

Binstock ML, Mundy GR (1980) Effects of calcitonin and glucocorticoids in combination in hypercalcemia of malignancy, *Ann Intern Med* **93**: 269–72.

Black K, Garret IR, Mundy GR (1991) Chinese hamster ovarian cells transfected with the murine interleukin-6 gene cause hypercalcemia as well as cachexia, leukocytosis and thrombocytosis in tumor-bearing nude mice, *Endocrinology* **128**: 2657–9.

Boyce BF, Aufdemorte TB, Garrett IR et al (1989) Effects of interleukin-1 on bone turnover in normal mice, *Endocrinology* **125**: 1142–50.

Breslau NA, McGuire JL, Zerwekh JE et al (1984) Hypercalcemia associated with increased serum calcitriol levels in three patients with lymphoma, *Ann Intern Med* **100**: 1–7.

Budayr AA, Nissenson RA, Klein RF et al (1989) Increased serum levels of a parathyroid hormone-like protein in malignancy-associated hypercalcemia, *Ann Intern Med* **11**: 807–12.

Bunn PA, Schechter GP, Jaffe E et al (1983) Clinical course of retrovirus associated adult T cell lymphoma in the United States, *N Engl J Med* **309**: 257–64.

Cozzolino F, Torcia M, Aldinucci D et al (1989) Production of interleukin-1 by bone marrow myeloma cells, *Blood* **74**: 380–7.

Davies M, Hayes ME, Mawer EB et al (1985) Abnormal vitamin D metabolism in Hodgkin's lymphoma, *Lancet* **i**: 1186–8.

Delmas PD (1992) Clinical use of biochemical markers of bone remodeling in osteoporosis, *Bone* **13**: S17–S21.

Durie BGM, Salmon SE, Mundy GR (1981) Relation of osteoclast activating factor production to the extent of bone disease in multiple myeloma, *Br J Haematol* **47**: 21–30.

Farhangi M, Merlini G (1986) The clinical implications of monoclonal immunoglobulins, *Semin Oncol* **13**: 366–79.

Fetchick DA, Bertolini DR, Sarin PS et al (1986) Production of 1,25-dihydroxyvitamin D_3 by human T-cell lymphotrophic virus-I transformed lymphocytes, *J Clin Invest* **78**: 592–6.

Feyen JHM, Elford P, Dipadova FE et al (1989) Interleukin-6 is produced by bone and modulated by parathyroid hormone, *J Bone Miner Res* **4**: 633–8.

Firkin F, Seymour JF, Watson AM et al (1996) Parathyroid hormone-related protein in hypercalcemia associated with haematological malignancy, *Br J Haematol* **94**: 486–92.

Gailani S, McLimans WF, Mundy GR et al (1976) Controlled environment culture of bone marrow explants from human myeloma, *Cancer Res* **36**: 1299–304.

Garrett IR, Durie BGM, Nedwin GE et al (1987) Production of the bone resorbing cytokine lymphotoxin by cultured human myeloma cells, *N Engl J Med* **317**: 526–32.

Gilles J, Roodman GD, Reddy SV et al (1993) Osteoclast expression of interleukin-6 (IL-6) is 100-fold greater than that of osteoblasts, *J Bone Miner Res* **8** (Suppl 1): no 201.

Girasole G, Jilka RL, Passeri G et al (1992) 17β-Estradiol inhibits interleukin-6 production by bone marrow-derived stromal cells and osteoblasts in vitro. A potential mechanism for the antiosteoporotic effect of estrogens, *J Clin Invest* **89**: 883–91.

Gowen M, Wood OD, Ihrie EJ et al (1983a) An interleukin-1 like factor stimulates bone resorption in vitro, *Nature* **306**: 378–80.

Gowen M, Meikle MC, Reynolds JJ (1983b) Stimulation of bone resorption in vitro by a non-prostanoid factor released by human monocytes in culture, *Biochem Biophys Acta* **762**: 471–4.

Gowen M, Nedwin G, Mundy GR (1986) Preferential inhibition of cytokine stimulated bone resorption by recombinant interferon gamma, *J Bone Miner Res* **1**: 469–74.

Horton JE, Raisz LG, Simmons HA et al (1972) Bone resorbing activity in supernatant fluid from cultured human peripheral blood leukocytes, *Science* **177**: 793–5.

Ishimi Y, Miyaura C, Jin CH et al (1990) IL-6 is produced by osteoblasts and induces bone resorption, *J Immunol* **145**: 3297–303.

Jilka RL, Hangoc G, Girasole G et al (1992) Increased osteoclast development after estrogen loss-mediation by interleukin-6, *Science* **257**: 88–91.

Josse RG, Murray TM, Mundy GR et al (1981) Observations on the mechanism of bone resorption induced by multiple myeloma marrow culture fluids and partially purified osteoclast activating factor, *J Clin Invest* **67**: 1472–81.

Kawano M, Tanaka H, Ishikawa H et al (1989) Interleukin-1 accelerates autocrine growth of myeloma cells through interleukin-6 in human myeloma, *Blood* **73**: 2145–8.

Kukla LJ, Abramson EC, McGuire WP et al (1984) Cisplatinum treatment for malignancy-associated humoral hypercalcemia in an athymic mouse model, *Calcif Tissue Int* **36**: 559–62.

Lazor MZ, Rosenberg LE (1964) Mechanisms of adrenal-steroid reversal of hypercalcemia in multiple myeloma, *N Engl J Med* **270**: 749.

Linkhart TA, Linkhart SG, MacCharles DC et al (1991) Interleukin-6 messenger RNA expression and interleukin-6 protein secretion in cells isolated from normal human bone: regulation by interleukin-1, *J Bone Miner Res* **6**: 1285–94.

Lokhorst HM, Lamme T, de Smet M et al (1994) Primary tumor cells of myeloma patients induce interleukin-6 secretion in long-term bone marrow cultures, *Blood* **84**: 2269–77.

Lowik CWGM, Vanderpluijm G, Bloys H et al (1989) Parathyroid hormone (PTH) and PTH-like protein (Plp) stimulate interleukin-6 production by osteogenic cells. A possible role of interleukin-6 in osteoclastogenesis, *Biochem Biophys Res Commun* **162**: 1546–52.

Manning LS, Berger JD, O'Donoghue HL et al (1992) A model of multiple myeloma: culture of 5T33 murine myeloma cells and evaluation of tumorigenicity in the C57BL/KaLwRij mouse, *Br J Cancer* **66**: 1088–93.

McSheehy PMJ, Chambers TJ (1986) Osteoblastic cells mediate osteoclastic responsiveness to parathyroid hormone, *Endocrinology* **118**: 824–8.

Michigami T, Dallas SL, Mundy GR et al (1997) Interactions of myeloma cells with bone marrow stromal cells via $\alpha_4\beta_1$ integrin — VCAM-1 is required for the development of osteolysis, *J Bone Min Res* **12** (Suppl): 104.

Minkin C (1973) Inhibition of parathyroid hormone stimulated bone resorption in vitro by the antibiotic mithramycin, *Calcif Tissue Res* **13**: 249–57.

Motokura T, Fukumoto S, Matsumoto T et al (1989) Parathyroid hormone-related protein in adult T-cell leukemia-lymphoma, *Ann Intern Med* **111**: 484–8.

Mundy GR, Martin TJ (1982) The hypercalcemia of malignancy: pathogenesis and management, *Metabolism* **31**: 1247–77.

Mundy GR, Wilkinson R, Heath DA (1983) Comparative study of available medical therapy for hypercalcemia of malignancy, *Am J Med* **74**: 421–32.

Mundy GR, Luben RA, Raisz LG et al (1974a) Bone-resorbing activity in supernatants from lymphoid cell lines, *N Engl J Med* **290**: 867–71.

Mundy GR, Raisz LG, Cooper RA et al (1974b) Evidence for the secretion of an osteoclast stimulating factor in myeloma, *N Engl J Med* **291**: 1041–6.

Mundy GR, Rick ME, Turcotte R et al (1978) Pathogenesis of hypercalcemia in lymphosarcoma cell leukemia—role of an osteoclast activating factor-like substance and mechanism of action for glucocorticoid therapy, *Am J Med* **65**: 600–6.

Ohsaki Y, Takahashi S, Scarcez T et al (1992) Evidence for an autocrine/paracrine role for interleukin-6 in bone resorption by giant cells from giant cell tumors of bone, *Endocrinology* **131**: 2229–34.

Pfeilschifter J, Chenu C, Bird A et al (1989) Interleukin-1 and tumor necrosis factor stimulate the formation of human osteoclast-like cells in vitro, *J Bone Miner Res* **4**: 113–18.

Radl J, Croese W, Zurcher C et al (1988) Multiple myeloma, *Am J Pathol* **132**: 593–7.

Raisz LG, Luben RA, Mundy GR et al (1975) Effect of osteoclast activating factor from human leukocytes on bone metabolism, *J Clin Invest* **56**: 408–13.

Ralston SH, Gardner MD, Dryburgh TJ et al (1985) Comparison of aminohydroxypropylidene diphosphonate, mithramycin and corticosteroids/calcitonin in treatment of cancer-associated hypercalcemia, *Lancet* **ii**: 907–10.

Roodman GD, Kurihara N, Ohsaki Y et al (1992) Interleukin 6. A potential autocrine/paracrine factor in Paget's disease of bone, *J Clin Invest* **89**: 46–52.

Rosenthal N, Insogna KL, Godsall JW et al (1985) Elevations in circulating 1,25 dihydroxyvitamin D_3 in three patients with lymphoma-associated hypercalcemia, *J Clin Endocrinol Metab* **60**: 29–33.

Ryzen E, Rude RK, Elbaum N et al (1983) Use of intravenous etidronate disodium in the treatment of hypercalcemia. In: Garattini S, ed, *Bone resorption, metastasis, and diphosphonates* (Raven: New York) 99–108.

Sabatini M, Boyce B, Aufdemorte T et al (1988) Infusions of recombinant human interleukin-1 α and β cause hypercalcemia in normal mice, *Proc Natl Acad Sci USA* **85**: 5235–9.

Schindler R, Mancilla J, Endres S et al (1990) Correlations and interactions in the production of interleukin-6 (IL-6), IL-1 and tumor necrosis factor (TNF) in human blood mononuclear cells: IL-6 suppresses IL-1 and TNF, *Blood* **75**: 40–7.

Siris ES, Sherman WH, Baquiran DC et al (1980) Effects of dichloromethylene diphosphonate on skeletal mobilization of calcium in multiple myeloma, *N Engl J Med* **302**: 310–15.

Snapper I, Kahn A (1971) *Myelomatosis* (Karger: Basel).

Stamp TCB, Child JA, Walker PG (1975) Treatment of osteolytic myelomatosis with mithramycin, *Lancet* **i**: 719–22.

Strumpf M, Kowalski MA, Mundy GR (1978) Effects of glucocorticoids on osteoclast-activating factor, *J Lab Clin Miner* **92**: 772–8.

Suda T, Testa NG, Allen TD (1983) Effects of hydrocortisone on osteoclasts generated in cat bone marrow cultures, *Calcif Tissue Int* **35**: 82–6.

Suki WN, Yium JJ, Von Minden M et al (1970) Acute treatment of hypercalcemia with furosemide, *N Engl J Med* **283**: 836–40.

Suzuki A, Takahashi T, Okuno Y et al (1994) Production of parathyroid hormone-related protein by cultured human myeloma cells, *Am J Hematol* **45**: 88–90.

Tabibzadeh SS, Santhanam U, Sehgal PB et al (1989) Cytokine-induced production of IFN-β_2/IL-6 by freshly explanted human endometrial stromal cells. Modulation by estradiol-17β, *J Immunol* **142**: 3134–9.

Thomson BM, Mundy GR, Chambers TJ (1987) Tumor necrosis factors alpha and beta induce osteoblastic cells to stimulate osteoclastic bone resorption, *J Immunol* **138**: 775–9.

Valentin-Opran A, Charhon SA, Meunier PJ et al (1982) Quantitative histology of myeloma induced bone changes, *Br J Haematol* **52**: 601–10.

Van Breukelen FJM, Bijvoet OLM, Van Oosterom AT (1979) Inhibition of osteolytic bone lesions by (3-amino-1-hydroxypropylidene)-1,1-bisphosphonate (APD), *Lancet* **i**: 803–5.

Warrell RP, Bockman RS, Coonley CJ et al (1984) Gallium nitrate inhibits calcium resorption from bone and is effective treatment for cancer-related hypercalcemia, *J Clin Invest* **73**: 1487–90.

Wener JA, Gorton SJ, Raisz LG (1972) Escape from inhibition of resorption in cultures of fetal bone treated with calcitonin and parathyroid hormone, *Endocrinology* **90**: 752–9.

Yoneda T, Mundy GR (1979a) Prostaglandins are necessary for osteoclast-activating factor production by activated peripheral blood leukocytes, *J Exp Med* **149**: 279–83.

Yoneda T, Mundy GR (1979b) Monocytes regulate osteoclast-activating factor production by releasing prostaglandins, *J Exp Med* **150**: 338–50.

Zaloga GP, Eli C, Medbery CA (1985) Humoral hypercalcemia in Hodgkin's disease, *Arch Intern Med* **145**: 155–7.

CHAPTER 9

Primary hyperparathyroidism

Primary hyperparathyroidism is due to excess and inappropriate production of PTH by the parathyroid glands. The hallmark of the disease is hypercalcemia. It is now an extremely common endocrine disease, particularly in the aging female population, and has a markedly variable clinical presentation that frequently confuses the clinician. The manifestations of the disease are due not just to the effects of PTH on the skeleton and kidneys, but also to 1,25 dihydroxyvitamin D_3, which is produced by the kidney in response to excess circulating concentrations of PTH. Most of the clinical features occur as a consequence of chronic hypercalcemia.

History

Primary hyperparathyroidism is an interesting and common condition. Although the disease has been recognized for almost 70 years, our notions of its incidence and prevalence in the general population, its natural history and its mode of presentation have undergone marked changes as methods for diagnosing the condition have changed and improved. It was first recognized as an uncommon condition, a "disease of bones and stones and abdominal groans occasionally complicated by psychological moans" (Albright and Reifenstein 1948). The early descriptions were greatly influenced by the methods of diagnosis that existed before the Second World War, and the mode of presentation (Figure 9.1). At that time, the disease presented as osteitis fibrosa cystica associated with hypercalcemia and recurrent renal stones. Since even in this day and age there are few patients with primary hyperparathyroidism who present with this clinical picture, it is not surprising that the disease is rarely recognized in this form. Since serum calcium became part of routine autoanalyzer measurements in the mid-1970s, it is only information after that time that can give accurate data on mode of presentation, epidemiology and frequency of this disease without bias by patient selection. At the present time, the major mode of presentation is the asymptomatic patient who has a routine determination of serum calcium for other reasons and is found unexpectedly to have hypercalcemia (Heath et al 1980; Mundy et al 1980). The disease occurs mainly in elderly females, the same patients who also develop postmenopausal osteoporosis. This is in contrast to the patients who present with osteitis fibrosa cystica or recurrent renal stones, who tend to be younger (more often between the ages of 20 and 50). The prevalence of primary hyperparathyroidism is probably about 1 : 1000, based on a study in which 26 000 consecutive serum calcium measurements were made (Boonstra and Jackson 1971).

Figure 9.1
Captain Charles Martell, the first patient with thoroughly documented primary hyperparathyroidism in the USA. (See Albright and Reifenstein (1948) for complete account.)

Pathology

Primary hyperparathyroidism may be due to a solitary parathyroid gland adenoma, hyperplasia of four parathyroid glands, or carcinoma of a parathyroid gland. A solitary parathyroid adenoma is by far the most common cause, being responsible for the clinical syndrome in approximately 85% of patients. Hyperplasia is responsible in the majority of the remaining patients. Carcinoma of the parathyroid gland is fairly rare, accounting for less than 1% of cases, with less than 200 cases so far reported in the world literature.

Adenoma

Most adenomas are composed of the chief cells of the parathyroid, and a few of transitional cells between chief cells and oxyphil cells. Rarely adenomas may be composed only of oxyphil cells. Parathyroid gland adenomas are usually between 0.5 and 5.0 g in weight, although occasional adenomas may weigh up to 10–20 g. (A normal parathyroid gland weighs 25–50 mg.) The largest adenomas usually secrete the most PTH and produce the most prominent clinical features. Adenomas usually consist of a homogeneous collection of chief cells, and are characteristically devoid of fat cells or prominent stromal elements, which helps the pathologist to distinguish an adenoma from normal tissue. In about 5–10% of patients, the adenoma may be in an abnormal location, such as in the thymus, within the thyroid, or in the mediastinum adjacent to the carotid sheath, the pericardium or in the retroesophageal space. Occasionally, a parathyroid cyst occurs within a hyperfunctioning adenoma. Nonfunctioning adenomas of the parathyroid gland probably occur, but their frequency is unknown.

Hyperplasia

Because hyperplasia is difficult to distinguish from adenoma histologically, and hyperplastic glands may vary considerably in size, there has been some confusion in distinguishing hyperplasia from single or multiple adenomas. However, if hyperplasia were more common, then patients treated by surgical removal of one abnormal gland should get recurrences of hypercalcemia more frequently. In reality, recurrence is fairly uncommon, occurring in less than 10% of all surgically treated cases. Most investigators believe that the presence of an adenoma in more than one gland is very rare (less than 2% of all cases).

Enlargement of all four parathyroid glands is almost always present in patients who have primary hyperparathyroidism associated with multiple endocrine neoplasia, but this enlargement is different in nature from the more straightforward hyperplasia that occurs in some patients with nonfamilial primary hyperparathyroidism. In familial multiple endocrine neoplasia Type 1, there may be an initial element of polyclonal hyperplasia followed later by monoclonal lesions due to deletion or mutation of a tumor suppressor gene found on chromosome 11. In familial multiple endocrine neoplasia Type 2, the picture is that of hyperplasia (Gagel 1989).

Carcinoma

Carcinoma of the parathyroid gland is rare. Estimates have been made in the literature that approximately 2% of all patients with primary hyperparathyroidism have a carcinoma of one of the parathyroid glands responsible, but this is clearly an overestimate since primary hyperparathyroidism has been recognized more frequently over the last 15 years, and the incidence of parathyroid carcinoma is apparently unchanged. Shane and Bilezikian (1982) noted that only a little over 100 patients had been described with this condition since 1938. Conservative estimates suggest that since every patient with parathyroid carcinoma comes to diagnosis eventually, probably only one patient with this condition for every 1000 or more patients with primary hyperparathyroidism exists. Parathyroid carcinoma can occur at any age and, although there is a slight female preponderance, it is relatively more common in males than benign primary hyperparathyroidism. Hypercalcemia is usually much more severe (>14 mg/dl in 70%) and "bone and stone disease" (nephrocalcinosis as well as nephrolithiasis) frequently coexist in these patients. The clinical course is usually prolonged. About 50% of patients survive for 5 years and one-third for 10 years. Occasionally these tumors metastasize, although local invasion and recurrence is more common. It may be difficult to distinguish between an adenoma and a carcinoma at the histologic level, and the diagnosis may be first made from the invasive or metastatic behavior of the tumor. Histologic features that are characteristic of a carcinoma include adherence to surrounding structures, capsular invasion by the parathyroid cells, and the presence of many mitotic figures, which are infrequent in nonmalignant adenomas. Carcinomas also frequently contain dense connective tissue strands or septra, which run through the tumor to disrupt the gland architecture. The tumor may be locally invasive, involving blood vessels. Spread is usually by lymphatics, but it may also involve liver, lungs, or bone by hematogenous spread. Patients die usually because of the effects of PTH excess, so surgical removal of lesions, whether primary or metastatic, may be warranted. Medical treatment with bisphosphonates, plicamycin or calcitonin and corticosteroids have all been shown to relieve symptoms by lowering the serum calcium. Radiation therapy has not been successful.

Multiple endocrine neoplasia Types 1 and 2 (MEN-1 and 2)

Primary hyperparathyroidism may occur in association with multiple endocrine neoplasia (MEN) Types 1 and 2. Type 1 is associated with pituitary adenomas and pancreatic adenomas. The pituitary adenomas may be growth-hormone secreting and associated with acromegaly or prolactinomas, causing the galactorrhea–amenorrhea syndrome. In MEN Type 2, primary hyperparathyroidism is associated with pheochromocytoma, medullary carcinoma of the thyroid and, in some cases, mucosal neuromas. It is a fairly uncommon association of MEN-2. It occurs more frequently in MEN-1, but usually becomes apparent after the age of 30 years, unlike the situation in familial hypocalciuric hypercalcemia (FHH), where hypercalcemia may be manifest from birth. These syndromes are discussed in more detail below.

Etiology

Parathyroid adenomas are monoclonal lesions (Arnold et al 1988). In contrast, nonfamilial primary hyperplasia is of polyclonal or multicellular origin. However, patients with familial MEN-1, which is associated with four-gland disease, may have monoclonal parathyroid lesions superimposed on polyclonal hyperplasia, as may occasional patients with long-standing secondary hyperparathyroidism due to end-stage renal disease.

The precise etiology of primary hyperparathyroidism is unknown, but it is probable that different mechanisms are responsible in the different types of primary hyperparathyroidism that are now being clarified. For example, a different mechanism is probably responsible for the monoclonal lesions that occur in parathyroid adenomas compared with the polyclonal or multicellular hyperplastic disease, which is more likely to be due to an extrinsic growth regulatory factor for parathyroid cells. Familial multiple endocrine neoplasia (FMEN) Types 1 and 2 are clearly due to different genetic mechanisms, which are currently being clarified.

Potential deletion or mutation of tumor suppressor genes

In 25% of patients with single parathyroid gland adenomas, there is a major deletion of chromosomal material from chromosome 11 (Arnold and Kim 1989; Friedman et al 1989; Bystrom et al 1990). This suggests that this portion of chromosome 11 may contain a tumor suppressor gene whose deletion by chromosomal loss (or loss of function possibly by mutation or rearrangement), may lead to development of a parathyroid gland adenoma. This region of chromosome 11 also contains the putative gene responsible for MEN-1 (Friedman et al 1989; Bystrom et al 1990). Other abnormalities that have been described include loss of heterozygosity on chromosome 11q13, 1P or M27B of the X chromosome. Deletions of the retinoblastoma tumor suppressor gene (rb) are also common in parathyroid carcinomas (Cryns et al 1994). Also found is allelic loss of the p53 gene in 33% of parathyroid cancers. Loss of heterozygosity has been described in some patients with MEN-1 on chromosome 11q13, as well as in parathyroid adenomas (Arnold et al 1988, 1989; Thakker et al 1989; Friedman et al 1990), and at the M27B region of the X chromosome (Arnold et al 1995). Retinoblastoma gene deletions occur frequently in parathyroid carcinomas (Cryns et al 1994).

Gene rearrangements involving PRAD1 oncogene

In a small subset (about 4%) of patients with parathyroid gland adenomas, there is a gene rearrangement in parathyroid cells that leads to insertion of an oncogene adjacent to the upstream regulatory region of the promoter for parathyroid hormone (Arnold et al 1989; Friedman et al 1990; Rosenberg et al 1991). This leads to overexpression of the oncogene (which is called PRAD1, for parathyroid adenomatosis gene) and subsequent increased parathyroid cell replication (Friedman et al 1990). PRAD1 is homologous to the family of cyclin genes that are important in regulating cell division. Since PRAD1 is on the long arm of chromosome 11 and PTH is on the short arm of the same chromosome, the gene rearrangement responsible for insertion of PRAD1 in the upstream regulatory region of PTH is a chromosome inversion. Since these tumors are almost always benign, this overexpression of PRAD1 and increased cell replication is not associated with local invasiveness or metastasis. However, the tumor cells remain under negative control by extracellular fluid calcium, thus limiting both their increased rates of continued replication and their overexpression of PTH (LeBoff et al 1985). How this balance between PRAD1 gene overexpression, causing both increased cell replication and PTH secretion, and negative feedback control by extracellular fluid calcium is determined remains unknown.

Other potential extrinsic etiologic agents

A growth factor for isolated bovine parathyroid cells is present in the plasma of many patients with FMEN-1 (Brandi et al 1988). This factor is similar in nature to basic fibroblast growth factor, and stimulates parathyroid endothelial cells. The source and precise nature of this factor remain unknown (see below).

Several other external stimuli have been linked to parathyroid gland hyperplasia. Prolonged hypocalcemia has long been known to cause secondary hyperparathyroidism and associated parathyroid gland hyperplasia. It has been suggested that hyperplastic glands associated with a history of prolonged hypocalcemia could become adenomatous (so-called "tertiary" hyperparathyroidism), although this has never been proved definitively. This syndrome has been described in patients with secondary hyperparathyroidism due to chronic renal failure, and it is probably a manifestation of persistent parathyroid cell secretory mass rather than a change in the pathology of the tissue from hyperplasia to an adenoma. After renal transplantation, patients may develop persistent hypercalcemia, which lasts for some months until the parathyroid glands slowly involute. Hypercalcemia in these circumstances does not necessarily mean a change in the underlying parathyroid gland histopathology.

Other factors have been implicated in the pathophysiology of primary hyperparathyroidism.

A history of previous irradiation is present in some patients. Several centers have suggested that up to one-third of patients have a previous history of neck irradiation (Katz and Braunstein 1983), and that a significant number of these patients who have received neck irradiation (up to 10%) are at risk from the development of primary hyperparathyroidism (Katz and Braunstein 1983). However, irradiation of the neck was frequently practiced in children after the Second World War, usually because of tonsillar problems, and so older patients with primary hyperparathyroidism might be expected often to have a history of neck irradiation, whether or not there is a direct link. Many secretagogues for PTH (other than calcium deficiency) have been described from both in vitro and in vivo experiments, but there is no current evidence that any of these factors is responsible for causing parathyroid adenomas to develop.

In primary hyperparathyroidism, serum concentrations of PTH are increased in the presence of hypercalcemia. This means that there is an abnormality in the normal mechanism by which extracellular fluid calcium controls PTH secretion by the parathyroid cells. On the other hand, a relationship between serum calcium and PTH secretion does persist since parathyroid hormone secretion from abnormal parathyroid tissue, either adenomatous or hyperplastic, may be altered by changes in the extracellular fluid calcium. It has long been argued whether in patients with primary hyperparathyroidism there is a change in the set-point in the abnormal parathyroid tissue whereby the parathyroid cell recognizes the extracellular fluid calcium in response to it, or, as appears more likely in many cases, the set-point for PTH release in response to serum calcium is normal, but the increased mass of cells associated with primary hyperparathyroidism by itself is sufficient to cause increased circulating PTH. Even in normal parathyroid cells, an increase in extracellular fluid calcium cannot completely suppress parathyroid hormone secretion. Thus, when there is a marked increase in the total secretory mass of parathyroid tissue, this basal nonsuppressible PTH may be sufficient to cause the clinical features of primary hyperparathyroidism irrespective of the plasma calcium.

This notion is supported by the report of Khosla et al (1993). These workers found that in both patients with familial benign hypocalciuric hypercalcemia and patients with primary hyperparathyroidism, the set-point is shifted to the right and superimposable. However, in patients with FHH, the PTH is suppressible at higher ionized calcium concentrations. In primary hyperparathyroidism, the set-point is also shifted to the right, but is associated with varying degrees of PTH secretion that is nonsuppressible by calcium, presumably related to increased parathyroid gland mass due to tumor.

Pathophysiology of familial multiple endocrine neoplasia Type 1 (FMEN-1)

Familial multiple endocrine neoplasia Type 1 is associated with a generalized parathyroid cell stimulation, leading to generalized glandular enlargement, which is polyclonal in nature. However, it is now well documented that monoclonal elements also occur in these lesions. The situation is thus very complex. It appears likely that both extrinsic growth factors as well as inherent cellular and genetic abnormalities may contribute to the neoplastic condition.

Parathyroid growth factor associated with FMEN-1

A growth factor that stimulates the replication of parathyroid gland cells freshly dispersed in culture has been identified in the serum of patients with MEN Type 1 (Brandi et al 1986, 1988). Although this factor has been linked to parathyroid gland hyperplasia in the FMEN-1 syndrome, it is apparently not present in most other patients with parathyroid gland hyperplasia. This factor may be related to the expanding fibroblast growth factor (FGF) family. The target cell appears to be the endothelial cell of the parathyroid gland vasculature. The parathyroid gland does not appear to be the source of this factor, since total parathyroid gland ablation does not remove it from the serum. The possible relationship of this parathyroid stimulant to the FGF family is interesting from two points of view. First, this factor stimulates parathyroid endothelial cells and the FGFs are powerful endothelial cell stimulants. Secondly, it suggests a possible relationship to the INT-2 oncogene. The predicted product of the INT-2 oncogene is homologous to basic FGF and recent findings suggest that the mutant gene in FMEN-1 is localized to the pericentric region of chromosome 11, a region that is near INT-2 (Peters et al 1983).

Tumor suppressor gene

Parathyroid tumors in more than half of the patients with FMEN-1 have a loss of chromosomal material from chromosome 11 (Larsson et al 1988; Friedman et al 1989; Thakker et al 1989; Bystrom et al 1990; Radford et al 1990). Moreover, studies with linkage analysis have shown that the FMEN-1 gene can be linked to 11q12-q13 in kindreds with FMEN-1 (Bale et al 1989; Nakamura et al 1989). The situation is thus very confusing. It appears that the parathyroid lesions in FMEN-1 may have both polyclonal and monoclonal components. The polyclonal component may be related to the parathyroid gland growth factor found in the serum and the monoclonal component to genetic abnormalities in chromosome 11, possibly involving loss of a tumor suppressor gene. How or whether the extrinsic growth factor and the intrinsic genetic defect are associated remains unknown. One possibility is that the growth factor causes polyclonal hyperplasia, and later somatic mutation or chromosomal loss involving the critical gene locus for FMEN-1 leads to a superimposed monoclonal lesion.

Familial multiple endocrine neoplasia Type 2 (FMEN-2)

Parathyroid hyperplasia is the least common of the major components of the FMEN-2 syndromes, occurring in less than 10% of patients.

With linkage analysis studies utilizing restriction fragment length polymorphism, several groups have located the abnormality in FMEN-2A near the centromere on chromosome 10 (Gagel 1989). Other conditions related to neural crest differentiation, including familial medullary thyroid carcinoma (FMTC), without clinical manifestations of other features of the MEN-2 syndrome, but associated with Hirschsprung's disease, also arise from abnormalities of cells derived from the embyronic neural crest, which share the same genetic locus. The mechanism responsible may be similar to that demonstrated in hereditary retinoblastoma, with a "two-hit" process characterized by an inherited mutation in the first allele and a somatic mutation resulting in deletion of a second allele.

Recently, the RET proto-oncogene has been implicated in FMEN-2 syndromes. This proto-oncogene is a transmembrane tyrosine kinase expressed in medullary thyroid carcinoma and in pheochromocytomas. There were 20 out of 23 patients found to have missense mutations of this gene (Mulligan et al 1993), and in 19 of the 20 the same cysteine residue was affected, suggesting that this point mutation is the initiating event. This point mutation has not so far been detected in patients with MEN-2 associated with ganglioneuromatosis of the intestine and Marfanoid habitus, although these patients have also been mapped to the 10q11.2 region (Gardner et al 1993). The clinical phenotype can be predicted from knowledge of the location of the RET mutation (Hofstra et al 1994). This knowledge is now being used for children at risk within the first 2 years of life and for assigning gene carrier status to selected patients with near certainty.

Mode of presentation

The mode of presentation of primary hyperparathyroidism has changed dramatically in the last 20 years (Tables 9.1 and 9.2). Prior to that time, the most common modes of presentation were with recurrent renal stones or occasionally with the form of bone disease characteristic of primary hyperparathyroidism, namely osteitis fibrosa cystica. In most surveys prior to 1980, more than 75% of patients presented in this manner. However, with the advent of the autoanalyzer and routine measurement of serum calcium with other electrolytes, primary hyperparathyroidism is now diagnosed in the majority of patients as asymptomatic hypercalcemia (Figure 9.2). Most patients have blood drawn for reasons other than any suspicion of an abnormality of calcium metabolism, and hypercalcemia is found expectedly. The reasons for clinical presentation in an unselected series of 111 patients are shown in Table 9.2. About 10% of patients have more severe primary hyperparathyroidism characterized by serum calcium measurements greater than 12 mg/dl and urine calcium greater than 400 mg/g creatinine. A subset of these patients may have severe bone disease accompanied by anemia, increased erythrocyte sedimentation rate and weight loss.

Table 9.1 Age- and sex-distribution of primary hyperparathyroidism at time of presentation.[a]

Age (years)	Hellstrom and Ivemark (1962) (Sweden) 138 patients		Muller (1969) (Netherlands) 208 patients		Mallette et al (1974) (USA) 57 patients		Mundy et al (1980) 111 patients	
	Males	Females	Males	Females	Males	Females	Males	Females
0–19	1	1	2	1	—	2	—	—
20–29	1	4	8	5	—	—	—	2
30–39	8	9	7	8	9	4	—	—
40–49	8	21	10	13	14	18	2	5
50–59	7	23	8	19	9	23	5	11
60–69	3	12	4	14	9	9	6	6
70–79	—	2	1	2	2	4	8	38
>80	—	—	—	1	—	—	—	17
	28	72	39	64	42	58	21	79

[a] The numbers given are percentages of the total numbers of patients in that particular study. The percentages are rounded to the nearest whole number.

Table 9.2 Mode of presentation of primary hyperparathyroidism.[a]

Presentation	Hellstrom and Ivemark (1962) (Sweden) 138 patients	McGeown (1969) (UK) 177 patients	Watson (1974) (UK) 100 patients	Wang (1971) (US) 431 patients	Mundy et al (1980) 111 patients
Accidental (no symptoms)	—	3	14	1	57
Renal (stones or nephrocalcinosis)	79	72	47	55	7
Bone disease	20	17	13	21	—
Psychiatric disorder	—	—	2	1	5
Acute hypercalcemic syndrome	—	2	—	2	14
Gastrointestinal symptoms	—	4	12	12	4
Symptoms of hypercalcemia (lethargy, polyuria, etc)	—	2	8	4	8
Hypertension	1	—	4	1	5

[a] The numbers given are percentages of the total numbers of patients in that particular study. The percentages are rounded to the nearest whole number.

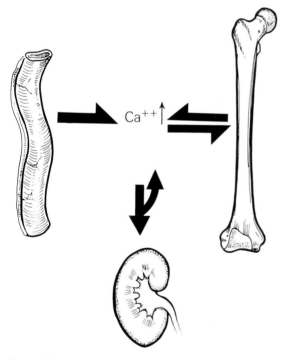

Figure 9.2

Pattern of abnormalities in calcium homeostasis in patients with primary hyperparathyroidism. These patients show increased bone turnover, increased renal tubular reabsorption of calcium, and increased gut absorption of calcium. The increase in the absorption of calcium from the gut is mediated by 1,25-dihydroxyvitamin D_3, which is produced in the renal tubules in response to PTH excess.

About 5–10% of patients with recurrent calcium-containing renal stones have primary hyperparathyroidism. For reasons that are not clearly understood, these patients usually do not have the bone disease of primary hyperparathyroidism (Albright and Reifenstein 1948; Hellstrom and Ivemark 1962). The renal calculi are usually calcium oxalate, calcium phosphate or mixed stones (Melick and Henneman 1958). Although it appears likely that recurrent renal stones are related to hypercalciuria in primary hyperparathyroidism, the precise reasons why these patients are particularly prone to recurrent renal stones are not clear. Moreover, although it seems that successful treatment (surgery) for primary hyperparathyroidism should affect the course of renal stone disease beneficially, this has not been well documented.

Patients with severe primary hyperparathyroidism, particularly those with parathyroid carcinoma, are also prone to nephrocalcinosis and renal failure. This occurs as a consequence of precipitation of calcium and phosphate in the renal tubular epithelium and in the renal interstitial tissue, and occurs more frequently in patients with osteitis fibrosa cystica.

Patients with primary hyperparathyroidism have a mild form of renal tubular acidosis due to the effects of parathyroid hormone on the proximal tubules of the kidneys to inhibit bicarbonate reabsorption. These patients also may have phosphaturia, aminoaciduria and glycosuria. In addition, hypercalcemia impairs the effects of

Figure 9.3

Radiograph of the clavicle of a patient with primary hyperparathyroidism showing the characteristic subperiosteal resorption and cystic destruction (arrow). These changes should be improved following successful parathyroid surgery. (Kindly supplied by Dr John Bilezikian.)

antidiuretic hormone on the distal tubules and collecting ducts of the kidney to cause water reabsorption, leading to inability to concentrate the urine (in effect, a form of nephrogenic diabetes insipidus).

Bone disease

Although the most common skeletal abnormality in patients with primary hyperparathyroidism is osteopenia (Dauphine et al 1975; Genant et al 1975), this is not apparent in many patients presenting with this disease in the 1990s. When osteopenia does occur, it may have the same radiologic appearance as osteoporosis. Since primary hyperparathyroidism most frequently presents in patients who are predisposed to postmenopausal osteoporosis, it may be hard to distinguish these two common conditions.

Primary hyperparathyroidism was first recognized as a characteristic and severe form of crippling bone disease known as osteitis fibrosa cystica (Mandl 1926; Bauer et al 1930; Albright and Reifenstein 1948) (Figures 9.3 and 9.4). This disease is characterized by a peculiar form of bone destruction associated with increased osteoclastic bone resorption (Figure 9.5) affecting not only endosteal bone surfaces but also periosteal surfaces. This is particularly marked in the acromio-clavicular joint, at the symphysis pubis, and in the sacroiliac joints. Subperiosteal resorption is seen most frequently along the radial

Figure 9.4

Radiograph of the skull with primary hyperparathyroidism, showing the "salt-and-pepper" skull, with mottling due to increased osteoclastic bone resorption. (Kindly supplied by Dr John Bilezikian.)

aspect of middle phalanges in the posterior–anterior view, and is frequently associated with erosions of the terminal tufts of the phalanges. The skull may have a mottled "salt and pepper" appearance. The distal thirds of the clavicles may show a distinctive tapering due to bone resorption. This type of bone resorption is frequently associated with cystic lesions known as brown tumors. Brown tumors are filled with osteoclasts and new woven bone, which is poorly mineralized. They usually resolve when primary hyperparathyroidism is surgically corrected. One sign frequently looked for in patients with bone disease and primary hyperparathyroidism is loss of the laminadura of the teeth. This occurs in most patients who have osteitis fibrosa cystica.

Primary hyperparathyroidism has been claimed recently (Silverberg et al 1995; Silverberg and Bilezikian 1996) to provide relative protection against trabecular bone loss. This can be distinguished by careful bone mineral density measurements of the axial skeleton, particularly at the hip and the forearm, which give the best measurement of cortical bone. The most simple interpretation of these results is that states of primary hyperparathyroidism are relatively catabolic for cortical bone and anabolic for vertebral bone. It is still not entirely clear what these findings mean with respect to the changes in bone remodeling that occur in this disease, or whether all patients can be categorized in this way.

Occasionally, patients with primary hyperparathyroidism may have osteosclerosis. This occurs particularly in the vertebrae, and is even more frequent in

Figure 9.5

Scanning electron microscopy of bone surface of a patient with primary hyperparathyroidism, showing characteristic resorption lacunae formed by osteoclasts stimulated by parathyroid hormone. (Kindly supplied by Professor Alan Boyde.)

patients with secondary hyperparathyroidism associated with chronic renal failure.

Patients with primary hyperparathyroidism almost always have an increase in bone turnover (Figure 9.6). There is an increase in osteoclastic bone resorption associated with new bone formation. The effects of parathyroid hormone on osteoblasts are extremely complex. In some patients, there is a primary increase in bone formation and marrow fibrosis. Whether this is a direct effect or indirect due to the production of local growth regulatory factors such as insulin-like growth factor I and transforming growth factor β in response to parathyroid hormone has not been adequately resolved.

Gastrointestinal symptoms

Gastrointestinal symptoms are common in patients with mild primary hyperparathyroidism. These include symptoms that may be related to hypercalcemia such as loss of appetite, anorexia, nausea and occasionally vomiting, but also may be symptoms caused by coexistent peptic ulcer disease and, in occasional patients, pancreatitis. Some patients have constipation. Primary hyper-

Figure 9.6

Histologic sections of bone in a patient with primary hyperparathyroidism and osteitis fibrosa cystica. Note evidence of increased osteoclastic bone resorption (curved arrow), with marrow fibrosis and increased osteoblast activity (straight arrow).

parathyroidism is probably not related directly to the peptic ulcer disease, but the two conditions may occur together in patients who have multiple endocrine neoplasia Type 1 associated with Zollinger–Ellinson syndrome. In other patients with peptic ulcer disease, this may represent coincidental coexistence of two common conditions. In contrast, there is a clear association between primary hyperparathyroidism and acute pancreatitis. In occasional patients, acute pancreatitis is the presenting clinical feature (Cope et al 1957). It is directly related to the severity of the hypercalcemia, although it has been seen much more commonly in patients with primary hyperparathyroidism than patients with other forms of hypercalcemia, but the mechanism is unknown. However, in all patients with acute pancreatitis who have an elevated or even normal serum calcium, underlying primary hyperparathyroidism should be suspected. Patients with acute pancreatitis without any parathyroid abnormality usually present with hypocalcemia.

Neuromuscular and neuropsychiatric features

A whole spectrum of neuropsychiatric symptoms may be found in patients with primary hyperparathyroidism. These include lethargy, confusion, impaired mentation, emotional lability, depression, personality changes, psychomotor retardation, memory impairment, and occasional overt psychosis. Patients with primary hyperparathyroidism may recognize that they suffered from some of these milder symptoms after having successful surgery. In particular, people who have difficulty in coping with life situations may experience a greater ability to deal with the stress of living once a parathyroid adenoma has been successfully removed.

A few patients with primary hyperparathyroidism have been described with a specific neuromyopathic disorder (Patten et al 1974). This condition is characterized by atrophy of Type II muscle fibers, with microscopic findings characterized by denervation without accompanying inflammatory changes. The cause is unknown. The clinical features are weakness and easy fatigu-ability associated with atrophy of proximal muscle groups, particularly involving the lower extremity.

Occasional patients with primary hyperparathyroidism have articular changes. They may develop chondrocalcinosis, gout and degenerative joint disease. Occasionally, tendon avulsion has been described and rarely ankylosing spondylitis has been linked to primary hyperparathyroidism.

Although hypertension is frequently present in patients with primary hyperparathyroidism, particularly older patients, it is not clear whether it is directly related to primary hyperparathyroidism. This relationship may be similar to that seen with peptic ulcer disease and primary hyperparathyroidism. Hypertension in a patient with primary hyperparathyroidism may represent coincident occurrence of two common conditions.

Patients with hypercalcemia of any cause may experience pruritus, occasionally associated with skin necrosis due to precipitation of calcium and phosphate in the subcutaneous and epidermal tissues. Similarly, precipitation of calcium and phosphate crystals in the cornea may lead to band keratopathy. This can be seen microscopically or under the slit lamp. It is more common in conditions associated with phosphate retention such as vitamin D intoxication and sarcoidosis, and is frequently associated with renal failure.

Diagnosis of primary hyperparathyroidism

Since most patients with primary hyperparathyroidism have hypercalcemia at the time of presentation, the diagnosis of primary hyperparathyroidism usually means exclusion of other causes of hypercalcemia. (However, patients with primary hyperparathyroidism frequently undergo fluctuations in serum calcium. The serum calcium is normal on some occasions in at least 20% of patients with the condition.) Although the list of causes of hypercalcemia is long, 90% have either primary hyperparathyroidism or malignant disease (see Chapter 6). In the general population, primary hyperparathyroidism is more common than malignant disease as a cause of hypercalcemia. In contrast, in hospitalized populations, cancer is a more common cause.

There are features that certainly point to primary hyperparathyroidism as the diagnosis. Patients who are known to have been mildly hypercalcemic for a long period of time are much more likely to have primary hyperparathyroidism than malignancy, since the majority of patients with hypercalcemia of malignancy have advanced disease. The majority of patients with primary hyperparathyroidism are postmenopausal women, who are relatively asymptomatic. Primary hyperparathyroidism should certainly be suspected when hypercalcemia occurs in this situation. However, the disease may be difficult to diagnose, and particularly in those patients who have underlying cancer. There are numerous reported cases of both diseases occurring concurrently.

The majority of patients with primary hyperparathyroidism have normal renal function and a mild hyperchloremic acidosis (Wills and McGowan 1964). This is accompanied by phosphaturia and hypophosphatemia. In patients who have hypophosphatemia and a serum chloride greater than 102 mM/l, primary hyperparathyroidism is by far the most likely diagnosis. The majority of patients with hypercalcemia of malignancy have a serum chloride of less than 98 mM/l.

The definitive test for primary hyperparathyroidism is the PTH radioimmunoassay. PTH radioimmunoassays have improved dramatically in recent years with the advent of the two-site or immunoradiometric assays (IRMA), which represent a significant advance (Nussbaum et al 1987; Silverberg et al 1989). Patients with primary hyperparathyroidism almost always have an increase in serum intact PTH as measured by the two-site IRMA, and the majority of patients with nonparathyroid malignancy have suppressed PTH (Figure 9.7). Suppression of serum PTH by this test indicates strongly that hypercalcemia is not

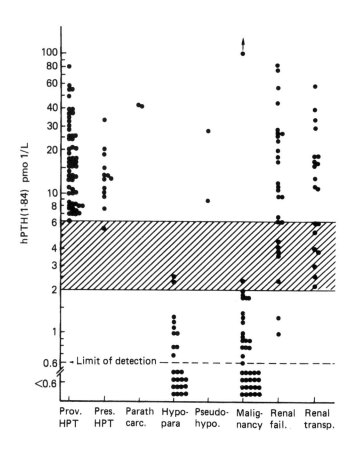

Figure 9.7

Parathyroid hormone concentrations in patients with the hypercalcemia of malignancy, primary hyperparathyroidism and other disorders of calcium homeostasis. (Reproduced from Blind et al (1988).)

PTH-mediated. Moreover, this test is less affected by changes in renal function than other radioimmunoassays that measure C-terminal, N-terminal or midregion areas of the parathyroid hormone molecule.

Bone markers are abnormal in many patients with primary hyperparathyroidism and correlate with states of bone turnover. Markers of both bone resorption (collagen crosslinks) and bone formation (osteocalcin, alkaline phosphatase) are increased proportionately.

Management of patients with primary hyperparathyroidism

One of the most difficult issues in the management of patients with primary hyperparathyroidism is what to do with the asymptomatic patient. Many asymptomatic patients may remain unchanged for many years. The problem is that there is no way of accurately predicting the natural course of the disease, and which patients will later develop complications that would be better avoided by prophylactic surgery. In a large prospective study from the Mayo Clinic of 134 patients, 50% of asymptomatic patients had no change in their clinical state over 5 years (Scholz and Purnell 1981). However, almost half of the rest of the patients eventually required surgery and the other half were lost to follow-up. For these reasons, the indications for treatment are arbitrary and are greatly influenced by key factors such as the availability of a competent surgeon experienced in parathyroid surgery, the medical condition of the patient and the ease of follow-up management. If hyperplasia is suspected, then surgery should be avoided if possible. An NIH Consensus Conference was held on the diagnosis and management of the patient with asymptomatic primary hyperparathyroidism (NIH 1990, 1991). These patients were defined as patients with primary hyperparathyroidism without symptoms or signs commonly attributable to the disease. Without data and with advice from a series of selected experts, this conference concluded that decisions about surgical and medical management could be made only on clinical judgement and a case-by-case basis. Moreover, there were no specific clinical signs or laboratory criteria that could be used to identify patients who were likely to develop complications if not treated surgically. Recommendations were that indications for surgery should be a markedly elevated serum calcium (>11.5 mg/dl), a previous episode of life-threatening hypercalcemia, reduced creatinine clearance, the presence of kidney stones, a markedly elevated 24-hour urine calcium excretion, or a reduced bone mass.

When cortical bone density measured at the forearm is greater than 2 standard deviations below the mean value for age-matched individuals, neck exploration may be indicated and should be considered seriously. However, there is no data to document that these recommendations for surgery are absolute, and they should be regarded as guidelines rather than firm indications. Moreover, there are other considerations such as the wishes of the patient (some patients may wish surgery, some may prefer to avoid it), the age of the patient, the presence of coexistent illness and, probably most importantly, the availability of a skilled and experienced surgeon.

However, some argue that essentially everybody with primary hyperparathyroidism should have surgery provided their medical condition permits surgical intervention. The key issue may be whether the patient has a solitary adenoma (85%) or multiple gland disease, and this is impossible to know prior to surgery in most patients. In the hands of an experienced surgeon (surgeons who are removing at least 10 parathyroid adenomas per year), the surgical treatment of solitary adenoma should be 100% successful. This is the experience at centers of excellence in the management of this disease. However, the success rate falls in every surgeon's hands when more than one gland is involved, and particularly if the surgeon is not performing this operation frequently. For patients who require a second operation because of persistent or recurrent hyperparathyroidism, the surgical cure rate is still approximately 90% with state-of-the-art localization techniques and experienced endocrine surgeons. About 25% of these patients will be left with persistent hypocalcemia.

If it is decided that the patient should not have surgery, then a reasonable plan of management must be designed to follow the patient carefully and watch for any change in clinical state that will require surgery. A reasonable approach is measurement of serum calcium every 6 months and a more careful evaluation of the patient including abdominal radiographs, measurement of urine calcium excretion, creatinine clearance, a bone mass measurement quantitative digital radiography every 1–2 years, with particular attention to cortical bone, and abdominal radiographs to look for renal stones. Patients should be asked to avoid dehydration, immobilization and diuretics, all of which could exacerbate mild hypercalcemia.

Medical therapy

Medical therapy for the treatment of primary hyperparathyroidism is not entirely satisfactory. Available agents include oral phosphate, bisphosphonates, estrogen, plicamycin and calcitonin, and glucocorticoids. Estrogens and progestins may be used successfully in postmenopausal women. This was first shown by Gallagher and Nordin (1972), but has been confirmed by Marcus et al (1984), and Selby and Peacock (1986). The mechanism by which estrogen lowers the serum calcium in these patients is unknown. Bisphosphonates have also been used successively (Shane et al 1981). However, they are unlikely to be effective long term, even when the more potent new bisphosphonates such as risedronate are used (Reasner et al 1993). Our experience is that they are unlikely to have long-term beneficial effects of keeping the serum calcium within the normal range for prolonged periods. Oral phosphate has been used in some patients for periods of years in controlling the serum calcium (Mundy et al 1983), but there is an inevitable risk of renal stones and even of nephrocalcinosis unless the therapy is very carefully monitored and renal function followed. Calcitonin and glucocorticoids or plicamycin should only be used in patients where other agents are not satisfactory, or where medical therapy is required and nothing else is available, such as parathyroid carcinoma (Singer et al 1970; Au 1975; Binstock and Mundy 1980). The identification of the calcium sensor in the parathyroid glands has coincided with the development of drugs that mimic the actions of calcium on this receptor to block PTH secretion. One of these is NPS-R-568 and encouraging results have been reported in limited numbers of patients with primary hyperparathyroidism (Silverberg et al 1996).

Parathyroid gland localization (for review, see Turton and Miller 1996)

A physician managing a patient with primary hyperparathyroidism now has a choice of a number of localization procedures. These include ultrasound, QCT, magnetic resonance imaging, sestamibi scanning and arteriography or venography with venous sampling. Localization is indicated for the following reasons: (1) reoperation on a previously explored neck; (2) previous thyroid surgery; and (3) urgent hypercalcemia (where the gland may be visualized). The success rate with these procedures is in the range of 80–90%, possibly a little more with sestamibi scanning, although experience is still accumulating. This is not as effective as an experienced surgeon, who will localize abnormal parathyroid adenoma in 95–99% of patients. Preoperative localization is not a substitute for an experienced surgeon, and is not a reason not to explore the whole neck. There is no evidence that it significantly reduces the operation time or leads to fewer complications. The costs of localization procedures are significant. Ultrasound costs about US $300 and MRI US $1000, and sestamibi and QCT cost somewhere in between.

Ultrasound is probably the simplest and cheapest procedure. High resolution equipment is required and it is frequently used together with aspiration biopsy (using cytology or radioimmunoassay). Although the sensitivity is approximately 70% without prior surgery, it is markedly improved to over 90% when it is combined with either MRI or sestamibi scanning. An adenoma is characterized by decreased echogenicity, but hyperplasia is very difficult to diagnose.

The greatest advancement in this field over the last 10 years is sestamibi scanning, and there have been a myriad of reports, mostly anecdotal and uncontrolled, extolling the virtues of this technique over the past 3 years. It detects the solitary parathyroid adenoma in more than 90% of patients. However, experience is still limited and early results with every new technique are always reported with superlatives. It has replaced thallium technetium scanning, which is now not indicated. Sestamibi is a cardiac imaging agent and can be used in two ways, either as the single agent "double-phase" technique with an early delayed view, or with simultaneous thyroid scanning and subtraction. Sestamibi is particularly useful in the localization of ectopic glands including those in the mediastinum.

For those patients in whom preoperative localization is indicated but noninvasive localization studies have failed to detect the site of the abnormal gland, arteriography and venous sampling may be performed. Arteriography is helpful in approximately 40% of patients and venous sampling in over 90%. However, arteriography provides more precise localization of an adenoma.

Surgery for primary hyperparathyroidism

There remains considerable variability in the surgical approach to patients with primary hyperparathyroidism from center to center. The surgical approach may depend on the level of suspicion that multigland disease is present, although in most patients this remains unknown until the time of surgery (and, in some, even after that). One change from over 20 years ago is that most of the leading surgeons in this field now recommend that all four glands should be identified and biopsied. Enlarged or abnormal glands should be removed, and normal glands left. If all four parathyroid glands are enlarged, then $3\frac{1}{2}$ glands should be removed and either the residual tissue left in the neck or engrafted intramuscularly at an ectopic site.

In patients who are treated surgically, the postoperative course is usually very simple. Patients may leave the hospital the following day. In patients with solitary adenomas, essentially 100% should be cured if treated by an experienced surgeon. In more complicated situations such as multigland disease, some patients may develop hypocalcemia due to parathyroid damage or recurrent hypercalcemia. Patients should be seen every 6–12 months following surgery with repeat measurements of serum calcium and parathyroid hormone. Bone mineral density can be performed annually. Occasional patients develop the "hungry bone" syndrome, particularly if they have had severe bone disease and hypercalcemia preceding surgery. These patients can be managed by calcium and vitamin D therapy. In those patients in whom it is anticipated, vitamin D therapy can be begun from the time of surgery.

The intra- and postoperative management of patients with primary hyperparathyroidism is a complex subject beyond the scope of this text. It is considered in detail elsewhere (Mundy 1990).

References

Albright F, Reifenstein EC (1948) *The parathyroid glands and metabolic bone disease: selected studies* (Williams and Wilkins: Baltimore).

Arnold A, Kim HG (1989) Clonal loss of one chromosome 11 in a parathyroid adenoma, *J Clin Endocrinol Metab* **69**: 496–9.

Arnold A, Staunton CE, Kim HG et al (1988) Monoclonality and abnormal parathyroid hormone genes in parathyroid adenomas, *N Engl J Med* **318**: 658–62.

Arnold A, Kim HG, Gaz RD et al (1989) Molecular cloning and chromosomal mapping of DNA rearranged with the parathyroid hormone gene in a parathyroid adenoma, *J Clin Invest* **83**: 2034–40.

Arnold A, Brown MF, Urena P et al (1995) Monoclonality of parathyroid tumors in chronic renal failure and in primary parathyroid hyperplasia, *J Clin Invest* **95**: 2047–53.

Au WYW (1975) Calcitonin treatment of hypercalcemia due to parathyroid carcinoma—synergistic effect of prednisone on long-term treatment of hypercalcemia, *Arch Intern Med* **135**: 1594–7.

Bale SJ, Bale AE, Stewart K et al (1989) Linkage analysis of multiple endocrine neoplasia type 1 with int2 and other markers on chromosome 11, *Genomics* **4**: 320–2.

Bauer W, Albright F, Aub JC (1930) A case of osteitis fibrosa cystica (osteomalacia?) with evidence of hyperactivity of the parathyroid bodies, *J Clin Invest* **8**: 229–48.

Binstock ML, Mundy GR (1980) Effects of calcitonin and glucocorticoids in combination in hypercalcemia of malignancy, *Ann Intern Med* **93**: 269–72.

Blind E, Schmidt-Gayk H, Scharla S et al (1988) Two-site assay of intact parathyroid hormone in the investigation of primary hyperparathyroidisim and other disorders of calcium metabolism compared with a midregion assay, *J Clin Endocrinol Metab* **67**: 353–60.

Boonstra CE, Jackson CE (1971) Serum calcium survey for hyperparathyroidism, *Am J Clin Pathol* **55**: 523–6.

Brandi ML, Aurbach GD, Fitzpatrick LA et al (1986) Parathyroid mitogenic activity in plasma from patients with familial multiple endocrine neoplasia Type 1, *N Engl J Med* **314**: 1287–93.

Brandi ML, Marx SJ, Aurbach GD et al (1988) Familial multiple endocrine neoplasia type 1: a new look at pathophysiology, *Endocrinol Rev* **8**: 341–405.

Bystrom C, Larsson C, Blomberg C et al (1990) Localization of the MEN1 gene to a small region within chromosome 11q13 by deletion mapping in tumors, *Proc Natl Acad Sci U S A* **87**: 1968–72.

Cope O, Culver PJ, Mixter CG et al (1957) Pancreatis, diagnostic clue to hyperparathyroidism, *Ann Surg* **145**: 857–63.

Cryns VL, Thor A, Xu HJ et al (1994) Loss of the retinoblastoma tumor-suppressor gene in parathyroid carcinoma, *N Engl J Med* **330**: 757–61.

Dauphine RT, Riggs BL, Scholz DA (1975) Back pain and vertebral crush fractures: an unemphasized mode of presentation for primary hyperparathyroidism, *Ann Intern Med* **83**: 365–7.

Friedman E, Sakaguchi K, Bale AE et al (1989) Clonality of parathyroid tumors in familial multiple endocrine neoplasia type 1, *N Engl J Med* **321**: 213–18.

Friedman E, Bale AE, Marx SJ et al (1990) Genetic abnormalities in sporadic parathyroid adenomas, *J Clin Endocrinol Metab* **71**: 293–7.

Gagel R (1989) The pathogenesis and clinical course of multiple endocrine neoplasia, type 2a. In: Kleerekoper M, Krane SM, eds, *Clinical disorders of bone and mineral metabolism* (Mary Ann Liebert: New York) 563–71.

Gallagher JC, Nordin BEC (1972) Treatment with oestrogens of primary hyperparathyroidism in postmenopausal women, *Lancet* **i**: 503–7.

Gardner E, Papi L, Easton DF et al (1993) Genetic linkage studies map the multiple endocrine neoplasia Type-2 Loci to a small interval on chromosome 10q11.2, *Hum Mol Genet* **2**: 241–6.

Genant HK, Baron JM, Struas FH et al (1975) Osteosclerosis in primary hyperparathyroidism, *Am J Med* **59**: 104–13.

Heath H III, Hodgson SF, Kennedy MA (1980) Primary hyperparathyroidism: incidence, morbidity, and potential economic impact in a community, *N Engl J Med* **302**: 189–93.

Hellstrom J, Ivemark BI (1962) Primary hyperparathyroidism, *Acta Chir Scand* **294** (Suppl): 1–133.

Hofstra RM, Landsvater RM, Ceccherini I et al (1994) A mutation in the RET proto-oncogene associated with multiple endocrine neoplasia type 2B and sporadic medullary thyroid carcinoma, *Nature* **367**: 375–6.

Katz A, Braunstein GD (1983) Clinical, biochemical, and pathologic features of radiation-associated hyperparathyroidism, *Arch Intern Med* **143**: 79–82.

Khosla S, Ebeling PR, Firek AF et al (1993) Calcium infusion suggests a set-point abnormality of parathyroid gland function in familial benign hypercalcemia and more complex disturbances in primary hyperparathyroidism, *J Clin Endocrinol Metab* **76**: 715–20.

Larsson C, Skogseid B, Oberg K et al (1988) Multiple endocrine neoplasia type 1 gene maps to chromosome 11 and is lost in insulinoma, *Nature* **332**: 85–7.

LeBoff MS, Shoback D, Brown EM et al (1985) Regulation of parathyroid hormone release and cytosolic calcium by extracellular calcium in dispersed and cultured bovine and pathological human parathyroid cells, *J Clin Invest* **75**: 49–57.

Mallette LE, Bilezikian JP, Heath DA et al (1974) Primary hyperparathyroidism: clinical and biochemical features, *Medicine* **53**: 127–46.

Mandl F (1926) Therapeutischer Versuch bei einem Falle von Ostitis Fibrosa Generalisata mittels Exstirpation eines Epithelkorperchen Tumors, *Zentralbl Chir* **53**: 260–4.

Marcus R, Madvig P, Crim M et al (1984) Conjugated estrogens in the treatment of postmenopausal women with hyperparathyroidism, *Ann Intern Med* **100**: 633–40.

McGeown MG (1969) Sex, age and hyperparathyroidism, *Lancet* **i**: 887–8.

Melick RA, Henneman PH (1958) Clinical and laboratory studies of 207 consecutive patients in a kidney stone clinic, *N Engl J Med* **259**: 307–14.

Muller H (1969) Sex, age and hyperparathyroidism, *Lancet* **i**: 449–50.

Mulligan LM, Kwok JB, Healey CS et al (1993) Germ-line mutations of the RET proto-oncogene in multiple endocrine neoplasia type 2A, *Nature* **363**: 458–60.

Mundy GR (1990) *Calcium homeostasis: hypercalcemia and hypocalcemia*, 2nd edn (Martin Dunitz: London).

Mundy GR, Cove DH, Fisken R (1980) Primary hyperparathyroidism: changes in the pattern of clinical presentation, *Lancet* **i**: 1317–20.

Mundy GR, Wilkinson R, Heath DA (1983) Comparative study of available medical therapy for hypercalcemia of malignancy, *Am J Med* **74**: 421–32.

Nakamura Y, Larsson C, Julier C et al (1989) Localization of the genetic defect in multiple endocrine neoplasia type 1 within a small region of chromosome 11, *Am J Hum Genet* **44**: 751–5.

NIH (1990) NIH Consensus Development Conference Statement: Diagnosis and management of asymptomatic primary hyperparathyroidism, *Ann Int Med* **114**: 593–7.

NIH (1991) NIH Consensus Development Conference Statement: Diagnosis and management of asymptomatic primary hyperparathyroidism, *J Bone Miner Res* **6** (Suppl 2): S9–S13.

Nussbaum SR, Zahradnik RJ, Lavigne JR et al (1987) Highly sensitive two-site immunoradiometric assay of parathyrin, and its clinical utility in evaluating patients with hypercalcemia, *Clin Chem* **33**: 1364–7.

Patten BM, Bilezikian JP, Mallette LE et al (1974) Neuromuscular disease in primary hyperparathyroidism, *Ann Intern Med* **80**: 182–93.

Peters G, Brookes S, Smith R et al (1983) Tumorigenesis by mouse mammary tumor virus: evidence for a common region for provirus integration in mammary tumors, *Cell* **33**: 369–77.

Radford DM, Ashley SW, Wells SA et al (1990) Loss of heterozygosity of markers on chromosome 11 in tumors from patients with multiple endocrine neoplasia syndrome type 1, *Cancer Res* **50**: 6529–33.

Reasner CA, Stone MD, Hosking DH et al (1993) Acute changes in calcium homeostasis during treatment of primary hyperparathyroidism with risedronate, *J Clin Endocrinol Metab* **77**: 1067–71.

Rosenberg CL, Kim HG, Shows TB et al (1991) Rearrangement and overexpression of D11S287E, a candidate oncogene on chromosome 11q13in benign parathyroid tumors, *Oncogene* **6**: 449–54.

Scholz DA, Purnell DC (1981) Asymptomatic primary hyperparathyroidism. 10 year prospective study, *Mayo Clinic Proc* **56**: 473–8.

Selby PL, Peacock M (1986) Ethinyl estradiol and norethindrone in the treatment of primary hyperparathyroidism in postmenopausal women, *N Engl J Med* **314**: 1481–5.

Shane E, Bilezikian JP (1982) Parathyroid carcinoma: a review of 62 patients, *Endocrinol Rev* **3**: 218–26.

Shane E, Baquiran DC, Bilezikian JP (1981) Effects of dichloromethylene diphosphonate on serum and urinary calcium in primary hyperparathyroidism, *Ann Intern Med* **95**: 23–7.

Silverberg SJ, Bilezikian JP (1996) Extensive personal experience: evaluation and management of primary hyperparathyroidism, *J Clin Endocrinol Metabol* **81**: 2036–40.

Silverberg SJ, Shane E, De La Cruz et al (1989) Skeletal disease in primary hyperparathyroidism, *J Bone Miner Res* **4**: 283–91.

Silverberg SJ, Gartenberg P, Iacoba TP et al (1995) Longitudinal measurements of bone density and biochemical studies in anbroated hyperparathyroidism, *J Clin Endocrinol Metab* **80**: 723–8.

Silverberg SJ, Thys-Jacobs S, Locker FG et al (1996) The effect of the calcimimetic drug NPS R-568 on parathyroid hormone secretion in primary hyperparathyroidism, *J Bone Miner Res* **11** (Suppl): no. 87.

Singer FR, Neer RM, Murray TM et al (1970) Mithramycin therapy of intractable hypercalcemia due to parathyroid carcinoma, *N Engl J Med* **283**: 634–6.

Thakker RV, Bouloux P, Wooding C et al (1989) Association of parathyroid tumors in multiple endocrine neoplasia type 1 with loss of alleles on chromosome 11, *N Engl J Med* **321**: 218–24.

Turton DB, Miller DL (1996) Recent advances in parathyroid imaging, *Trends Endocrinol Metab* **7**: 163.

Wang CA (1971) Surgery of the parathyroid glands, *Adv Surg* **5**: 109–27.

Watson L (1974) Primary hyperparathyroidism, *Clin Endocrinol Metab* **3**: 215–35.

Wills MR, McGowan GK (1964) Plasma-chloride levels in hyperparathyroidism and other hypercalcaemic states, *Br Med J* **i**: 1153–6.

CHAPTER 10

Paget's disease of bone

Paget's disease of bone was first described as a case report of a single patient (Figure 10.1) (Paget 1877), although it is now recognized to be a very common disorder of the elderly with variable clinical expression. Paget called the disease osteitis deformans, but it is now universally referred to as Paget's disease of bone. It is a disease of antiquity, having been found in mummies in Egyptian tombs as well as in Neanderthal man.

Epidemiology

Paget's disease occurs most commonly in people with a northern European ethnic background. It is very commonly seen in the United Kingdom, western Europe and Australasia (Kanis 1991). There is a striking prevalence of this disease in the Manchester area of England and in one community in Italy. Paget's disease in Manchester has been linked to dog ownership (O'Driscoll and Anderson 1985). It is also common in the Anglo-American population who have their ethnic origins in western Europe. It is rare in Scandinavia, Asia and Africa, but does occur in African-Americans, albeit less commonly than in Anglo-Americans. It is very rare in some countries in Latin America, and extremely uncommon in Mexican-Americans.

It is predominantly a disease of the elderly. It is uncommon below the age of 40, but has been described rarely in teenagers. Sixty percent of patients are male.

There have long been questions of whether there is a specific hereditable pattern in Paget's disease. This may vary in different countries. In Spain, it is possible that up to 40% of patients have a family history of the disease, whereas in the UK about 15% of patients have affected relatives, but in Germany and Holland a positive family history is much less common. Paget's disease has been described in monozygotic twins, but since it is a very common disorder it is hard to determine whether this is coincidental. A history of Paget's disease in first-degree relatives is present in 12% of patients overall, compared with only 2% of controls, and there is an even stronger hereditary element in certain families. In some families, 40% of members have an affected first-degree relative (Morales-Piga et al 1995), and transmission occurs in an autosomal dominant pattern. However, it should be noted that in some of these cases, the bone disease may not be characteristic of Paget's disease, and may represent either a variant or a distinct bone disease. Clustering of patients with Paget's disease has been noted in some communities. Some studies have suggested weak associations with certain HLA antigens, but these have not been consistently found (Singer et al 1985; Foldes et al 1987). Recently, a locus on 18q has been identified by linkage analysis studies of several families in both the United Kingdom and the United States with a combined LOD score of approximately 9.0 (LOD

Figure 10.1

Drawing by Paget of the first patient described with Paget's disease, demonstrating all the clinical features of the advanced disease including increase in size of the head, bowing of the lower extremities due to deformity, and eventual development of osteosarcoma in the forearm.

Pathophysiology

Paget's disease of bone is a disorder of excessive but disordered bone remodeling (Figure 10.2). Rates of bone remodeling may be enhanced up to 20-fold, and there is an increase both in osteoclastic bone resorption and new bone formation. However, the coupling between bone formation and resorption is imperfect. The bone formation is excessive, irregular, chaotic and there is a mixture of both woven and lamellar bone, which probably reflects the rapidity of the process.

There is convincing evidence that the primary abnormality appears to be in the osteoclast. The disease is inhibited by antiosteoclastic drugs. When patients with Paget's disease are treated with antiosteoclastic drugs there is a fall in markers of bone resorption, such as urine hydroxyproline, before a change in markers of bone formation, such as serum alkaline phosphatase. Moreover, the osteoclast nuclei contain inclusion bodies that have been linked to a viral etiology (see below).

The pagetic osteoclast does indeed have a characteristic phenotype (Figure 10.3). These cells are very large, and contain increased numbers of nuclei compared with normal osteoclasts. They also show increased tartrate resistant acid phosphatase activity compared with normal osteoclasts, and seem to be exquisitely sensitive to some osteotropic hormones such as calcitonin (Kukita et al 1990).

score of 3.0 is needed to establish linkage). This locus is closely linked to that reported for familial expansile osteolysis, a rare bone dysplasia that has many features of Paget's disease (Hughes et al 1994).

Characteristics of Paget's Disease

1. Grossly distorted bone remodeling
2. Greatly increased bone resorption
3. Abundant new bone formation
4. 1° abnormality resides in osteoclast

Figure 10.2

Abnormalities in bone remodeling seen in patients with Paget's disease.

PAGETIC OSTEOCLASTS

1. Increased in number and size
2. Contain viral nuclear inclusions
3. Express viral antigens
4. Contain viral transcripts

Figure 10.3

Characteristic abnormalities in the osteoclasts of patients with Paget's disease, showing very large multinucleated cells, and associated with increased bone formation, marrow fibrosis and vascularity.

As indicated above, bone formation is also abnormal in Paget's disease (Figure 10.4). However, it is likely that this increase in bone formation occurs as a consequence of prior increases in resorption. The new bone that is formed in Paget's disease is disorganized in structure with immature woven collagen matrix of irregular pattern (reflecting increased production of both woven and lamellar bone). There is also an increase in vascular fibrous tissue throughout the marrow cavity. The osteoblasts and fibroblasts are morphologically normal. Occasionally, reparative granulomas (collections of inflammatory cells) are found in the marrow. The increase in vascularity of the bone is associated with increased arteriovenous shunting and enhanced local blood flow through the bone. This may cause an increase in local warmth over the affected bones and a high output cardiac state.

Although any bone may be involved in patients with Paget's disease, the bones most frequently involved are the vertebrae, skull, pelvis, axial skeleton, proximal ends of the long bones and tibiae. The pagetic lesion may occur as a single localized lesion or as multiple lesions. The lesions are usually patchy and irregular. Many workers have noted that although existing lesions may expand in size, new lesions do not tend to occur.

Evidence for an abnormal microenvironment in Paget's disease

Recent studies by Roodman and colleagues suggest that the bone marrow microenvironment in which the osteoclast forms may be abnormal in patients with Paget's disease (Figure 10.5). In part this may be explained by the production of the

Paget's Normal

Figure 10.4

Structure of bone in a patient with Paget's disease showing distorted architecture. (Kindly supplied by Dr David Dempster.)

cytokine interleukin-6, which is expressed by pagetic osteoclasts and may be responsible for the increase in osteoclast formation that is apparent in this disease, even away from focal sites of disease activity (Roodman et al 1991). However, other factors as well may be involved. There certainly appears to be increased generation of osteoclasts, and this is demonstrated by an increase in numbers of CFU-GM, the precursor for the osteoclast (as well as the formed elements of the blood) (Demulder et al 1991) (Figures 10.6 and 10.7).

Etiology

The cause of Paget's disease remains unknown. There is no convincing evidence to support concepts that Paget's disease is a disorder of hormonal regulation of bone metabolism, is a benign neoplasm of bone, or is a chronic inflammatory condition. Most current evidence suggests that Paget's disease occurs as a result of a slow virus infection. However, although viruses of the measles family have been implicated for more than 15 years, there is still no proof of a direct cause and effect relationship. This viral hypothesis arose from morphologic observations of nuclei of pagetic osteoclasts (Rebel et al 1974). These nuclei contain inclusion bodies (Figure 10.8), which are characteristic of persistent viral infection (Rebel et al 1974, 1976), and are a finding that has been confirmed many times since (Mills and Singer 1976; Gherardi et al 1980; Vacher-Lavenu et al 1981; Harvey et al 1982). They are microfilamentous structures of 150 Å diameter, with a lucent core of 50–70 Å. They are confined to the nuclei of osteoclasts. Although similar inclusion bodies are occasionally seen in other conditions such as giant cell tumors of bone and in osteopetrosis, they always occur in the abnormal osteoclasts of patients with Paget's disease. They have the appearances of an RNA virus related to the paramyxovirus family. These inclusion bodies resemble the inclusion bodies found in other virus-related diseases such as subacute sclerosing panencephalitis and measles. Since this viral family can cause certain slow viral diseases, it is conceivable that an infection in early life could lead to later development of the characteristic bone disease that occurs in the elderly

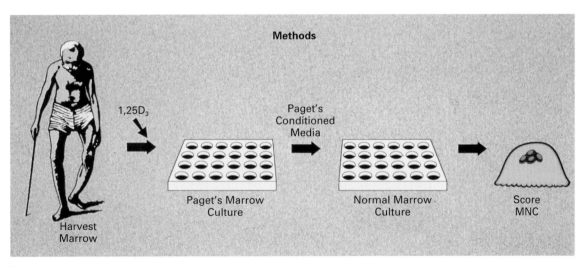

Figure 10.5

Methods used by Roodman and colleagues to study pathophysiology of abnormality in bone remodeling in Paget's disease at the in vitro level. Marrow mononuclear cells from patients with Paget's disease are cultured and studied for their functional and morphologic abnormalities.

Figure 10.6

Characteristics of multinucleated osteoclast-like cells found in prolonged marrow cultures from patients with Paget's disease described by Roodman and colleagues. (Kubita et al 1990.)

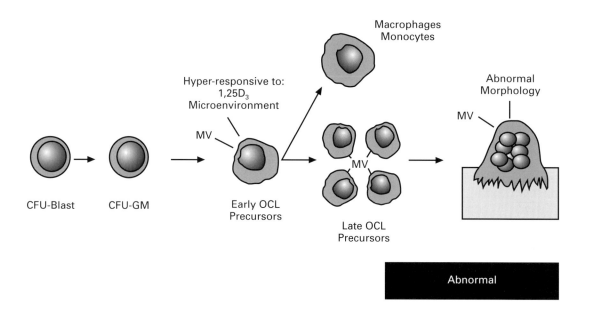

Figure 10.7

Model for abnormalities in cells in the osteoclast lineage and Paget's disease, derived from studies of Roodman and colleagues.

(Dayan 1973). Moreover, there have been suggestions that osteoclasts from pagetic patients express the measles virus and respiratory syncytial virus nucleocapsid antigens as detected by immunohistochemistry (Gherardi et al 1980; Vacher-Lavenu et al 1981), and measles virus RNA is expressed in pagetic osteoclasts (Basle et al 1986, 1987). Another paramyxovirus that has been implicated is canine distemper virus. Segments of this or a closely related virus appear to be expressed in osteoclasts and some other bone cells from patients with Paget's disease

Figure 10.8

Osteoclasts in patients with Paget's disease contain characteristic intranuclear inclusion bodies, suggesting infection with members of the paramyxovirus family. (Reproduced from Rebel et al (1976).)

studied in the Lancashire area of England (O'Driscoll and Anderson 1985; O'Driscoll et al 1990). However, these findings have not been observed by all workers (Barker and Detheridge 1985; Stamp et al 1986).

It has been reported that the peripheral blood mononuclear cells in patients with Paget's disease contain nuclear caspid antigen, similar to the mature multinucleated cells, and distinct from the peripheral blood cells from normal individuals (Reddy et al 1995). This suggests first that the abnormality in Paget's disease is present in early osteoclast progenitors, confirming results that we have found before (Kukita et al 1990; Roodman et al 1991), and in addition confirms that the osteoclast precursor circulates in the peripheral blood. However, cells of the osteoclast lineage are not the only cells in Paget's disease that contain measles virus transcripts. They are also detectable in erythroid progenitors and in pluripotent hematopoietic cells. Roodman has postulated that the virus may infect multipotent hematopoietic progenitors, but that the virus may become defective and the defective viral transcripts are passed on to many of the progeny of these pluripotent cells (Roodman 1996). However, osteoclasts, which are cells incapable of self-renewal, may contain the complete virus.

The morphologic findings suggestive of viral infection are a primary driving force in the search for the cause of Paget's disease. A viral infection could explain some of the features. For example, the enormous size and multinuclearity of the abnormal osteoclasts could occur as a consequence of viral infection. Viruses may enhance syncytial formation, which is a characteristic of the pagetic osteoclast. This increase in osteoclast size and presumably activity may lead to enhanced production of local growth regulatory factors, which stimulate bone formation.

However, it is important to realize that no virus has yet been definitively identified, and there is no proof that these viral inclusion bodies do not represent merely an epiphenomenon rather than the primary cause of the disease. Demonstration that the virus is responsible for Paget's disease will require characterization and isolation of the virus, and the demonstration that cells infected with this virus develop the characteristic phenotype of the pagetic osteoclast.

The viral hypothesis for the etiology of Paget's disease has recently been reviewed (Roodman 1994).

There is a clear genetic predisposition to Paget's disease. There is familial aggregation of the disease, which has been noted by many authors. Approximately one-third of patients have first-degree relatives with the disease, possibly inherited as an autosomal dominant. In preliminary studies, Leach et al (1996) have mapped the locus to chromosome 18q. Moreover, the more severe the disease then the greater the chance a first-degree relative will develop the disease. The mechanism responsible is unknown.

Clinical features (DeDeuxchaisnes and Krane 1964)

The majority of patients with Paget's disease (probably 90%) are asymptomatic. It cannot be discerned in any particular patient when the disease begins, or how long it has been present. The disease is usually diagnosed by X-rays that are taken for some other reason or by routine measurement of serum alkaline phosphatase, which is measured as part of a routine blood test, and is found unexpectedly to be increased.

The most common complaint in symptomatic patients is bone pain. There are a number of different types of bone pain in Paget's disease. The most common is local bone pain over the lesions. This is associated with underlying involvement of bone with Paget's disease, and the abnormality can usually be seen on bone scans or X-rays. The pain is usually dull, aching and often nocturnal. The cause is unknown, but it may be related to expansion pressure on the periosteum, or associated hyperemia. Less common causes of pain are radicular pain due to nerve root compression or nerve entrapment secondary to osseous overgrowth, or related conditions such as degenerative joint disease. Degenerative joint disease is common in the elderly, is even more common in Paget's disease and most frequently involves the hip joints.

Deformity is frequent in patients with advanced Paget's disease. It is caused by abnormal bone architecture secondary to the disordered bone remodeling. It is often worsened by weight-bearing. The most common deformities are seen in the skull and lead to an increase in skull size (notable in Paget's original patient), lateral bowing of the long bones (such as the humerus, radius, femur or tibia), and dorsal kyphosis. Other clinical features such as angioid streaks in the retina have been described, but are unusual. It is not clear that these are specific to Paget's disease.

Complications of Paget's disease

Fracture

Possibly the most common complication of Paget's disease is fracture. This occurs most frequently in weight-bearing bones such as the femur or tibia. It usually occurs after trivial injury or possibly even spontaneously. Although it is said that these fractures heal well because of good blood supply, in practice failure to unite and impaired bone healing are a common problem. These patients should be treated vigorously with bisphosphonates (or calcitonin). Fractures through sclerotic lesions do worst.

Nerve entrapment

Nerve entrapment occurs because of increased bone formation at the site of the lesion, which leads to nerve compression if diseased bone involves a nerve foramen or canal. It is most frequently seen with the auditory nerve, but may involve other cranial nerves. Rarely, spinal cord compression occurs as a consequence of narrowing of the spinal canal.

Deafness

Patients with Paget's disease may have impaired hearing either because of conduction deafness, nerve deafness due to auditory nerve compression or a combination of both. Auditory nerve compression occurs when Paget's disease involves the petrous temporal bone and compresses the VIIIth cranial nerve. This may exacerbate underlying nerve deafness, which is common in the elderly with or without Paget's disease. Conduction deafness due to otosclerosis is commonly found in patients with Paget's disease.

Cardiac failure

It remains controversial whether Paget's disease itself can cause cardiac failure directly. More likely, Paget's disease may exacerbate underlying cardiac decompensation. Cardiac failure is due to arteriovenous shunting through bone (and possibly skin and subcutaneous tissue) leading to a high cardiac output state, which may be enough to precipitate failure in a patient with underlying cardiac disease.

Hypercalcemia

Hypercalcemia was described many years ago by Albright in three immobilized patients. Hypercalcemia is rare in patients with Paget's disease. When it does occur, a careful search for coexistent primary hyperparathyroidism should be instituted. It is possible in retrospect that this may have been the explanation in Albright's patients.

Sarcomatous transformation

Although this is a much feared complication, it is fortunately very rare. It probably occurs in fewer than 1% of all patients. The great majority of nonpagetic osteosarcomas occur before the age of 20, whereas pagetic sarcomas are most frequent in the seventh decade. Sarcomas occur most frequently in patients with widespread longstanding disease. It is often multifocal, and occurs most frequently in the humerus and skull, or occasionally in the vertebrae. The distribution of osteosarcoma is different from the distribution of Paget's disease. The sarcomatous lesion may be an osteosarcoma, fibrosarcoma or chondrosarcoma, or any combination of these. It is an extremely malignant lesion and prognosis is very poor, with only 2% of patients surviving 5 years.

Renal calculi

Hypercalciuria and nephrolithiasis are probably slightly more frequent in pagetic patients.

Laboratory evaluation

Serum calcium, phosphate, alkaline phosphatase

Serum calcium and phosphate are usually normal in patients with Paget's disease. Serum alkaline phosphatase may be increased, reflecting increased new bone formation. The serum alkaline phosphatase concentration depends on both the extent and activity of the disease. Urine hydroxyproline is also increased in patients with Paget's disease, and reflects bone resorption. Newer markers of bone resorption, such as deoxypyridinoline crosslinks, are also increased, and these have replaced measurements of urine hydroxyproline.

X-rays

Paget's disease can usually be diagnosed from the characteristic radiologic features. It is characterized by:

- increased bone resorption with features of widespread radiolucent areas of patchy distribution; and
- increased localized bone formation represented by irregular cortical thickening and sclerosis, trabecular sclerosis and occasionally increased irregular width of the bones (Figure 10.9).

The patterns of X-ray changes may be characteristic. The skull frequently shows a "cotton-wool" appearance of alternating bone formation with resorption (Figure 10.10). Occasionally there is an ax-head shaped resorptive area known as "osteoporosis circumscripta", which is characteristic of Paget's disease. If an expanding irregular radiolucent defect occurs in the skull of pre-existing Paget's disease, then malignant transformation should be suspected. In the pelvis, a characteristic radiologic appearance is sclerosis along the ileopectineal line. In the vertebrae, the appearance may be confused with an osteoblastic metastasis. An osteoblastic metastasis is characterized by trabecular sclerosis without cortical thickening, and tends to lead to vertebral collapse, in contrast to Paget's disease where cortical thickening and

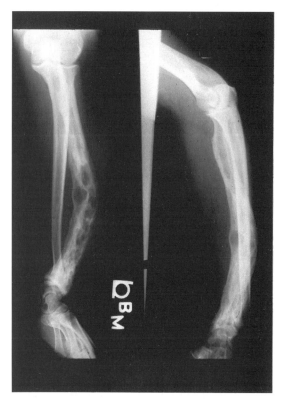

Figure 10.9

X-ray of the leg of a patient with Paget's disease showing marked lateral bowing, a characteristic abnormality of the tibiae.

Figure 10.10

X-ray of the skull of a patient with Paget's disease showing markedly increased bone formation with increase in size of the calvarium.

expansion of the vertebrae are more characteristic. However, the distinction may be very difficult.

Bone scan

The bone scan shows a characteristic increased uptake of isotope at sites of disease activity (Figure 10.11). The intensity of isotope uptake corresponds approximately to activity of the disease and reflects bone formation. The appearance of multifocal but discrete areas of increased uptake is characteristic of Paget's disease. The bone scan is nonspecific, but may be useful to determine if symptoms such as bone pain correspond to underlying bone disease. Bone scans also provide a guide to the overall extent of the disease.

Bone biopsy

Bone biopsy is not required in routine cases where the disease can be diagnosed by characteristic X-rays and bone scan. It may be indicated for diagnosis in patients with localized disease in whom definitive diagnosis is not possible from the X-ray, and can be particularly helpful if malignancy is suspected. Paget's disease may be present in the iliac crest biopsy even when bone is radiologically normal. There is some morphologic evidence that there is an increase in bone remodeling even in radiologically normal areas of bone, which may reflect increased production of osteotropic cytokines by pagetic osteoclasts.

Treatment modalities in Paget's disease

The goals of treatment in Paget's disease are to reduce pain and increase mobility. It still remains unclear whether treatment reduces pre-existing deformity or improves nerve compression. The

Figure 10.11

Bone scan of a patient with Paget's disease showing the disease to be multifocal, but comprising discrete lesions predominantly in the axial skeleton.

major indication for surgery is pain, but inhibitors of bone resorption should also be considered in preparation for elective surgery (to reduce bleeding), for prolonged immobilization (to prevent hypercalcemia), and for the prevention of local progression and future complications (for example, in a younger patient with an osteolytic lesion in a long bone, even if asymptomatic). The only drugs with proven efficacy are those that are specific inhibitors of osteoclastic bone resorption. These include calcitonin, bisphosphonates, plicamycin and probably gallium nitrate.

Calcitonin

Calcitonin has been used in the therapy of Paget's disease for approximately 20 years (Bijvoet and Jansen 1967; Haddad et al 1970; Woodhouse et al 1971). Any form of calcitonin is efficacious. It can be administered subcutaneously, intramuscularly or even intranasally. In the United States, the form most frequently used is salmon calcitonin given as a subcutaneous injection. A common therapeutic schedule is to use 100 IU three times weekly for one month followed by 50 IU three times weekly. However, there is little evidence that this schedule is any better than daily injections of 50–100 IU. Responses can be monitored by measurement of serum alkaline phosphatase, urine hydroxyproline or urinary deoxypyridinoline crosslinks. It may take 4–8 weeks for an objective response to decide a particular drug is ineffective, although most patients will show a subjective (pain improvement) response in the first 2 weeks. Two-thirds of patients will respond well with pain relief or a change in biochemical parameters. About one-half of the responders will later relapse on treatment. The cause of this relapse is unclear, and although antibodies to calcitonin have been implicated, it may be more complex. It is likely that the pagetic osteoclast becomes unresponsive to calcitonin after prolonged exposure. Calcitonin is a very safe, non-toxic drug. Occasional patients develop nausea shortly after injection, but this may be avoided by the use of promethazine together with calcitonin before bedtime. Treatment for Paget's disease is indicated in patients with severe pain and progressive deformity. Efficacy for nerve compression or complications such as cardiac failure is not well established, although beneficial effects have been reported. The major disadvantage with the use of calcitonin is that it is expensive and must be administered by subcutaneous injection. The use of intranasal calcitonin would obviate the latter problem.

Bisphosphonates

Bisphosphonates are extremely effective in the treatment of Paget's disease of bone (Smith et al 1971) (Figures 10.12 and 10.13). All the bisphosphonates have proven to be efficacious in this condition. Etidronate has been available for many years (Altman et al 1973), and although it is currently the only orally available bisphosphonate in the United States, it is also the bisphosphonate

Figure 10.12

Effects of bisphosphonates in Paget's disease showing marked reduction in osteoclast number and activity. (Kindly supplied by Dr Pierre Meunier.)

Figure 10.13

Effects of bisphosphonates in Paget's disease, showing improvement in the chaotic bone architecture following reduction in bone resorption. (Kindly supplied by Dr John Bilezikian.)

with the most significant side effects. In doses of greater than 10 mg/kg body weight per day for prolonged periods, etidronate may cause osteomalacia and susceptibility to fracture. Newer bisphosphonates do not have this side effect in doses that inhibit osteoclastic bone resorption. There is now very wide experience with the use of clodronate and pamidronate in Paget's disease. Anderson and colleagues have advocated the use of large doses of pamidronate, which they believe may cure the condition (Cantrill and Anderson 1990). There are multiple regimens for using pamidronate. One reasonable regimen is to use a 60 mg infusion to be repeated when symptoms recur (possibly every 3 months). Another is to treat monthly with an infusion of 30–60 mg, with the goal of reducing pain and normalizing the serum alkaline phosphatase. Alendronate has recently been approved by the FDA for use in Paget's disease of bone. It has a similar spectrum of activity as pamidronate, but has the additional advantage that it can be used orally in doses of 40 mg per day. However, care should be taken when it is administered to avoid the possibility of upper gastrointestinal mucosal operation. Moreover, it probably should be avoided in patients who have underlying gastrointestinal disease. Other newer bisphosphonates, such as ibandronate, tiludronate, risedronate and zoledronate are probably all equally as effective as pamidronate and alendronate.

Other agents that are likely to be effective in Paget's disease are plicamycin (Ryan et al 1970) and gallium nitrate. However, the newer bisphosphonates are likely to make these agents obsolete for this condition. Plicamycin is an antitumor antibiotic, which is given by intravenous infusion in low doses in Paget's disease. It has been shown to produce good results in small numbers of patients in uncontrolled studies. However, it is a cytotoxic drug with side effects that are potentially important in elderly patients. It certainly has potential for nausea, vomiting, diarrhea, bone marrow suppression, hepatocellular toxicity and renal failure. Because of potential toxicity its routine use cannot be recommended without evidence that its efficacy is greater than that of bisphosphonates or calcitonin. Gallium nitrate is an effective inhibitor of osteoclastic bone resorption. It also must be given by infusion or injection. Although it may not have the same spectrum of toxicity as plicamycin, it is inconvenient to administer to patients with Paget's disease (Bockman et al 1989). However, to obtain an important place in treatment, it would need to be shown that it has advantages over the newer bisphosphonates or calcitonin, which are not yet apparent.

References

Altman RD, Johnston CC, Khairi MRA et al (1973) Influence of disodium etidronate on clinical and laboratory manifestations of Paget's disease of bone, *N Engl J Med* **289**: 1379–84.

Barker DJP, Detheridge FM (1985) Dogs and Paget's disease, *Lancet* **ii**: 1245.

Basle MF, Fournier JG, Rozenblatt S et al (1986) Measles virus RNA detected in Paget's disease bone tissue by in situ hybridization, *J Gen Virol* **67**: 907–13.

Basle MF, Rebel A, Fournier JG et al (1987) On the trial of paramyxoviruses in Paget's disease of bone, *Clin Orthop Rel Res* **217**: 9–15.

Bijvoet OLM, Jansen A (1967) Thyrocalcitonin in Paget's disease, *Lancet* **ii**: 47–52.

Bockman R, Warrell R, Bosco B et al (1989) Treatment of Paget's disease of bone with low-dose subcutaneous gallium nitrate, *J Bone Miner Res* **4** (Suppl 1): no 199.

Cantrill JA, Anderson DC (1990) Treatment of Paget's disease of bone, *Clin Endocrinol* **32**: 507–18.

Dayan AD (1973) Progressive multifocal leukoencephalopathy. In: Whitty CWM, Hughes JTC, MacCallum FO, eds, *Virus diseases and the nervous system* (Blackwell: Oxford) 199.

DeDeuxchaisnes CN, Krane S (1964) Paget's disease of bone: clinical and metabolic observations, *Medicine* **43**: 233–66.

Demulder A, Singer F, Roodman GD (1991) Granulocyte macrophage progenitors (CFU-GM) are abnormal in Paget's disease, *J Bone Miner Res* **6** (Suppl): no 433.

Foldes J, Shamir S, Scherman L et al (1987) Histocompatibility antigens and Paget's disease of bone, *Calcif Tissue Int* **41** (Suppl 2): 59.

Gherardi G, LoCascio V, Bonucci E (1980) Fine structure of nuclei and cytoplasm of osteoclasts in Paget's disease of bone, *Histopathology* **4**: 63–74.

Haddad JG, Birge SJ, Avioli LV (1970) Effects of prolonged thyrocalcitonin administration on Paget's disease of bone, *N Engl J Med* **283**: 549–55.

Harvey L, Gray T, Beneton MNC et al (1982) Ultrastructural features of the osteoclasts from Paget's disease of bone in relation to a viral aetiology, *J Clin Pathol* **35**: 771–9.

Hughes AE, Sherman AM, Weber JL et al (1994) Genetic linkage of familial expansile osteolysis to chromosome 18q, *Hum Mol Genet* **3**: 359–61.

Kanis JA (1991) *Pathophysiology and treatment of Paget's disease of bone* (Carolina Academic Press/Martin Dunitz: London).

Kubita A, Chenu C, McManus LM et al (1990) Atypical multinucleated cells form in long term marrow cultures from patients with Paget's disease, *J Clin Invest* **85**: 1280–6.

Leach RJ, Singer FR, Lewis TB et al (1996) Evidence of a locus for Paget's disease of bone on human chromosome 18Q, *J Bone Miner Res* **11** (Suppl 1): no 19.

Mills BG, Singer FR (1976) Nuclear inclusions in Paget's disease of bone, *Science* **194**: 201–2.

Morales-Piga AA, Rey-Rey JS, Corres-Gonzales J et al (1995) Frequency and characteristics of familial aggregation in Paget disease of bone, *J Bone Miner Res* **10**: 663–70.

O'Driscoll JB, Anderson DC (1985) Past pets and Paget's disease, *Lancet* **ii**: 919–21.

O'Driscoll JB, Buckler MM, Jeacock J et al (1990) Dogs, distemper and osteitis deformans: a further epidemiological study, *Bone Mineral* **11**: 209–16.

Paget J (1877) On a form of chronic inflammation of bones (osteitis deformans), *Medico-Chirurgical Transactions of London* **60**: 37–63.

Rebel A, Malkani K, Basle M (1974) Anomalies nucléaires des osteoclastes de la maladie osseuse de Paget, *Nouv Presse Med* **3**: 1299.

Rebel A, Malkani K, Basle M et al (1976) Osteoclast ultrastructure in Paget's disease, *Calcif Tissue Res* **20**: 187–99.

Reddy SV, Singer FR, Roodman GD (1995) Bone marrow mononuclear cells from patients with Paget's disease contain measles virus nucleocapsid messenger ribonucleic acid that has mutations in a specific region of the sequence, *J Clin Endocrinol Metab* **80**: 2108–11.

Roodman GD (1994) Biology of the osteoclast in Paget's disease, *Semin Arthritis Rheum* **23**: 235–6.

Roodman GD (1996) Paget's disease and osteoclast biology, *Bone* **19**: 209–12.

Roodman GD, Kurihara N, Ohsaki Y et al (1991) Interleukin-6 a potential autocrine/paracrine factor in Paget's disease of bone, *J Clin Invest* **89**: 46–52.

Ryan WG, Schwartz TB, Northrop G (1970) Experiences in the treatment of Paget's disease of bone with mithramycin, *JAMA* **213**: 1153–7.

Singer FR, Mills BG, Park MS et al (1985) Increased HLA-DQWI antigen pattern in Paget's disease of bone, *Clin Res* **33**: 574A.

Smith R, Russell RGG, Bishop M (1971) Diphosphonates and Paget's disease of bone, *Lancet* **i**: 945–7.

Stamp TCB, Mackney PH, Kelsey CR (1986) Innocent pets and Paget's disease, *Lancet* **ii**: 917.

Vacher-Lavenu M, Louvel A, Daudet-Monsac M et al (1981) Inclusion tubulofilamenteuse intranucléaires dans les cellules multiinuclées des tumeurs a cellules géantes des os. Étude ultrastructurale d' une série de 31 tumeurs, *C R Séances Acad Sci Paris* **293**: 639.

Woodhouse NJW, Reiner M, Bordier P et al (1971) Human calcitonin in the treatment of Paget's bone disease, *Lancet* **i**: 1139–43.

CHAPTER 11

Osteopetrosis

Osteopetrosis is the bone disease caused by impaired osteoclastic bone resorption. Since an impairment of osteoclastic bone resorption could be due to decreased osteoclast formation or to decreased capacity of preformed osteoclasts to resorb bone, the disorder may be caused by multiple molecular mechanisms, and represents a number of separate inherited bone defects in the different types. It is characterized by an increase in bone mass that impairs normal bone marrow function (hematopoiesis) (Figure 11.1). The bone disorder has heterogeneous pathophysiology, but in all types there is a generalized increase in radiodensity, which has led to the term marble bone disease to describe the X-ray appearance. Impaired osteoclast function causes impaired removal of osseocartilaginous matrix, and a subsequent increase in cancellous and cortical bone volumes, usually with disorganized architecture and incomplete mineralization. The calcified cartilage and bone that are formed during endochondral bone formation are not removed by osteoclasts, and persist into adult life. The excess bone matrix may obliterate the marrow cavity, and in specific locations may encroach on nerve foramina and lead to neural disturbances. The bones are usually fragile, despite their increased radiodensity, and fracture easily. When first described, the disease was called marble bone disease, although the bone is clearly of increased fragility. However, in view of the bone fragility, "chalk bone disease" is a term that has sometimes been used.

Figure 11.1
Histology of a vertebral body from a mouse with osteopetrosis, showing accumulation of osseocartilaginous tissue in the marrow cavity and reduction in normal marrow elements.

Pathophysiology

There is a multitude of different causes of osteopetrosis, but the primary underlying mechanism is the same—a failure of normal osteoclastic bone resorption during bone remodeling. Osteopetrosis has been better characterized in animal models than it has in humans (Table 11.1). Studies in animal models of osteopetrosis have provided information not just on this uncommon

Table 11.1 Characteristics of various forms of osteopetrosis.

	Mouse						Rat			Rabbit	Human	
	gl	mi	oc	op	src-	fos	ia	op	tl	os	Juvenile	Adult
Osteoclasts:												
Number	↓	↓	↓	↓↓	nl	↓↓	↑↑	↓↓	↓↓	↓	↑↓	?
Ruffled border	+	-	-	+	-	?	-	?	?	-	±	?
Cured by bone marrow transplants	+	+	-	-	+	?	+	+	-	?	±	?
Genetic transmission	R	R	R	R	R	R	R	R	R	R	R	D

R, autosomal recessive; D, autosomal dominant.

Table 11.2 Some insights into osteoclast biology from studies in osteopetrosis.

- Osteoclast precursors are present in marrow and spleen
- Defect in M-CSF expression in op/op mouse
- Defect in carbonic anhydrase II expression in human variant of osteopetrosis
- Src tyrosine kinase deficiency causes osteopetrosis
- Fos deficiency causes a switch in the mononuclear phagocyte lineage from osteoclasts to macrophages

disease, but also have provided much information about normal osteoclast biology (Table 11.2). At least 10 animal forms are known, six in the mouse, three in the rat and one in the rabbit. Human forms of osteopetrosis have generally been less well characterized, with the notable exception of carbonic anhydrase Type II deficiency (Sly et al 1985). It is still unclear whether any of the well characterized murine models occur in humans. Table 11.1 shows the known animal models of osteopetrosis. Possibly the best characterized animal model is op/op osteopetrosis in the mouse. In this model, there is a defect in the coding region of the CSF-1 (colony-stimulating factor 1) gene, with subsequent impaired production of biologically active CSF-1 (Felix et al 1990; Wiktor-Jedrzejczak et al 1982, 1990; Yoshida et al 1990; Kodama et al 1991). The result is a decrease in osteoclast formation, particularly during the neonatal period. CSF-1 production by stromal cells is required for normal osteoclast formation. The disease can be cured by treating animals with CSF-1. Two of the most recently described forms of osteopetrosis in mice have been caused by the introduction of null mutations into the germ line by homologous recombination, with subsequent impaired production of the known proto-oncogenes c-src (Soriano et al 1991) and c-fos (Johnson et al 1992; Wang et al 1992). In src deficiency osteopetrosis, there is an impairment of osteoclast action (Boyce et al 1992) (Figures 11.2–11.4). The defect is within the osteoclast lineage (Lowe et al 1993) (Figures 11.5 and 11.6). Thus, this abnormality is very different from what is seen in the op/op mouse, where the defect is in cells separate from the osteoclasts. Fos-deficient osteopetrosis is characterized by a decrease in osteoclast formation due to an intrinsic abnormality in differentiation in the osteoclast lineage (Grigoriadis et al 1994).

Examples of osteoporosis occurring in genetically engineered mice are increasing. Mice lacking the hematopoietic transcription factor PU.1 (Tondravi et al 1997) and NF_kB (Franzoso et al 1997) have severe osteoporosis due to failure of osteoclast formation.

Figure 11.2
Demonstration that in src mutants with impaired expression of src tyrosine kinase, there is failure of normal osteoclastic bone resorption and osteopetrosis. (Reproduced from Boyce et al (1992).)

Figure 11.4
Transmission electron micrograph of osteoclasts in src mutants with osteopetrosis. Note the absence of formation of the ruffled border in the src-deficient mutant compared with the normal wild-type control. (Reproduced from Boyce et al (1992).)

Figure 11.3
Decreased osteoclastic bone resorption in the calvaria of mice with src-deficient osteopetrosis. Note, however, that osteoclasts, albeit nonfunctional, do form in this disease. Both src-deficient mice and normal mice were treated with parathyroid hormone-related protein. (Reproduced from Boyce et al (1992).)

Figure 11.5
Effects of transplantation of fetal liver containing osteoclast precursors to src-deficient mutant mice, demonstrating rescue from the osteopetrotic phenotype. (Reproduced from Lowe et al (1993).)

Recently, there has been further progress in identifying the responsible mechanisms in the mi form of murine osteopetrosis. The mi mouse has normal osteoclast numbers, and the disease can be cured by bone marrow transplantation. The mi gene has been identified as a novel basic helix-loop-helix leucine zipper transcription factor (Weilbaecher et al 1997). Its role in osteoclast function is currently being investigated.

There are at least nine forms of osteopetrosis that occur in humans. The best characterized from a pathophysiologic point of view is one that is very rare, carbonic anhydrase Type II deficiency. In these patients, renal tubular acidosis and cerebral calcification occur together with osteopetrosis (Sly et al 1985), and is caused by variable missense mutations.

Figure 11.6

Demonstration that in src-deficient mutant mice transplanted with fetal liver containing osteoclast precursors, normal osteoclasts appear on bone surfaces forming characteristic resorption lacunae. (Reproduced from Lowe et al (1993).)

There are a number of other forms of osteopetrosis that occur in humans and have not been distinguished pathophysiologically, but are clearly different on clinical grounds. A particularly malignant childhood form, inherited as an autosomal recessive trait, is characterized by severe bone marrow failure in the first year of life and usually a poor prognosis. The children are blind, severely anemic and have profound frontal bossing. The more benign form presents during adult life (often during the second decade) and is inherited as an autosomal dominant trait. In this adult variety, bone marrow failure does not occur, but the patients are prone to fracture, increased skeletal radiodensity, and encroachment on cranial nerves at the base of the skull.

Recently, it has been suggested that there may also be an abnormality in the osteoblast phenotype in vitro in patients with osteopetrosis. This report was based on observations of osteoblast behavior in primary culture of cells obtained from two patients (Lajeunesse et al 1996). Bone formation appears adequate in most patients and animals with the disease, as exemplified by the accumulation of osseous tissue in the marrow space.

Lessons for bone cell biology from studies of osteopetrosis

Osteopetrosis is the disease of the incompetent, or nonfunctional, osteoclast. Since the different causes of the clinical phenotype are inherited as genetic disorders, clarification of molecular mechanisms underlying each osteopetrotic variant has not only provided insights into the causes of the disease, but more importantly has indicated specific molecular mechanisms required for normal osteoclastic bone resorption. Some examples of specific genes whose expression is now known to be an absolute requirement for normal osteoclastic bone resorption from studies of humans and rodents with osteopetrosis, are the c-src proto-oncogene (Soriano et al 1991), the c-fos proto-oncogene (Johnson et al 1992; Wang et al 1992), the Type II isoenzyme of carbonic anhydrase (Sly et al 1985), and monocyte–macrophage colony-stimulating factor (M-CSF) (and, by extension, the M-CSF receptor) (Yoshida et al 1990). As more of the genetic abnormalities responsible for causing variants of osteopetrosis are clarified, so too will key molecular mechanisms known to be essential for normal osteoclastic bone resorption.

Studies in osteopetrosis by Walker and Loutit of 20 years ago have also provided insights into the origin of the osteoclasts (Table 11.2). Parabiosis experiments and marrow and spleen transplantation of normal osteoclast precursors into osteopetrotic mice have shown that the osteoclast precursor is a circulating hematopoietic cell resident in marrow and spleen (Walker 1972, 1973, 1975; Ash et al 1980; Loutit and Nisbit 1982). These particular studies represented a turning point in osteoclast biology, and focused the attention of many researchers on the osteoclast as a first cousin of the monocyte–macrophage family and formed elements of the blood, with a common multipotent progenitor. All studies on osteoclast formation in vitro by marrow and spleen mononuclear cell precursors date from these landmark observations.

Clinical features

Osteopetrosis is uncommon. There are approximately only 500 cases reported in the world literature, although the disease was first described 100 years ago. The frequency is less than 1 in 20 000 and probably closer to 1 in 500 000.

There are probably at least nine distinct variants of osteopetrosis that occur in humans, but in the absence of more detailed knowledge of pathophysiology these are difficult to classify. The common childhood form of the disease usually results in death during the first 2 years of life. In contrast, the common adult form is mild and does not usually impair life expectancy. The rare childhood form of the disorder associated with carbonic anhydrase II deficiency is not characterized by severe extramedullary hematopoiesis and bone marrow failure, and although it is compatible with long survival, renal tubular acidosis may shorten life expectancy.

Bone marrow failure, characterized by obliteration of the marrow cavity by osseocartilaginous matrix, is the striking feature of the childhood form. The consequences of bone marrow failure are anemia, leukopenia and thrombocytopenia. Although compensatory extramedullary hematopoiesis occurs in the liver and spleen, the children frequently die during infancy from effects of leukopenia and thrombocytopenia such as infection or bleeding. If patients with this form of the disease survive into adult life, they suffer from anemia, recurrent fractures and hepatosplenomegaly. Some have symptoms due to encroachment on cranial nerves, such as deafness or blindness, and most who survive have growth retardation. This is characteristic of the severe childhood variant. In the more benign adult form of the disease, sufficient marrow cavity is present for unimpaired normal hematopoiesis, and the major symptomatology in these patients comes from their increased susceptibility to fractures of long bones. However, many of these patients are asymptomatic, and the disease may be recognized accidentally when an X-ray is taken for some reason unrelated to the disease.

The precise reasons that osteopetrotic bones are fragile are not clear. Despite their increased radiologic density, the bones are more likely to fracture. Possibly the relative increase in woven bone is an important factor. There is a failure of both primary modeling and subsequent Haversian and cancellous bone remodeling. Although the bones are more susceptible to fracture, healing proceeds normally because in most cases osteoblast function appears to be unimpaired.

Despite the fragility of the bones, deformity is usually not prominent. When present, it is characterized by thickening of the shafts of the long bones so that the bones develop broad or club-shaped ends. The disease may be patchy in some bones, with some segments of bone appearing normal and some sections sclerotic on X-rays. This occurs most frequently in the vertebral bodies and the metacarpals for unknown reasons. The skull and pelvis show a uniform increase in bone density, and the long bones show obliteration of the marrow cavity by dense compact bone. Failure of resorption of cortical bone may result in obliteration of osseous foramina and entrapment of nerves, particularly the cranial nerves.

Differential diagnosis

A number of other diseases may be associated with an increase in bone density, and an X-ray appearance of diffuse sclerosis. This appearance is sometimes loosely referred to as osteopetrosis, but this term should be reserved for the disorder caused by a defect in osteoclast function, and osteosclerosis is a better term to describe these other disorders. Particular characteristics of osteopetrosis are that the bone disease is generalized, and often dates back to childhood. Other conditions that occasionally may be confused with osteopetrosis include osteoblastic metastases, pyknodysostosis and fluorosis. Osteoblastic metastases occasionally occur around metastatic tumor deposits. These are most common in carcinomas of the prostate or breast, but also occur occasionally in patients with hematologic neoplasms such as Hodgkin's disease or myeloma. (Most patients with myeloma have discrete osteolytic lesions.) Bones affected by osteoblastic metastases are also more fragile and susceptible to fracture than normal bones, despite the increase in radiologic density. Van Buchem's disease, or hyperostosis corticalis generalisata, is characterized by thickening of cortical bone and is probably due to increased bone formation rather than to impairment of bone resorption. This condition is also inherited, although the mode of transmission is unclear.

The skull is primarily involved. Engelmann's disease, or progressive diaphyseal dysplasia, is characterized by localized cortical thickening and is a rare autosomal dominant disorder.

Pyknodysostosis is a very rare autosomal recessive disorder in which, although there is increased remodeling of the cancellous bone, cortical bone may be of increased density. There is frequently hypoplasia of the mandible and clavicle and resorption of the terminal phalanges of the fingers. The patients are usually very short, and the bones are susceptible to fracture. The X-ray appearance of many of the bones resembles that of osteopetrosis. This condition has recently been associated with deficiency of the osteoclast enzyme, cathepsin K (Bossard et al 1996), and may in fact be a form of true osteopetrosis.

Recently, a syndrome of painful osteosclerosis occurring in patients who have been positive for hepatitis C has been identified (Whyte et al 1996). Some, but not all, of these patients are intravenous drug abusers.

Excess fluoride ingestion for many years causes generalized osteosclerosis, the formation of osteophytes, and calcification of ligaments. Endemic fluorosis is seen in some parts of the world where the drinking water contains enormous amounts of fluoride, such as India and South Africa. It does not occur with the much smaller amounts that are added to drinking water to prevent dental caries in many communities in the United States. It occurs occasionally in patients with osteoporosis who are treated with fluoride therapy. Fluorotic bone is radiologically dense but is poorly mineralized and characterized radiologically by excess osteoid. Fluoride stimulates osteoblast activity, but the mineral phase of the new bone that is formed in increased amounts is defective, and the bone is brittle.

Treatment

No treatment is necessary for the benign adult form of osteopetrosis. Autosomal recessive infantile osteopetrosis has been treated recently with bone marrow transplantation, which has resulted in good responses in the short term in a few patients to date. This procedure was first tried only a few years ago, so the long-term results are not yet known. Overall, it results in a survival rate of about 45% at 2 years. The mortality due to transplant complications is high. However, there is evidence in some of the survivors, at least for a few years, of normal osteoclastic bone resorption. With better understanding of the genetic disorder, it is hoped that it will be possible to distinguish those patients who have a primary defect in the osteoclast lineage, since they should respond best to marrow transplantation. It cannot be expected to work in those patients in whom the defect is in an accessory cell required for osteoclastic bone resorption (such as occurs in murine op/op osteopetrosis).

Some children with severe osteopetrosis have been treated successfully with large doses of 1,25-dihydroxyvitamin D_3 in combination with γ-interferon (Key et al 1995), and this has led to an improvement in survival rates. Glucocorticoids may be used to reduce splenic size and improve pancytopenia.

References

Ash P, Loutit JF, Townsend KM (1980) Osteoclasts derived from haematopoietic stem cells, *Nature* **283**: 669–70.

Bossard MJ, Tomaszek TA, Thompson SK et al (1996) Proteolytic activity of human osteoclast cathepsin K—expression, purification, activation and substrate identification, *J Biol Chem* **271**: 12 517–24.

Boyce BF, Yoneda T, Lowe C et al (1992) Requirement of pp60$^{c\text{-}src}$ expression of osteoclasts to form ruffled borders and resorb bone, *J Clin Invest* **90**: 1622–7.

Felix R, Cecchini MG, Fleisch H (1990) Macrophage colony stimulating factor restores in vivo bone resorption in the op/op osteopetrotic mouse, *Endocrinology* **127**: 2592–4.

Franzoso G, Carlson L, Xing L et al (1997) Requirement for NF$_k$B in osteoclast and B-cell development, *Genes and Development* **11**: 3482–96.

Grigoriadis AE, Wang ZQ, Cecchini MG et al (1994) c-fos: a key regulator of osteoclast–macrophage lineage determination and bone remodeling, *Science* **266**: 443–8.

Johnson RS, Spiegelman BM, Papaloannou V (1992) Pleiotropic effects of a null mutation in the c-fos proto-oncogene, *Cell* **71**: 577–86.

Key LL, Rodriguez RM, Willi SM et al (1995) Long-term treatment of osteopetrosis with recombinant human interferon gamma, *N Engl J Med* **332**: 1594–9.

Kodama H, Yamasaki A, Nose M et al (1991) Congenital osteoclast deficiency in osteopetrotic (op/op) mice is cured by injections of macrophage colony stimulating factor, *J Exp Med* **173**: 269–72.

Lajeunesse D, Busque L, Menard P et al (1996) Demonstration of an osteoblast defect in two cases of human malignant osteopetrosis, *J Clin Invest* **98**: 1835–42.

Loutit JF, Nisbit NW (1982) The origin of osteoclasts, *Immunobiology* **161**: 193–203.

Lowe C, Yoneda T, Boyce BF et al (1993) Osteopetrosis in src deficient mice is due to an autonomous defect of osteoclasts, *Proc Natl Acad Sci USA* **90**: 4485–9.

Sly WS, Whyte MP, Sundaram V et al (1985) Carbonic anhydrase II deficiency in 12 families with the autosomal recessive syndrome of osteopetrosis with renal tubular acidosis and cerebral calcification, *N Engl J Med* **313**: 139–45.

Soriano P, Montgomery C, Geske R et al (1991) Targeted disruption of the c-src proto-oncogene leads to osteopetrosis in mice, *Cell* **64**: 693–702.

Tondravi MM, Mckercher SR, Andersen K et al (1997) Osteoporosis in mice lacking haematopoietic transcription factor PU.1, *Nature* **386**: 81–4.

Walker DG (1972) Congenital osteopetrosis in mice cured by parabiotic union with normal siblings, *Endocrinology* **91**: 916–20.

Walker DG (1973) Osteopetrosis cured by temporary parabiosis, *Science* **180**: 875.

Walker DG (1975) Bone resorption restored in osteopetrotic mice by transplants of normal bone marrow and spleen cells, *Science* **90**: 784–5.

Wang ZQ, Ovitt C, Grigoriadis AE et al (1992) Bone and haematopoietic defects in mice lacking c-fos, *Nature* **360**: 741–5.

Weilbaecher K, Hememsath TJ, Tashjian AH et al (1997) Micropthalmia: a central regulator of osteoclast development, *Proceedings of Keystone Symposium*, Santa Fe, NM, no 314.

Whyte MP, Teitelbaum SL, Reinus WR (1996) Doubling skeletal mass during adult life: the syndrome of diffuse osteosclerosis after intravenous drug abuse, *J Bone Miner Res* **11**: 554–8.

Wiktor-Jedrzejczak W, Ahmed A, Szczylik C et al (1982) Hematological characterization of congenital osteopetrosis in op/op mouse, *J Exp Med* **156**: 1516–27.

Wiktor-Jedrzejczak W, Bartocci A, Ferrante AWJ et al (1990) Total absence of colony-stimulating factor 1 in the macrophage-deficient osteopetrotic (op/op) mouse, *Proc Natl Acad Sci USA* **87**: 4828–32.

Xing L, Franzoso G, Siebenlist U et al (1997) Targeted disruption of the P50 and P52 subunits of NF_kB transcription factor leads to failure of osteoclast formation and osteoporosis, *J Bone Min Res* **12**: 133.

Yoshida H, Hayashi S, Kunisada T et al (1990) The murine mutation osteopetrosis is in the coding region of the macrophage colony stimulating factor gene, *Nature* **345**: 442–4.

CHAPTER 12

Osteomalacia and rickets

Definition of osteomalacia

Osteomalacia is the bone disorder that results from impaired mineralization of newly formed bone. The result is excess unmineralized bone matrix (known as osteoid tissue). Osteomalacia occurs by a variety of different causes including a lack of vitamin D, impairment of vitamin D metabolism, or due to a lack of calcium or phosphorus at the site of mineralization of newly formed bone. Before puberty, vitamin D-deficiency osteomalacia is referred to as rickets and is characterized by failure of calcification and overgrowth of cartilage at the growth plate, with resultant impairment of endochondral ossification and stunted growth. The causes of rickets/osteomalacia are shown in Table 12.1.

Pathology of osteomalacia

The definitive diagnosis of osteomalacia is made by bone biopsy using undecalcified sections and labeling with tetracycline. A fluorescent antibiotic, tetracycline localizes at sites of mineralization so that when sequential courses of tetracycline are given before bone biopsy, rates of bone mineralization can be assessed. Other histological parameters that are quantified in a bone biopsy and are relevant to the diagnosis include the relative volume of osteoid tissue (that is, the volume of bone tissue that is nonmineralized), the relative osteoid surface, and the osteoid seam thickness.

The morphologic abnormalities in osteomalacia are the following.

- *Osteoid volume.* The normal osteoid volume is less than 5% of total bone volume. In osteomalacics, the value is typically 20–75%. All patients with pseudofractures have greater than 20% osteoid volume.

- *Relative osteoid surfaces.* The normal value is below 20–30% of the total bone surface. This can extend up to 100% in patients with osteomalacia. Osteoclasts will not resorb the unmineralized osteoid seams, but rather burrow under them and remove the adjacent calcified matrix.

- *Osteoid seam thickness.* In early stages, osteoid seam thickness may be normal but bone turnover, osteoid surface and volume may be increased. In intermediate and later stages, osteoid seam width increases (>15 μm) and mineralized bone formation falls dramatically.

- *Osteoblast surfaces.* The osteoblast surface correlates very closely with the osteoid seam thickness. In normals this is below 40% of the total bone surface. In osteomalacia it is below 5%, with an absolute decrease in osteoblast-covered surfaces. In some patients, particularly those with renal failure, there may be low turnover (or aplastic) osteomalacia.

Table 12.1 Causes of osteomalacia

- Vitamin D Deficiency

    Dietary lack – rare in developed countries because of supplementation of diet with vitamin D; however, may occur in elderly and alcoholics in association with other mechanisms

    Poor sunlight exposure

    Gut malabsorption (vitamin D is a fat-soluble vitamin) and fat malabsorption (steatorrhoea) leads to vitamin D deficiency

    Anticonvulsant therapy (these drugs stimulate liver metabolism of vitamin D to inactive metabolites and cause a decrease in serum 25-hydroxyvitamin D)

    Chronic liver disease, and particularly primary biliary cirrhosis

    Chronic renal disease due to impaired formation of 1,25-dihydroxyvitamin D by kidneys, and to circulating inhibitors of mineralization found in uraemic state

- Vitamin D-dependent osteomalacia

    Type I — inherited deficiency of the 1-hydroxylase enzyme necessary for conversion of 25-hydroxyvitamin D to 1,25-dihydroxyvitamin D

    Type II — inherited inability of target organs to respond to vitamin D

- Hypophosphataemic

    Excess ingestion of aluminum hydroxide gels which decrease phosphate absorption

    Sex-linked hypophosphataemia (inherited phosphate transport abnormality, with renal phosphate wasting)

    Tumour osteomalacia (some tumours, particularly mesenchymal tumours, produce a humoral factor that causes renal phosphate wasting)

    Other renal tubular disorders, such as Fanconi's syndrome

- *Mineralization lag time.* The tetracycline antibiotics localize at sites of mineralization in bone and are fluorescent. Rates of bone mineralization can be assessed by giving two courses of tetracycline 10 days apart and then taking a bone biopsy. Two separated bands of tetracycline fluorescence will be seen allowing estimation of the bone mineral accretion rate over that 10-day period. In normal adults, the distance separating the fluorescent bands averages 1 μm for every day between the courses of tetracycline administration. In osteomalacia there may be no label, there may be a single fluorescent line or there may be very close double lines indicating a decreased mineralization rate. In Paget's disease, hyperthyroidism or thyrotoxicosis (all diseases in which there may be excess osteoid tissue), the mineralization rate is increased, so that the two lines of tetracycline fluorescence are more widely separated than normal.

Nutritional rickets/osteomalacia

Nutritional rickets almost never occurs in the United States, since milk and dairy products are fortified with vitamin D. However, rickets may occur in infants in the third world and in countries in western Europe, such as the United Kingdom, where immigrants from Asia are particularly susceptible. This occurs particularly in the setting of a woman who wears traditional Asian clothing during pregnancy, eats a diet which is deficient in vitamin D and then breast feeds an infant for prolonged periods. Breast milk is low in vitamin D. The use of chappatti flower in the diet may also be a factor in the pathogenesis of calcium and vitamin D malabsorption.

When rickets occurs in the infant, it has a classical clinical picture of severe bone pain, bone deformities, X-ray changes at the epiphyses and abnormal serum chemistry (increased alkaline phosphatase, hypocalcemia and hypophosphatemia). Children with rickets may suffer severe bone pain, but the pain in osteomalacia tends to be more diffuse. The growth of children is stunted. Bone deformities are characteristic of rickets, and include prominence of the costochondral junction, also called the rachitic rosary, and Harrison's groove, the deformity that is due to softening and indentation of the lower ribs. In children with severe rickets, there is indentation of the sternum, kyphoscoliosis, lateral bowing of the lower limbs, softening of the calvaria (craniotabes) and frontal bossing. Posterior flattening of the skull and widening of the cranial sutures are common. There may be delayed eruption of permanent dentition together with enamel defects.

Vitamin D deficiency-related osteomalacia in adults is usually multifactorial. For example, it may occur in an institutionalized elderly person with impaired liver or renal function resulting in abnormal vitamin D metabolism, lack of sunlight exposure and poor diet. It may also occur in alcoholics, but again multiple factors may be involved including malabsorption, pancreatic disease and poor dietary intake. Patients with nutritional rickets and severe osteomalacia may be hypocalcemic, but this is not present in all adults with osteomalacia. The hypocalcemia may be manifested by hypotonia and tetany as well as muscle weakness. Tetany is more common in children than it is in adults. Vitamin D deficiency in adults is also accompanied by muscle weakness and tenderness, particularly involving the proximal muscles of the lower extremities associated with hypotonia. Patients may have generalized bone pain, and occasionally present with spontaneous fractures. Pain in the hip may be due to a pseudofracture of the femoral neck. Patients may have a waddling gait related to proximal myopathy, which improves after treatment with vitamin D.

In children with nutritional rickets, the epiphyses show gross demineralization, together with a "cupping" deformity and loss of epiphyseal definition with a coarse trabecular pattern. In adults, there may be a diffuse osteopenia and in occasional patients pseudofractures (Looser's zones). These represent lines of rarefaction at sites where arteries cross bones, such as below the glenoid fossa, the scapula, the pubic rami and the ribs.

In the majority of patients with rickets, the serum chemistry is abnormal (Table 12.2). However, in some adults, osteomalacia may be present but there is no discernible abnormality in the serum calcium, phosphorus or alkaline phosphatase. When there is malabsorption or dietary lack of vitamin D, serum calcium is decreased or at the lower limit of normal, serum phosphorus is markedly decreased due to secondary hyperparathyroidism, and urine calcium excretion is also decreased. In these patients, secondary hyperparathyroidism occurs as a consequence of hypocalcemia, and there is subsequent increased bone turnover. In patients with rickets or osteomalacia due to chronic renal disease, impairment of glomerular filtration leads to phosphate retention so that serum calcium is low because of impaired formation of 1,25-dihydroxyvitamin D_3 and impaired gut absorption of calcium, but serum phosphorus is high. In patients with rickets or osteomalacia due primarily to a renal phosphate leak, serum calcium concentrations may be normal but the serum phosphorus concentration is decreased. Parathyroid secretion rates are normal and bone turnover is low.

The diagnosis of rickets may be suspected from the presence of a painful deforming bone disease that is associated with characteristic abnormalities of serum chemistry. In patients with malabsorption or dietary deficiency of vitamin D, serum 25-hydroxyvitamin D_3 is an important measurement since it reflects the major transport form of vitamin D in the circulation. It is also a good parameter of gut absorption of vitamin D. X-rays may be diagnostic in children with rickets, who develop a characteristic expansion of the epiphy-

Table 12.2 Serum chemistry in different types of osteomalacia

Vitamin D Deficiency	Secondary Hyperparathyroidism	Chronic Renal Disease	Renal Phosphorus Leak
calcium ↓ phosphate ↓ (with normal kidneys)	serum calcium (normal or subnormal) ↓ urine calcium ↓ phosphate ↓↓	glomerular filtration rate ↑ phosphate ↑ calcium ↓ (due to impaired formation of 1,25-(OH)2 vitamin D)	serum phospate ↓ serum calcium normal

seal plates leading to cupping of the adjacent long bones and a fuzzy indistinct appearance of the epiphysis, and also in some adult patients with osteomalacia who develop pseudofractures. However, pseudofractures are uncommon, and in patients in whom osteomalacia is suspected on clinical or radiological grounds, it may be necessary to perform a bone biopsy for a definitive diagnosis.

Children or adults with vitamin D deficient rickets or osteomalacia should be treated with ergocalciferol (vitamin D in oil) given either orally or intramuscularly. In infants, doses may be 10 000–50 000 IU/month intramuscularly, or 1500–5000 IU/day orally. Intramuscular medication is probably best in those patients with steatorrhea and malabsorption. The available vitamin D preparations are shown in Table 12.3.

Gastrointestinal and hepatic disorders

Osteomalacia occurs frequently in patients with gastrointestinal diseases that either lead to malabsorption of fat soluble vitamins, impairment of vitamin D metabolism or interference with the use of enterohepatic circulation of vitamin D. This occurs in the setting of gluten enteropathy, celiac disease and other diseases of the gut leading to malabsorption such as Crone's disease of the small bowel, and is frequent after surgical procedures that involve resection of large areas of the stomach or intestines. Osteomalacia and rickets also occur frequently after biliary obstruction, particularly in primary biliary cirrhosis, and in chronic pancreatitis, due to impaired intestinal absorption of vitamin D and calcium. In many patients with longstanding gastrointestinal disorders, the development of osteomalacia may be insidious and remain undiagnosed for many months or years. On the other hand, if osteomalacia is recognized because of changes in the serum chemistry, or skeletal aches and pains that lead to a biopsy-proven diagnosis, this may lead to recognition of previously unsuspected malabsorption due to celiac or Crone's disease.

Chronic renal failure

Patients with chronic renal failure frequently develop osteomalacia for reasons that are multiple and complex. These patients have a mixture of bone diseases including osteomalacia, low turnover osteoporosis and osteofibrosa due to secondary hyperparathyroidism. The pathophysiology is complex. In part, it is due to impaired gastrointestinal absorption of calcium due to impaired production of 1,25-dihydroxyvitamin D_3 by the failing kidneys, but there are additional factors that interfere with calcium absorption, which are still not completely understood, and with bone mineralization. The secondary hyperparathyroidism is due to impaired calcium absorption, which leads to hypocalcemia. In many patients, the defect in mineralization is related to aluminum intoxication. In the past, this was due predominantly to patients undergoing hemodialysis with water containing high concentrations of aluminum. This leads to a low turnover type of osteomalacia, and is associated with the deposition of aluminum at the mineralization front. Some of these patients may be triggered effectively by desferrioxamine. These patients have reduced parathyroid gland response with relatively low parathyroid hormone concentra-

Table 12.3 Vitamin D metabolites used in the treatment of vitamin D depletion states

Nonproprietary Name	Abbreviation	Effective Daily Dose	Time for Reversal of Toxic Effects (Days)
Ergocalciferol	Vitamin D_3	1–10 mg	17–60
Calcifediol	25-$(OH)D_3$	0.05–0.5 mg	7–30
Dihydrotachysterol		0.1–1 mg	3–14
Alfacalcidol	1α-$(OH)D_3$	1–2 µg	5–10
Calcitriol	1,25-$(OH)_2D_2$	0.5–1 µg	2–10

tions. They do poorly if treated with parathyroidectomy for the hypercalcemia, which is typically present in aluminum-related osteomalacia. In these patients there is an accumulation of lamellar osteoid, which occupies most of the trabecular surfaces. There is also a dramatic reduction in the number of bone cells, osteoclasts and osteoblasts. More than 90% of patients with this histologic picture have stainable aluminum at the bone osteoid interface. This interface is scalloped due to evidence of previous osteoclastic bone resorption. These patients have the classic clinical features of renal bone disease, and they are indistinguishable from patients with other types of osteomalacia. When aluminum is the etiologic factor, there may be an associated encephalopathy. The serum PTH concentrations may be relatively low in these patients, and the serum alkaline phosphatase concentrations are determined by the amount of osteoid tissue present. Despite this, many of these patients are hypercalcemic, and the hypercalcemia is difficult to manage. Measurements of serum aluminum concentrations are not as reliable for diagnosis as assessment of the stainable aluminum at the bone osteoid interface in bone biopsy assessment. This condition is best recognized by bone biopsy with double tetracycline labeling.

Some of these patients with aluminum-related bone disease may be treated effectively by desferrioxamine.

Aluminum bone disease has been a major problem in patients with chronic renal failure, particularly those on dialysis. It presents a picture that can be readily suspected by the presence of aplastic bone disease with high aluminum content, and the patient with mild hypercalcemia and hyperparathyroidism but relatively little increase in alkaline phosphatase.

Patients with renal bone disease associated with osteomalacia should be assessed for aluminum intoxication and treated when necessary with desferrioxamine, and dialyzed with water of low aluminum content. The commonest cause of aluminum intoxication currently is administration of aluminum-containing phosphate binders, and for this reason aluminum-containing antacids should be avoided. Patients with osteomalacia without evidence of aluminum intoxication should be treated with 1,25-dihydroxyvitamin D_3 or a potent analog. This may serve the purpose of not only correcting calcium malabsorption, but also reducing parathyroid hormone secretion and limiting secondary hyperparathyroidism.

There are some patients with renal bone disease that do not have this dramatic reduction in bone cells. Rather they have evidence of increased bone turnover and hyperparathyroidism as part of the histologic features. Some of these patients may have aluminum staining as the mineralization front, but the more cellular aspect of the histologic picture leads to diagnosis of mixed uremic osteodystrophy.

Other causes of rickets/osteomalacia

Patients may develop rickets or osteomalacia for causes other than vitamin D deficiency or phosphate deficiency. Aluminum intoxication causes a special form of osteomalacia in patients with renal failure. Aluminum intoxication occurs usually in patients with chronic renal failure or patients taking chronic parenteral nutrition and is associated with an aplastic form of osteomalacia, characterized by low bone turnover and a decreased bone–osteoblast interface. Patients receiving chronic parenteral nutrition who become osteomalacic may have been given preparations in which aluminum is contaminating the casein hydrolysate. Daily etidronate therapy for over 3 months in doses greater than 10 mg/kg body weight per day causes defective mineralization (Chapter 5).

Vitamin D-dependent osteomalacia

There is a group of syndromes associated with either abnormalities in conversion of 25-hydroxyvitamin D_3 to 1,25-dihydroxyvitamin D_3, or insensitivity of target organs to active vitamin D metabolites. In Type 1 vitamin D-dependent osteomalacia, there is deficiency of the 1-hydroxylase enzyme necessary for conversion of 25-hydroxyvitamin D_3 to 1,25-dihydroxyvitamin D_3 (Fraser et al 1973). This is an autosomal recessive disorder characterized by rickets, with low or undetectable serum 1,25-dihydroxyvitamin D_3 concentrations. These patients show no increase in serum 1,25-dihydroxyvitamin D_3 when treated with 25-hydroxyvitamin D_3, but respond very well to treatment with 1,25-dihydroxyvitamin D_3. The precise nature of the molecular defect responsible for this disorder has not been clarified. In Type II vitamin D-dependent osteomalacia, circulating concentrations of 1,25-dihydroxyvitamin D_3 are increased in the presence of rickets, and the patients have target organ resistance to the sterol (Liberman et al 1980; Marx et al 1984). This is apparent in the first 2 years of life. A number of kindreds with this condition have been described, and it is clear that there are different subgroups of this disorder, now recognized to represent different molecular mechanisms of target organ resistance. Some of these patients (about two-thirds) have ectodermal abnormalities including total alopecia, loss of the eyebrows, and dental anomalies including hypoplasia with cone-shaped teeth due to enamel deformities. In these patients, a series of point mutations in the vitamin D receptor have been described (Hughes et al 1988), some in the DNA binding domain (leucine zipper) and some in the hormone binding domain. The site of these mutations determines the nature of impaired vitamin D receptor function, which may be represented by decreased hormone binding to the receptor, decreased affinity of the hormone for the receptor, deficient nuclear localization of the receptor, or decreased activation of target genes by hormone-receptor complexes.

Hypophosphatemic rickets

Hypophosphatemic rickets is also known as sex-linked hypophosphatemia, phosphate diabetes, or vitamin D-resistant rickets (from its first description by Albright et al (1937) over 60 years ago). It is an inherited condition in which rickets usually develops in early life, and is associated with growth retardation and bowing deformities of the legs; the hypophosphatemia does not respond to vitamin D therapy. Unlike most patients with other forms of rickets or osteomalacia, the patients are healthy, and are not hypocalcemic. Also unlike patients with vitamin D deficiency rickets, they do not have enamel hypoplasia of the teeth. The classic triad in hemizygous male patients comprises (1) hypophosphatemia; (2) lower limb deformities; and (3) stunted growth. Patients present with hypophosphatemia from an early age, but the deformities are not apparent before they become weight-bearing. Patients have normal serum calcium concentrations with a low serum phosphate concentration due to increased urine phosphate excretion. Serum alkaline phosphatase is usually increased. The morphologic abnormality of bone is distinct from that of calcium deficiency rickets, since in this syndrome there is no secondary hyperparathyroidism or increased osteoclast activity. A characteristic feature is the hypomineralized periosteocytic lesions (Marie and Glorieux 1983). These also occur in the Hyp mutation in mice, and are probably due to an abnormality in osteoblast–osteocyte function. The plasma 1,25-dihydroxyvitamin D_3 concentration may be decreased or inappropriately normal (in the presence of hypophosphatemia). The reason for this failure of increase in 1-hydroxylase activity in the renal tubular cells is unexplained. The basic defect is phosphate depletion, probably due to a primary defect in renal tubular function, and therapy for this condition involves aggressive use of oral phosphate and a vitamin D metabolite, usually calcitriol. This combination will prevent the short stature and deformities if started early. In older patients with established deformities and short stature, the gains are less. The clinical features of this condition are very similar to those of oncogenic osteomalacia described below.

A closely related condition has been observed in mice, namely the Hyp mutation, and this has been studied extensively as a model for the human disease (Eicher et al 1976). In Hyp mice, there is an abnormality in the brush border area of the proximal convoluted tubules of the kidney (Tenenhouse et al 1978). It is possible that the condition could be due to increased production of a hypophosphatemic factor, and there is some experimental support for this idea (Bonjour et al 1982; Nesbitt et al 1992). The responsible gene has been mapped to the distal part of the short arm of the X chromosome (Thakker et al 1987; Francis et al 1995).

Oncogenic osteomalacia

Rickets or osteomalacia develops in some patients with tumors. Although there are only about 100 reported cases in the world literature, this syndrome may in fact be far more common than is usually thought. The syndrome is characterized by the clinical features of hypophosphatemic rickets/osteomalacia occurring in the presence of a tumor, which is usually a benign mesenchymal tumor and abates when the tumor is excised or ablated. The tumor produces an (as yet) unidentified factor that causes phosphate wasting from the kidneys, due to an impairment of renal tubular phosphate reabsorption. The syndrome of oncogenic osteomalacia mimics hypophosphatemic rickets/osteomalacia very closely, other than for the presence of the tumor. Tumors are usually benign and slow growing, and are most commonly of mesenchymal cell origin. Tumors that have been associated with this syndrome include sclerosing hemangiomas, ossifying or non-ossifying mesenchymal tumors, hemangiopericytoma, giant cell tumors, osteoid osteomas, chondromas, cavernous hemangiomas, but also more malignant tumors such as breast cancer, prostate cancer, and oat cell carcinoma have been associated with this syndrome (Hosking et al 1975; Dent and Gertner 1976; Dent and Stamp 1978; Lyles et al 1980; Taylor et al 1984; Leehey et al 1985; Murphy et al 1985; Shaker et al 1995). It is possible that if patients with these malignant tumors lived longer, manifestations of osteomalacia may be more apparent. However, the presence of Looser's zones in a terminally ill patient should arouse suspicion of this diagnosis. Drezner (1996) has provided a table of all the patients reported in the literature. The presence of rickets depends on the age of the patient. Most present before mid-life, and about 10% are children.

The pathogenesis of this syndrome is unknown. The most likely explanation is that the tumor produces a factor ("phosphotonin") that acts systemically to alter phosphate transport in the renal tubules, and causes phosphate wasting. In fact, tumor extracts from these patients have been shown to contain such biological activity. It is possible that there is more than one factor that can be responsible for this syndrome. However, it has not been possible to identify any such factor or factors definitively as yet. Part of the reason is that these tumors are usually not possible to establish in long-term cell culture, so a renewable source of the putative factor is not available, and as a result complete identification has not been possible (Cai et al 1994). In essentially all patients, there is also decreased renal 1-hydroxylase activity for 25-hydroxyvitamin D_3 metabolites, and decreased circulating 1,25-dihydroxyvitamin D_3 concentrations, for reasons that are unclear in the face of hypophosphatemia. These are corrected with surgical ablation of the tumor.

The differential diagnosis may not be as straightforward as first appears. The tumors may be very small, occult, slow growing and be present for years before they are identified. In adults in whom the tumor is hard to find, the diagnosis may be confused with adult-onset hypophosphatemic osteomalacia, which the syndrome can resemble almost identically. Of course, detection of a benign occult tumor in a patient with hypophosphatemia does not prove that the tumor is causing the hypophosphatemia.

The best treatment is tumor removal. In those patients in whom this is not possible, or the tumor recurs, treatment with calcitriol (which is frequently depleted) will increase renal phosphate reabsorption, and oral phosphate therapy (2–4 g/day) replenishes losses of this ion. This combination therapy may increase serum phosphorus levels, reduce renal phosphate losses and enhance bone healing (Drezner and Feinglos 1977; Lobaugh et al 1984).

References

Albright F, Butler AM, Bloomberg E (1937) Rickets resistant to vitamin D therapy, *Am J Dis Child* **54**: 529.

Bonjour JP, Caverzasio J, Muhlbauer R et al (1982) Are 1,25(OH)$_2$D$_3$ production and tubular phosphate transport regulated by one common mechanism which would be defective in X-linked hypophosphatemic rickets? In: Norman AW, Schaefer K, Herrath DV, Grigoleit HG, eds, *Vitamin D, chemical, biochemical and clinical endocrinology of calcium metabolism* (Watler de Gruyter: Berlin, New York) 427–33.

Cai Q, Hodgson SF, Kao PC et al (1994) Brief report: inhibition of renal phosphate transport by a tumor product in a patient with oncogenic osteomalacia, *N Engl J Med* **330**: 1645–9.

Dent CE, Gertner JM (1976) Hypophosphatemic osteomalacia in fibrous dysplasia, *Q J Med* **45**: 411–20.

Dent CE, Stamp TCB (1978) Vitamin D rickets and osteomalacia. In: Avioli LV, Krane S, eds, *Metabolic bone disease*, Vol 1 (Academic Press: New York) 237.

Drezner MK (1996) Tumor-induced rickets and osteomalacia. In: Favus MJ, ed, *Primer on the metabolic bone diseases and disorders of mineral metabolism* (Lippincott-Raven: New York) 319–25.

Drezner MK, Feinglos MN (1977) Osteomalacia due to 1,25-dihydroxycholecalciferol deficiency. Association with a giant cell tumor of bone, *J Clin Invest* **60**: 1046–53.

Eicher EM, Southard JL, Scriver CR et al (1976) Hypophosphatemia: mouse model for human familial hypophosphatemic (vitamin D-resistant) rickets, *Proc Natl Acad Sci U S A* **73**: 4667–71.

Francis F, Henning S, Korn B et al (1995) A gene (PEX) with homologies to endopeptidases is mutated in patients with X-linked hypophosphatemic rickets, *Nat Genet* **11**: 150.

Fraser D, Kooh SW, Kind HP et al (1973) Vitamin D-dependent rickets: an inborn error of vitamin D metabolism, *N Engl J Med* **289**: 817–22.

Hosking DJ, Chamberlain MJ, Whortland-Webb WR (1975) Osteomalacia and carcinoma of prostate with major redistribution of skeletal calcium, *Br J Radiol* **48**: 451–6.

Hughes MR, Malloy PJ, Kieback DG et al (1988) Point mutations in the human vitamin D receptor gene associated with hypocalcemia rickets, *Science* **242**: 1702–5.

Leehey DJ, Ing TS, Daugiradas JT (1985) Fanconi syndrome induced with a non-ossifying fibroma of bone, *Am J Med* **78**: 708–10.

Liberman UA, Halase A, Samuel R et al (1980) End-organ resistance to 1,25-dihydroxycholecalciferol, *Lancet* **i**: 504–6.

Lobaugh B, Burch WM, Drezner MK (1984) Abnormalities of vitamin D metabolism and action in the vitamin D resistant rachitic and osteomalacic diseases. In: Rumar R, ed, *Vitamin D* (Martinus Nijhoff: Boston, MA) 665–720.

Lyles KW, Berry WR, Haussler M et al (1980) Hypophosphatemic osteomalacia: association with prostatic carcinoma, *Ann Intern Med* **93**: 275–8.

Marie PJ, Glorieux FH (1983) Relation between hypomineralized periosteocytic lesions and bone mineralization in vitamin D resistant rickets, *Calcif Tissue Int* **35**: 443–8.

Marx SJ, Liberman UA, Eli C et al (1984) Hereditary resistance to 1,25-dihydroxyvitamin D_3, *Recent Prog Horm Res* **40**: 589–620.

Murphy P, Wright G, Rai GS (1985) Hypophosphatemic osteomalacia induced with prostatic carcinoma, *Br Med J* **290**: 1945.

Nesbitt T, Coffman TM, Griffiths R et al (1992) Crosstransplantation of kidneys in normal and Hyp mice. Evidence that the Hyp mouse phenotype is unrelated to an intrinsic renal defect, *J Clin Invest* **89**: 1453–9.

Shaker JL, Brickner RC, Divgi AB et al (1995) Case report: renal phosphate wasting, syndrome of inappropriate antidiuretic hormone and ectopic corticotropin production in small cell carcinoma, *Am J Med Sci* **310**: 38–41.

Taylor HC, Fallon MD, Velasco ME (1984) Oncogenic osteomalacia and inappropriate antidiuretic hormone secretion due to oat-cell carcinoma, *Ann Intern Med* **101**: 786–8.

Tenenhouse HS, Scriver CR, McInnes RR et al (1978) Renal handling of phosphate in vivo and in vitro by the X-linked hypophosphatemic male mouse (Hyp/Y). Evidence for a defect in the brush border membrane, *Kidney Int* **14**: 236–44.

Thakker RV, Read AP, Davies KE et al (1987) Bridging markers defining the map position of X-linked hypophosphatemic rickets, *J Med Genet* **24**: 756–60.

CHAPTER 13

Osteoporosis

Definition of osteoporosis

Osteoporosis is a metabolic bone disease in which there is both a decrease in the amount of normally mineralized bone and disturbance in bone microarchitecture so that the risk of fractures occurring in the absence of trauma or in response to trivial trauma (for example, a fall from a standing height or even less) is increased, or such fractures have already occurred (Figure 13.1).

Osteoporosis has been defined recently by a study group at the World Health Organization (WHO) who have proposed diagnostic guidelines based on bone mass measurements in Caucasian women. It should be emphasized that this functional or operational definition is limited to this group of people.

- *Severe osteoporosis*
  Bone mineral density (BMD) greater than 2.5 standard deviation (SD) below the mean value of peak bone mass in young normal women together with the presence of fractures.

- *Osteoporosis*
  BMD greater than 2.5 SD below the mean value of peak bone mass in young normal women.

- *Low bone mass (or osteopenia)*
  BMD between 1 SD and 2.5 SD below the value of peak bone mass in young normal women.

- *Normal*
  BMD not more than 1 SD below the value of peak bone mass in young normal women.

Figure 13.1

Clinical appearance of a patient with severe osteoporosis, associated with dorsal kyphosis and crush fracture of the lumbar vertebrae obvious on lateral spine X-ray. (Kindly supplied by Dr Louis Avioli.)

It should be emphasized that this operational definition is not meant to be used as an indication for intervention, although that is how it commonly tends to be used. The analogy that is often used for the value of this approach is hypertension, where a practical definition of normal systolic and diastolic blood pressure is used for assessment of hypertension, but other features such as history, physical examination and laboratory tests are also important in consideration of the patient's state.

Prevalence of osteoporosis and its importance as a public health problem

The prevalence of osteoporosis is not as precisely known as many texts suggest (Eastell et al 1991; Kanis 1993). The difficulty lies in the precise diagnosis of the disease. The definition provided by the WHO Study Group would mean it affects one in three postmenopausal Caucasian women, and 75 million people in Europe, Japan and the United States combined. Its costs are astronomical—probably 30 billion dollars annually.

A major area of controversy has been in the diagnosis of vertebral fractures. The precise incidence of vertebral fracture is uncertain because these fractures are often asymptomatic and may be inapparent to the patient. In addition, there are varying definitions for what constitutes a vertebral fracture (Melton et al 1989; Eastell et al 1991). In the absence of a single widely accepted criterion for diagnosis, some workers rely on a percent change in posterior height of a vertebra, others on changes in ratios of anterior–posterior diameters (Kanis 1993). However, the location of the vertebra is clearly important in these considerations since the vertebrae vary in their normal shape and dimensions down the thoracic and lumbar spine and in the presence of deformity. It is possible that only one-third of patients with vertebral fracture seek medical attention as a consequence of the fracture (Cooper and Melton 1992; Johnell 1993). Most patients are over the age of 60, and the ratio of women to men is 5:1. There are an estimated 1.5 million Americans who develop osteoporotic fractures each year involving predominantly the hip and spine. Although there is controversy over criteria for the diagnosis of vertebral fracture, no such doubt exists for hip fracture, which is the most serious consequence of osteoporosis. There are over 250 000 hip fractures each year in the United States, and possibly 1.5 million world-wide. This is likely to increase two to five-fold by the year 2050 at current estimates, by which time more than half may occur in people living in Asia. The economic cost of this disease to the United States health care system currently is greater than 10 billion dollars annually.

As the numbers of people in the elderly population increase in the United States, the number of patients who can be expected to suffer from osteoporosis will correspondingly increase. It is estimated that by year 2025, there will be 60 million Americans over the age of 65. In these terms alone, it can be readily appreciated that osteoporosis is a public health problem that is going to become increasingly more important.

Terminology

The definition of osteoporosis proposed based on bone mineral density measurements has operational advantages, but also some disadvantages. Degenerative joint disease and osteophyte formation may cause artifacts. Measurement of bone mineral density does not assess morphology and there are other bone diseases that can potentially mimic the X-ray or DEXA (dual energy X-ray absorptiometry) picture of osteoporosis. One of these is osteomalacia, a different type of bone disorder that may also present with a similar radiologic appearance to osteoporosis and with pathologic fractures. Osteomalacia is a disease of bone caused by failure of mineralization of newly formed or remodeling bone and results in an excess of unmineralized bone matrix (called osteoid tissue). The same disorder in children is known as rickets. In children the bone disorder is most prominent at the growth plate, because the epiphyses are not yet fused and cartilage overgrowth occurs to produce characteristic deformities and radiologic changes such as expansion of the growth plate, separation of the distal epiphysis from the diaphysis, and splaying of the ends of the diaphysis. Osteomalacia and rickets are most frequently due to vitamin D deficiency, but may also be due to phosphate depletion.

As noted above, some clinicians use the term osteopenia to describe decreased mineralized bone mass. Osteopenia is a generic term, which is useful because it does not presuppose any particular bone pathology for the decrease in bone mineral density. Osteopenia (decreased bone mineral density) may be due to osteoporosis, osteomalacia, primary hyperparathyroidism, or malignant disease, all of which may cause generalized bone loss. Osteopenia is a major risk factor for osteoporotic fracture.

Pathophysiology of age-related bone loss and osteoporosis

In order to comprehend the pathogenesis of osteoporosis, it is necessary to understand the natural history of the skeleton and the characteristics of age-related bone loss. These changes are of two types: the changes in bone mass that occur with advancing age, and the specific changes in cancellous bone microarchitecture that occur in the vertebral bodies and the necks of femora of the osteoporotic. Both are important for the increased fragility at these sites.

Pathophysiology of osteopenia

The natural history of the skeleton and the changes in bone mass that occur with age have been considered in Chapter 1.

The changes in bone mass with age are illustrated in Figure 1.1. Bone mass reaches a maximum after linear growth stops, begins to fall at about 30 and declines to half its maximum value by age 80 or 90. Women have less bone mass at their peak than men and show an accelerated phase of bone loss for 10 years after the menopause. This loss involves endosteal and Haversian resorption and loss of cancellous bone, particularly in the vertebrae, without replacement by new bone.

The low bone mass which is common with advancing age is due to a combination of suboptimal peak bone mass attained in early adult life, and to increased rates of bone loss that occur after middle age. Osteoporotic bones are prone to fracture because of low bone mass, architectural abnormalities both at the micro and macro levels, and acute trauma. The relative importance of each of these in the causation of osteoporotic fracture depends on the site of the fracture.

Attainment of peak bone mass

Peak bone mass, which is attained in early adult life, is dependent primarily on genetic factors (Mundy 1994, 1995), but is also influenced considerably by dietary calcium intake during adolescence and physical activity (Johnston et al 1992). Genetic factors have been obvious since there are differences in peak bone mass in various ethnic groups. For example, the black population have greater peak bone mass than Caucasians, who in turn have greater peak bone mass than Orientals, particularly the Japanese.

In early 1994, an original article was published in *Nature* that attracted an enormous amount of attention. This work suggested that in a population of Australian twins, there was a relationship between polymorphisms in the vitamin D receptor gene and the development of peak bone mass (Morrison et al 1994). The authors suggested that these polymorphisms in the vitamin D receptor gene could account for 75% of the genetic influence on bone mass. This was a finding that created a great deal of attention, particularly from the world lay press, many of whom reported that the "osteoporosis gene" had been discovered. The article was received with great interest by the bone field, and over the following 2 years there were many studies and much research with claims either confirming or disputing these findings.

It has long been known that peak bone density is predominantly due to genetic influences. However, the precise mechanism for which genes are involved in this presumably polygenetic effect has been unclear. The study by Morrison et al (1994) showed that there were polymorphisms in the vitamin D receptor gene that could account for up to 75% of the effects on peak bone mass. They based their studies predominantly on monozygotic and dizygotic twins and in fact showed that there was a much tighter correlation in bone density with these polymorphisms in monozygotic twins than in dizygotic twins, and there was a clear dose effect.

This finding attracted a lot of controversy. Many found it inherently unlikely that one single candidate gene could be so important in the development of peak bone mass. Over the subsequent two years there were a spate of papers, several of which suggested that polymorphisms in the vitamin D receptor are correlated with bone mass (Spector et al 1994; Yamagata et al 1994), but the majority of which found no association (Hustmyer et al 1994; Garnero et al 1995; Jorgensen et al 1996). Most of these studies were done in patients with the disease rather than in twins. The pros and cons for the two points of view were discussed in two recent back-to-back editorials in the *Journal of Bone and Mineral*

Research (Eisman 1995; Peacock 1995). The situation has been clarified a little at the World Congress in Osteoporosis in May 1996, when it was revealed that further studies on the normal Australian twins did not confirm the earlier findings. In summary, it appears most likely that the vitamin D receptor gene is a determinant of peak bone mass, although not as important as first suggested.

Vitamin D receptor polymorphisms are not the only polymorphisms that have been linked to peak bone density. There have also been suggestions that other genes, including interleukin-6, transforming growth factor β, the estrogen receptor and Type I collagen may be part of the polygenic picture. There is no question that the tremendous interest provoked by the article by Morrison et al (1994) has led to a large amount of work in this important area. For a candidate gene to be a convincing candidate as a major genetic component of peak bone mass, it needs to be shown that the polymorphisms are correlated with bone mass in a number of different populations, and that there is a demonstrable clearcut link between the polymorphism and altered function of the gene products that could be correlated with bone mass.

Rates of bone loss with advancing age

Figure 13.2 shows the factors that affect peak bone mass (genetic and environmental factors) and the factors that cause progressive loss of bone mass after middle life (aging, menopause, environmental factors).

Bone loss occurs in all individuals after middle life. The mechanisms of bone loss are multifactorial. They are due to complicated changes in bone cell activity during bone remodeling. These cellular changes depend on the major factor that is operative at any point in time. The major factors causing bone loss after middle life include sex hormone deficiency, disuse, and calcium and vitamin D deficiency. The rates of bone loss following abrupt hormonal withdrawal are exponential, whereas the rates of loss due to disuse or calcium and vitamin deficiency are more gradual (Heaney 1993). Since sex hormone withdrawal is usually abrupt in women, this is the reason that women suffer a rapid phase of accelerated bone loss after the menopause, whereas men lose bone slowly in parallel with a more gradual decline in sex hormone production. The losses of bone associated with the menopause are probably greater in cancellous bone than in cortical bone. It has been estimated that about two-thirds of the bone loss in older women can be ascribed to the menopause, and about one-third to aging (Riggs et al 1981). Although not all workers might agree with these estimates, there is no disagreement on the major role that estrogen deficiency plays in bone loss in women. The importance of other factors such as disuse, and dietary calcium and vitamin D deficiency will be considered below.

Christiansen and colleagues have long favored the view that rates of bone loss after the

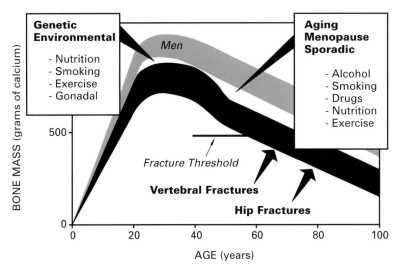

Figure 13.2

Important factors influencing attainment of peak bone mass and influence rates of bone loss in later adult life.

menopause are important, but that there is value in distinguishing the "fast losers" from the "slow losers" in decision making with respect to choice of treatment. This group has followed over 180 women over 15 years, and stratified them into fast and slow losers based on measurements of serum and urine markers of bone turnover, and correlated these findings with the risk of fracture and bone mass (Riis et al 1996). The concept is important for several reasons. If fast losers can be predicted, then this will be important in the selection of appropriate therapy as well as in predicting the natural history of the disease.

The other concept that is now being re-examined is that of fast and slow bone turnover, and the notion that low turnover is common in the aged. There is now greater appreciation that the rates of bone turnover may be increased even in the elderly. Garnero et al (1996) showed that rates of bone turnover may remain high in elderly women when followed carefully by measurement of bone markers. Those with the highest bone turnover have the lowest bone mass. Greenspan et al (1994) have shown that femoral bone loss, as assessed by careful studies in elderly women over the age of 65, may continue at high rates into the eighth decade, and cannot be predicted by measurement of spinal bone mineral density alone. Although it is not entirely clear as yet what the effects of these concepts will be on selection of therapy and management of patients, it seems likely that they will ultimately have some bearing.

Pathophysiology of osteoporotic fracture

Osteoporotic fractures occur most commonly in the hip and the vertebral bodies. They also occur at the wrist. Osteoporotic fractures occur because of low bone mass, architectural abnormalities in the skeleton and acute trauma. The factors responsible for peak bone mass and the rate of bone loss after middle life have been considered earlier. Here we will consider disturbances in bone architecture, femoral neck geometry and falls.

Bone microarchitecture

Bone loss associated with advanced age and estrogen deficiency in women is accompanied by a disturbance of bone microarchitecture (Parfitt et al 1983; Parfitt 1984, 1987). There is focal perforation of cancellous bone plates caused by osteoclastic resorption, leading to loss of connectivity of these horizontal plates (or "struts"), and the presence of "unconnected" vertical rods and bars dispersed throughout the marrow cavity (Figures 13.3–13.5). This has two important consequences. First, it places the remaining cancellous bone at a major structural disadvantage and increases the

Figure 13.3

Abnormality in cancellous bone that occurs in the vertebral bodies of patients with osteoporosis associated with aging, compared with normals. (Reproduced from Dempster et al (1986).)

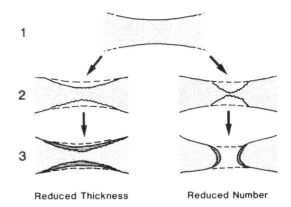

Figure 13.4

Mechanisms proposed by Parfitt for thinning (left) and complete perforation (right) of trabecular bone plates that occur in patients with osteoporosis associated with increased osteoclastic bone resorption. (Reproduced from Parfitt (1987).)

Normal | Osteoporosis

Figure 13.5

Summary of the pathogenetic abnormalities in patients with osteoporosis. There are three major findings: (1) thinning and fragmentation of the trabecular bone plates (there is some debate over whether thinning of the trabeculae occurs); (2) endosteal bone resorption leading to decreased cortical bone width; and (3) increased porosity of the Haversian canals, due to decreased osteoblast activity.

chances of compression or crush fractures in those bones that are rich in cancellous bone, such as the vertebral bodies. Unconnected vertical rods are liable to buckle and fracture, particularly if further thinned by states of high bone turnover. The mean thickness of cancellous bone plates is approximately 100–150 µm, whereas osteoclasts cause resorption defects of 50–100 µm during normal remodeling. Parfitt has suggested that focal perforations in cancellous bone plates could be due to increased osteoclast activity (caused by so-called "killer" osteoclasts), or to normal osteoclastic resorption defects occurring in relatively thin plates, an event that would be increased in frequency when activation of remodeling sites is increased (for example, by estrogen deficiency after the menopause) (Parfitt 1981). Secondly, it causes the (at least) theoretical situation where there is no basis of support for new bone formation to occur, even if osteoblasts can be stimulated to make new bone. The vertebral fracture rate can be inhibited either by reducing rates of bone remodeling, which reduces erosion of the vertical rods, or by factors that stimulate bone formation leading to thickening of the rods. It is possible (although not proven) that these changes in connectivity of horizontal struts that occur in older women can be corrected by formation-stimulating agents (Figure 13.5).

Femoral neck geometry

There is some evidence to suggest that patients with particularly long femoral necks, as assessed by the length of the hip axis, are more likely to fracture the hip (Faulkner et al 1993). This measurement has increased by one standard deviation in New Zealanders between 1950 and 1990. This is an inherited and congenital trait and cannot be corrected by any known agents.

Falls

Acute trauma is almost certainly a more important factor leading to fractures at the hip or the wrist than in the vertebrae. Factors that increase the risk of falls such as the use of medications, and in particular sedatives, decrease muscle strength and may impair vision. Concomitant disease should be reduced as much as possible to reduce the need for unrelated medications (Cummings and Nevitt 1994; Tinetti et al 1994). Fractures are most likely to occur at those skeletal sites with the greatest proportions of trabecular bone.

Factors that influence bone loss during aging

Nonhormonal

Bone cell senescence

Although there is no direct evidence, it appears likely that age-related bone loss is due in part to decreased functional capacity of bone cells associated with the aging process, which results in impaired bone formation relative to bone resorption. Several histomorphometric studies have shown that in elderly individuals the cavities formed by resorbing osteoclasts are incompletely filled by osteoblasts after the completion of a remodeling cycle. This abnormality is known as decreased mean wall thickness (Darby and Meunier 1981). It could theoretically be due to decreased capacity of osteoblasts to form new bone due to an inherent cellular defect or to decreased production of local growth regulatory factors (coupling factors) required to stimulate normal new bone formation. It is likely that both are important. However, the fact that fractures heal in the elderly does show that osteoblasts can function normally in the old, albeit often more slowly than in the young.

Diet

There is very convincing evidence to link dietary calcium deficiency with osteoporosis. Calcium deficiency in animals such as cats, rodents and dogs causes osteoporosis (Heaney et al 1982). Calcium balance studies in osteoporotic patients have consistently revealed that these patients are in negative calcium balance, with dietary calcium intake insufficient to account for calcium losses in feces, urine and sweat (Heaney et al 1982). Calcium absorption from the gut declines in all individuals with aging for multiple reasons, including changes in the gut epithelium, decreased vitamin D receptor content in gut epithelium, and decreased synthesis and/or responsivity to vitamin D (Gennari 1993). Normal young individuals can adapt by increasing the fractional absorption of calcium by the gut, but this capacity is reduced in the elderly (Slovik et al 1981; Heaney et al 1982). Since early data came mainly from cross-sectional rather than longitudinal studies, it is not surprising that there have been some disagreements on how much dietary calcium is required to prevent negative calcium balance. Some have suggested it should be 550 mg/day (Nordin et al 1979), whereas others have estimated that postmenopausal women require 1500 mg/day (Heaney et al 1978). More recently, several studies have shown that children receiving modest calcium supplements during the preteen years achieve higher peak bone mass than those with unsupplemented diets (Johnston et al 1992). After middle age, increasing calcium intake has minimal effects in the first 5 years after the menopause, but much greater effects thereafter.

Dietary calcium deficiency has also been implicated as a pathogenetic factor by other data. Dietary calcium intake is less in females than in males at all ages, and particularly in adolescent females, in whom calcium intake is not sufficient to maintain normal calcium balance. Moreover, epidemiologic studies in Hungary have revealed that populations with low dietary calcium intakes suffer increased incidence of hip fracture and have decreased cortical bone mineral density, as measured by cortical metacarpal thickness (Matkovic et al 1979). Exactly how dietary calcium deficiency could cause bone loss is unclear. It is possible that secondary hyperparathyroidism, occurring as a consequence of dietary calcium deficiency, causes cortical bone loss and increased bone turnover. This has been reinforced by recent studies showing that calcium and vitamin D supplements decrease hip fracture rates in the elderly and suppress plasma PTH concentrations (Chapuy et al 1992). Alternatively, since evidence exists that estrogen may stimulate 1,25-dihydroxyvitamin D_3 production, increased calcium requirements following the menopause could be due to estrogen deficiency, leading to decreased production of 1,25-dihydroxyvitamin D_3, which would cause decreased gut absorption of calcium (Riggs et al 1981).

Calcium deficiency and secondary hyperparathyroidism are common in osteoporotic patients, and can be reduced by increasing the calcium in the diet to the order of 1000–1500 mg elemental calcium per day. Calcium intake in the elderly tends to be low because of vitamin D deficiency, decreased skin synthesis of vitamin D, decreased gut vitamin D receptors, decreased renal conversion of 25-hydroxyvitamin D_3 to 1,25-

dihydroxyvitamin D_3 and decreased dietary intake of vitamin D. Calcium absorption from the gut can be improved by therapy with either vitamin D or active vitamin D metabolites, and the combination of vitamin D and calcium has been shown to decrease hip fracture rates (Chapuy et al 1992). Vitamin D deficiency is found or suspected in patients who are institutionalized, who are very old and who live in climates where there is little exposure to sunlight. Active vitamin D metabolites may also be used to increase calcium absorption, but they are more likely to lead to hypercalciuria and are more expensive.

Not everyone agrees that the effects of dietary calcium are important. Increasing calcium intake in the diet by supplementation can lead to increased bone growth in adolescence, although whether or not this has a lasting effect on bone mineral density is more controversial. While there remains some uncertainty about the overall importance of calcium intake, it is safe to prescribe calcium intakes of 1000–1500 mg/day, which are certainly not harmful. Moreover, in the elderly population, particularly those who are institutionalized and at risk for vitamin D deficiency, there is little to contraindicate supplementing vitamin D in the diet by 400 IU/day. However, more active vitamin D metabolites increase the risk of vitamin D toxicity and hypercalcemia in the elderly.

Protein malnutrition is occasionally present in patients with osteoporosis. Protein malnutrition is usually associated with alcoholism, malabsorption or nephrotic syndrome in most Western societies. Excess alcohol intake may be an independent factor impairing bone remodeling, and particularly osteoblast function (see below). High protein diets can cause a negative calcium balance, probably because of renal calcium losses associated with impaired renal tubular calcium reabsorption (Heaney et al 1982). There is a high prevalence of osteoporosis in patients with lactase deficiency (Newcomer et al 1978), which is possibly related to decreased tolerance to dairy foods and subsequent dietary calcium lack.

Ethnic influences

There are quite marked differences in the prevalence of osteoporosis in different ethnic groups. Osteoporosis is much less common in African-Americans (Trotter et al 1960) and in Mexican-Americans (Bauer 1986) than in Caucasians or Asians. The reasons for these differences are not clear. However, since bone mineral density shows a higher concordance between monozygotic twins than dizygotic twins, genetic factors are likely to be important (Smith et al 1973). In African-Americans, it appears likely that peak bone mass is greater (Cohn et al 1977). Bone mass and osteoporotic hip fracture are poorly correlated in Japanese, possibly because cultural differences lead to stronger musculature of the pelvic girdle in traditional Japanese, and subsequent decreased propensity to fall.

The studies of Eisman and colleagues (Kelly et al 1991; Morrison et al 1992) have focused attention on genetic influences that affect peak bone mass, and possibly also on rates of bone loss. This group has suggested that changes in vitamin D receptor function may be one of the major determinants in the genetic component of peak bone mass. However, other genes are also likely to be important (for more detailed discussion, see earlier).

Environmental influences

Epidemiologic evidence suggests that tobacco intake, alcoholism and inadequate sunlight are associated with increased propensity to osteoporosis (Daniell 1976; Seeman et al 1983). Moreover, increased coffee ingestion, and particularly caffeine intake, has been linked to osteoporosis (Daniell 1976). Inadequate sunlight exposure causes decreased formation of vitamin D, which in turn would decrease calcium absorption from the gut. The importance of marginal vitamin D deficiency in the pathogenesis of osteopenia associated with aging is probably greater in Europe than it is in the US, where sunlight and fortified foods make vitamin D deficiency very rare.

Physiologic stresses and illnesses

Pregnancy and lactation may have a protective effect on the skeleton, since patients with multiple pregnancies seem less prone to later development of osteoporosis. There is, however, a small subset of patients who suffer a severe and reversible form of osteoporosis during pregnancy (discussed later). Obesity is also protective. Immobilization, and even lack of physical exercise, predispose people to bone loss (discussed later). Bone mass is directly related to lean muscle mass (Cohn et al 1977). As muscle mass declines, so too does bone mass (Thompson et al 1986). The importance of physical exercise and maintenance of muscle mass is supported by many studies showing that regular physical exercise is good for muscle mass (Aloia et al 1978; Smith et al 1981; Krolner et al 1983).

Pregnancy and lactation are associated with severe demands on the maternal skeletal and calcium homeostasis, which are poorly understood. It is likely that there is a rapid and transient loss of bone during lactation, which is reversible with weaning (Sowers 1996). This area needs more investigation.

Hormonal

Gonadal hormones

Osteoporosis has been associated with the postmenopausal state since Fuller Albright noted over 40 years ago that 40 of his 42 patients with osteoporosis were postmenopausal females. In recent years, it has been clearly shown that there is accelerated loss of bone, occurring immediately after the time of the menopause, which lasts for about 10 years but is relatively much greater in the first 2–3 years (Lindsay et al 1976, 1980). This rapid phase of bone loss is reversed by estrogen therapy during these years. The precise mechanism by which estrogen deficiency increases bone resorption is still not clear (see Chapter 5).

Parathyroid hormone

Parathyroid hormone secretion is probably normal in many patients with osteoporosis. In a subset of patients, plasma PTH is increased (Riggs et al 1973; Gallagher et al 1980). These patients often have so-called Type II osteoporosis, characterized by older age and propensity to osteoporotic hip fracture. The senile secondary hyperparathyroidism and risk of hip fracture can be reduced by increasing oral calcium and vitamin D intake (Chapuy et al 1992).

Recently, Harms et al (1989) suggested that PTH is secreted in a pulsatile manner in normal individuals, with bursts of about 6–8 pulses per hour. This has been verified by several other groups (Kitamura et al 1990; Samuels et al 1993). Harms et al (1989) examined three males with idiopathic osteoporosis and suggested that these pulses of PTH secretion were lost in these individuals. This raises the possibility that nonpulsatile PTH secretion may be related to the bone loss associated with idiopathic osteoporosis. Since PTH causes different effects on bone cells when administered in a continuous manner compared with when it is administered in an intermittent manner, this is not an unreasonable hypothesis. However, we have been unable to confirm the findings of Harms et al (1989) that pulses of PTH secretion are lost in patients with osteoporosis (Samuels et al 1993).

The vitamin D–endocrine system

Most (but not all) studies have reported that circulating levels of 1,25-dihydroxyvitamin D_3 are decreased in elderly patients, including osteoporotics, by about 30% (Gallagher et al 1979; Tsai et al 1984). The reason for decreased 1,25-dihydroxyvitamin D_3 production is not entirely clear, although it is likely that vitamin D metabolism or production by the kidney is less efficient in the elderly (Armbrecht et al 1980). It is also possible that substrate availability is decreased because of dietary deficiency and decreased exposure to sunlight. Several studies have suggested that there is decreased 1,25-dihydroxyvitamin D_3 production in response to stimuli such as PTH in the elderly (Riggs et al 1981; Slovik et al 1981), although there is no convincing evidence that there is a difference between elderly patients with osteoporosis and those without osteoporosis.

As noted above, recent studies show that hip fractures can be reduced by increasing oral calcium and vitamin D intake in the institutionalized elderly (Chapuy et al 1992). The serum 25-hydroxyvitamin D_3 concentration should be greater than 80 nm/l. Hip fracture risk is increased dramatically if serum 25-hydroxyvitamin D_3 is less than 10 nm/l (Cummings et al 1993).

Calcitonin

Circulating calcitonin concentrations are less in the elderly than in the young and less in women than in men at any age (Heath and Sizemore 1977; Deftos et al 1980). Improvements in assay techniques (particularly plasma extraction) have cast some doubt on the age differences (Body and Heath 1983), although all workers agree that circulating concentrations of calcitonin in women are less than in men at any given age.

Local regulatory hormones or factors

Bone loss that occurs after middle life is characterized by an imbalance between bone resorption and bone formation, so that there is a relative increase in bone resorption over bone formation. This imbalance means that there is a disturbance in the coupling phenomenon that links resorption and formation, but the precise mechanism is entirely unknown. Since coupling is likely to involve local growth regulatory factors produced in the microenvironment of the remodeling unit, the secret to remodeling imbalance probably lies with abnormal local production of these factors, or abnormal responsivity of bone cells to them. These factors are discussed in more detail in Chapter 1.

Classification of osteoporosis

The traditional method for classifying osteoporosis has been to designate those patients without associated diseases as having primary osteoporosis, and those in whom osteoporosis occurs in association with other conditions as having secondary osteoporosis. This classification remains useful to the degree that it encourages clinicians to think of occult conditions that may occur in conjunction with osteoporosis. Several of the conditions frequently listed as secondary causes, such as thyrotoxicosis and myeloma, certainly cause osteopenia, but do not, in fact, cause osteoporosis with the same morphologic abnormalities when studied in detail as those seen in typical postmenopausal patients with primary osteoporosis. As Riggs and Melton point out (1986), the same pathophysiologic mechanisms responsible in primary osteoporosis could well be operative in many types of so-called secondary osteoporosis.

Primary osteoporosis

Senile or postmenopausal (involutional)

This is the most frequent type of osteoporosis and accounts for approximately 95% of all patients. It occurs most frequently in elderly white women. Riggs and co-workers at the Mayo Clinic have postulated that there are two distinct types of osteoporosis in the aging patient: Type I and Type II (Table 13.1) (Riggs et al 1981).

Table 13.1 Clinical types of osteoporosis.

	Type I	Type II
Eponym	Postmenopausal	Senile
Type of bone involved	Predominantly trabecular	Cortical and trabecular
Fractures	Vertebral	Hip/vertebral
Age incidence	55–65 years	>75 years
Sex incidence	Females/males 8 : 1	Females/males 3 : 1

Type I osteoporosis (also called accelerated osteoporosis)

This occurs in a subset (approximately 10%) of the female population within the first 20 years after menopause. These women have lost excessive amounts of cancellous bone, and frequently develop vertebral fractures. It is characterized by bone loss in excess of that associated with aging. The same syndrome occurs in men, but less than half as frequently as it does in women.

Type II osteoporosis

This occurs in older individuals, often over the age of 75 years, and is manifested by hip fractures as well as vertebral fractures. Rates of bone turnover are decreased and bone formation is impaired ("low-turnover" osteoporosis). It affects half the population of aging women and one-fourth the population of aging men. Bone loss is proportionate for both cortical and cancellous bone. This entity probably represents an exaggeration of age-related bone loss. This type of osteoporosis in old age is characterized by a form of secondary hyperparathyroidism, associated with low calcium absorption from the gut. Recent data suggest that treatment with calcium supplements and vitamin D may reduce both the secondary hyperparathyroidism and the propensity to hip fracture (Chapuy et al 1992).

Idiopathic

This unusual form of osteoporosis occurs in middle age and is relatively more frequent in men. There are infrequent reviews in the literature on this topic (Jackson 1958; Bordier et al 1973). It is usually associated with high bone turnover. It may be transient in nature, not lasting more than a few years. Recently, one group has found that monocytes derived from male patients with idiopathic osteoporosis constitutively produce more interleukin-1 than age-matched controls (Pacifici et al 1986). This finding is provocative and controversial, since not all others have been able to confirm it (Zarrabeitia et al 1991). More study will be required to confirm it and determine if other factors in addition to interleukin-1, which stimulates bone resorption, are produced by the monocytes of these patients. Harms et al (1989) have suggested that some of these patients have a disorder of pulsatile PTH secretion, although that has also not been confirmed by others.

Juvenile osteoporosis

Juvenile osteoporosis is less common than the other two forms of primary osteoporosis (Smith 1980). It occurs in both males and females during adolescence or in the 20s. The disease is very aggressive and is also associated with high bone turnover. Children with this condition are prone to metaphyseal fractures, particularly of the distal tibia. It tends to be transient and resolve spontaneously after puberty. The pathophysiology is entirely unknown. Any patient who presents with this form of osteoporosis should be evaluated very thoroughly for the presence of any of the associated conditions listed below. However, children with lymphomas or acute leukemia may also present with profound osteopenia of acute onset.

Secondary osteoporosis

This is osteoporosis associated with other medical conditions. The association between this group of conditions and the bone disease will now be reviewed.

Cushing's syndrome and steroid osteoporosis

Corticosteroid excess has long been known to be associated with a severe form of osteoporosis (Eisenhardt and Thompson 1939). This osteoporosis is frequently seen in patients treated with corticosteroids for prolonged periods (more than 3 months), particularly if they are postmenopausal women. Bone loss may occur very soon after the initiation of steroid therapy. It is a particularly striking feature of the rare form of Cushing's syndrome associated with macronodular hyperplasia of the adrenal glands, called Meador's syndrome.

Steroid osteoporosis is not common in patients treated with less than 10 mg of prednisone per day, but over one-third of patients will develop fragility fractures with prolonged use of higher doses. It involves predominantly cancellous bone, particularly of the vertebrae and ribs, and tends to spare cortical bone (Reifenstein 1956). The dominant effects on cancellous bone are particularly obvious when lumbar mineral density is assessed in the lateral projection by densitometry (Reid et al 1992). Delayed skeletal growth is characteristic of Cushing's syndrome in children. The effects of corticosteroids on the skeleton are most important when they are given to growing children or to postmenopausal women. The precise mechanism by which corticosteroids cause osteoporosis is unclear, since corticosteroids have multiple effects on bone cells (Mundy and Raisz 1974). Corticosteroids lead to an increase in bone resorption that is probably mainly indirect and mediated by parathyroid hormone. This is due to the effect of corticosteroids to inhibit calcium absorption from the gut, which leads to secondary hyperparathyroidism. Corticosteroids are also associated with decreased bone formation. This is almost certainly due to a direct effect of corticosteroids on osteoblasts to prevent their differentiation into more mature cells (Bressot et al 1979).

There is limited information on the morphologic effects of corticosteroids on the skeleton. Most information comes from well established or chronic cases of osteoporosis, which show a low turnover picture with primarily an impairment of bone formation. However, less is known of what happens in the first few months after initiation of corticosteroid therapy, and it is very possible that during this phase there is an increase in bone resorption, similar to that seen in immobilization osteoporosis. Clearly, more information is needed on the morphologic picture of corticosteroid osteoporosis.

Physicians treating patients with corticosteroids frequently do not pay enough attention to the possibility of osteoporosis occurring as a complication. Some studies have shown that less than 10% of the patients receiving large doses of corticosteroids long term are co-prescribed drugs to prevent or reverse bone loss. Part of the problem is that there are no generally accepted guidelines for prevention and treatment, as well as a lack of randomized controlled studies in patients with steroid osteoporosis. All the therapeutic agents used for postmenopausal osteoporosis have been tried. Of course, the problems with assessing the results of such studies are confounding variables such as the underlying disease over which corticosteroids are used, as well as the background bone mineral density of the patient before commencing therapy.

Thiazide diuretics may be useful to limit renal calcium losses and the propensity to develop nephrolithiasis. Obvious measures, such as reduction of steroid dosage as far as possible, are desirable. Alternate day therapy may be helpful, but this has not been documented. The drugs of choice are estrogen (if the patient is a postmenopausal female, and they are not contraindicated because of the underlying disease), bisphosphonates or calcitonin. Vitamin D and calcium supplementation have also been suggested (Hahn et al 1979, 1982), and work best when used prophylactically, particularly in postmenopausal Caucasian females at the initiation of high-dose corticosteroid therapy. Calcitonin, fluoride and pamidronate (Reid et al 1988) have also been tried with reports of success. Fluoride should not be given as sodium fluoride because of its propensity to cause irritation of the gastric mucosa. The bisphosphonate alendronate may be useful, but its propensity to cause mucosal irritation in patients taking corticosteroids is a concern until more information is available. Deflazocort is a synthetic steroid analog of prednisone, which is claimed to have lesser effects on bone cell and carbohydrate metabolism than other corticosteroids. The molecular mechanism responsible for the apparent bone-sparing effect is obscure.

A recent controlled study reported the effects of prophylactic use of calcitriol 0.6 µg/day and oral calcium supplementation (1000 mg/day) in patients beginning prednisone therapy (13.5 mg/day) (Sambrook et al 1993). Bone loss was prevented in the lumbar spine, but not in the hips or distal radius. Intranasal calcitonin potentiated the protective effect. However, hypercalcemia occurred in 25% of the patients. The limited efficacy and potential for side effects show that this is far from an optimal regimen.

This topic has been reviewed succinctly over the years in fine editorials by Baylink (1983) and Meunier (1993).

Chronic liver disease

Chronic liver disease is occasionally associated with osteopenia (Atkinson et al 1956). The mechanisms are likely to be multifactorial. Vitamin D metabolism is frequently impaired in patients with chronic liver disease. This may either lead to impairment of 25-hydroxylation and decreased circulating 25-hydroxyvitamin D_3 levels, or if obstruction of the biliary tract is present, then malabsorption of the fat soluble vitamins including vitamin D. However, in clinical practice it appears that impaired 25-hydroxylation is rarely of major clinical importance, and osteoporosis is more common in these patients than osteomalacia. Nevertheless, patients with chronic liver disease may also suffer from chronic pancreatic disease, particularly if alcoholism is responsible, and under these circumstances a component of malabsorption and osteomalacia is likely.

Turner's syndrome

Patients with Turner's syndrome suffer from lifelong hypogonadism and there is increased propensity to osteoporosis (Preger et al 1968). The mechanism is not known. It is not known whether they have decreased bone mass at maturity compared with normal ovulating women, but this appears likely.

Immobilization

Osteopenia occurs invariably in individuals who are immobilized or subjected to microgravity conditions, such as space flight. This type of osteopenia is frequently the result of immobilization following fractures, spinal cord lesions, strokes, and poliomyelitis, as well as space flight (Whedon and Shorr 1957; Mack and LaChance 1967; Birge and Whedon 1968; Panin et al 1971; Minaire et al 1974). Depending on the nature of the immobilization, it may involve the whole body or just segments of the skeleton. The major effects occur in weight-bearing bones. There appears to be an acute increase in both bone resorption and bone formation, although there is a relative increase in bone resorption that leads to a negative calcium balance involving the weight-bearing bones. Cancellous bone is involved predominantly. Over several months there is a gradual decrease in bone resorption and bone formation, so that eventually zero calcium imbalance ensues. Occasional immobilized patients, particularly those with the most rapid rates of bone turnover prior to immobilization (for example, in adolescent youths), develop hypercalciuria, and, less frequently, hypercalcemia (Plum and Dunning 1958). The precise pathophysiology of immobilization osteoporosis is unknown. It is possible the absence of weight-bearing alters bone cell function since it has been suggested for many years that there are piezoelectric forces present in bone that influence bone cell activity (Bassett 1968). However, immobilization also leads to a reduction in lean muscle mass, which in turn leads to a loss in bone mass. This type of osteoporosis usually takes 3–6 months to be detectable radiologically, although by this stage approximately 40% of bone mineral is lost (Minaire et al 1974). When more sensitive radiologic techniques, such as heel X-rays, are evaluated in astronauts following space flights, a striking difference is seen after just 2 weeks of microgravity conditions. This type of osteoporosis is usually reversible (at least partially) with remobilization. No treatment is known to be effective. Thiazide diuretics reduce the degree of hypercalciuria (Rose 1966), although it is unknown whether this makes any difference to the bone loss.

Heparin therapy

Heparin enhances the effects of PTH to stimulate osteoclastic bone resorption (Goldhaber 1965). It is not an important contributory factor in the osteopenia that may be present in some patients treated with heparin infusions for thromboembolic disease, although occasional cases have been reported (Griffith et al 1965; Jaffe and Willis 1965). However, a rare form of osteopenia associated with mastocytosis may be related to increased heparin production by mast cells (Chamus et al 1979). Mast cells are sometimes prominent in the bone marrow of patients with osteoporosis (Frame and Nixon 1968; Fallon et al 1980), but their etiologic significance is still uncertain.

Alcoholism

It has long been known that alcoholics are particularly predisposed to osteoporosis and alcohol is a clear risk factor in the development of osteoporosis, particularly in men (Seeman et al 1983). The mechanisms by which alcohol leads to osteoporosis are probably multiple. Alcoholism is frequently associated with both chronic liver disease and chronic pancreatic disease, both of which can lead to impairment in vitamin D metabolism and calcium malabsorption. Hypogonadism in males may also be a factor. Surprisingly, however, the limited studies of bone biopsy specimens by quantitative histomorphometry in alcoholics with osteopenia have not shown prominent mineralization defects or evidence of osteomalacia. Rather, they have shown low turnover osteoporosis with decreased osteoblast activity and decreased mean wall thickness (Bikle et al 1985).

The mechanisms by which alcohol affects bone cell function are obscure. Acute administration of alcohol leads to hypocalcemia in dogs, rats, and man (Kalbfleisch et al 1963; Peng et al 1972; Peng and Gitelman 1974; Baran et al 1980; Avery et al 1983). The relevance of this effect to osteopenia in chronic alcoholics is unclear, since it occurs only after short-term exposure. The mechanism is also unclear. Alcohol could cause osteopenia by directly suppressing osteoblast function, leading to decreased bone formation and collagen synthesis (de Vernejoul et al 1983), or indirectly by increasing secretion of adrenal corticosteroids. Acute ingestion of alcohol leads to a sharp rise in the plasma cortisol in normal patients (Rivier et al 1984; Valimake et al 1984). This is probably mediated by a direct effect on the hypothalamus to cause the release of corticotropin-releasing factor, and possibly also to a direct effect on the adrenal gland to release ethanol or acetaldehyde, the metabolic product of alcohol (Cobb et al 1979). It is also possible that alcohol could impair corticosteroid clearance by the liver. In recent years, there have been a number of reports of a syndrome occurring in chronic alcoholics resembling Cushing's syndrome. These patients have a sustained increase in corticosteroid production and evidence of impaired suppression by dexamethasone. This is usually reversible after alcohol is withdrawn. The bone biopsy appearance in Cushing's syndrome and alcoholic osteopenia is very similar.

Diabetes mellitus

It has long been argued whether osteopenia is a direct complication of diabetes mellitus.

The answer is still not known. Insulin is clearly a bone growth factor in vitro (Canalis et al 1977), and insulin deficiency could well be associated with decreased bone formation. However, patients with diabetes mellitus have many of the other risk factors that could lead to osteopenia, and it is difficult to know the relative significance of each in the individual patient. These include reduced physical activity, negative protein balance, renal disease and impaired gonadal function. On the other hand, obesity is common in many noninsulin-dependent diabetes mellitus, and this may be protective. Diabetics are prone to fracture, but this may at least in part be due to increased propensity to fall because of hypoglycemia, neuropathy or vascular disease. It is probable that insulin deficiency alone is not a major factor in the pathophysiology of osteopenia in diabetics.

Malabsorption

Patients with malabsorption syndrome, and particularly patients with primary biliary cirrhosis and other forms of chronic cholestasis, frequently develop osteopenia, but surprisingly have more prominent osteoporosis than osteomalacia (Sitran et al 1978; Adams and Mundy 1983). Usually, a combination of osteoporosis and osteomalacia is present, although osteoporosis typically is the predominant histologic abnormality. This does not seem to improve when osteomalacia is treated with vitamin D repletion. The pathogenetic factors responsible are unknown. If osteomalacia is an important component of the osteopenia of a patient with primary biliary cirrhosis, then clearly vitamin D therapy is warranted.

Osteogenesis imperfecta

Osteogenesis imperfecta represents a group of clinically heterogeneous inherited diseases of collagen metabolism that occur in approximately 1 in 20 000 live births. The disorders are due to a variety of point mutations in the Type I collagen gene that either decrease collagen synthesis or impair the stability of the collagen molecule (Shapiro and Rowe 1983). This results not only in decreased structural integrity of the bone matrix, but also in actual abnormalities in bone remodeling and particularly in bone formation for reasons that are not known. Approximately 100 separate mutations have been identified in the Type I collagen gene, which lead to either decreased collagen synthesis or impaired collagen function, both of which are characterized clinically by bone fragility. In some patients with subtle defects, the clinical manifestation of this condition may be osteoporosis (Spotila et al 1991). The frequency with which osteoporosis is the presenting clinical manifestation of subtle forms of osteogenesis imperfecta is currently unknown. The relationship between abnormal expression of Type I collagen and bone remodeling is discussed in more detail in Chapter 3.

Women with overt osteogenesis imperfecta are particularly susceptible to osteoporosis. It appears that there is a bimodal occurrence of fractures, with a peak frequency in fracture rate just before puberty and again after the menopause (Paterson et al 1984). The pubertal period often leads to improvement in symptoms and a decrease in fracture frequency. Patients with overt osteogenesis imperfecta have decreased bone mass at maturity, and as a consequence are probably more prone to develop osteoporosis during the postmenopausal period.

It appears possible that there is a significant subset of women with postmenopausal osteoporosis who, in fact, have underlying subtle osteogenesis imperfecta (Paterson et al 1984). Such a diagnosis could be suspected by the presence of a history of pathologic fractures during childhood, thin skin, higher rate of tooth loss than the average woman, blue sclerae, ligament laxity, and deafness, although the absence of these features does not exclude the diagnosis. The phenotype of these patients may be very similar to that of patients with familial idiopathic osteoporosis. In both conditions, osteoporosis may occur at a relatively young age and be associated with joint laxity and mild scoliosis. However, short stature, blue sclerae and deafness are features only of osteogenesis imperfecta. It seems reasonable to treat patients with osteogenesis imperfecta with estrogens following the menopause, since these patients clearly have increased risk for the development of osteoporotic fractures (Shapiro and Rowe 1984).

Anovulation in premenopausal women

Anovulation and amenorrhea of any cause will lead to bone loss in young women. Although most attention has been focused on excessive exercise, it is also true for anorexia nervosa, hyperprolactinemia, and treatment with gonadotropin releasing hormone agonists for endometriosis or uterine leiomyomata.

Exercise-induced amenorrhea is a relatively common condition. Estimates of frequency range from 3% to 10% of the total population of women who enter marathons to 30% to 50% of world-class athletes (Fricht et al 1978; Lutter and Cushman 1982). The mechanisms responsible are not clear, but it appears likely that extreme physical exercise (as well as dieting) is associated with a change in the pattern of release of gonadotropin releasing hormones from the hypothalamus characterized by decreased amplitude and decreased frequency of pulsatile hormone secretion, which in turn is associated with cessation of the normal menstrual cycle and a reduction in circulating estradiol levels (Fricht et al 1978; Lutter and Cushman 1982).

Several studies have shown that bone mineral density is reduced in amenorrheic athletes (Cann et al 1984; Drinkwater et al 1984; Marcus et al 1985). The type of athletic exercise is probably irrelevant, and the critical common denominator is anovulation. These women are particularly susceptible to fatigue fractures in, for example, the metatarsals or even tibiae in runners.

Exercise in small amounts is clearly beneficial to maintenance of bone mass. However, the studies referred to above indicate that women who exercise so excessively that they cease ovulation suffer from decreased bone mineral density and increased propensity to fractures (Cann et al 1984; Drinkwater et al 1984; Marcus et al 1985). Since athletes and particularly runners already have increased predisposition to stress fractures, this is a serious consideration for the female athlete who is amenorrheic. It remains to be shown whether this form of bone mineral loss is reversible. Elite female runners usually do not wish to be treated with estrogens, which are likely to change their body configurations and decrease their athletic performances. Patients with anorexia nervosa and patients with hyperprolactinemia from any cause who also are anovulatory suffer from similar osteopenia (Riggs et al 1982; Cann et al 1984; Drinkwater et al 1984; Rigotti et al 1984; Marcus et al 1985).

Pregnancy and lactation

A transient form of osteoporosis has been reported in small numbers of pregnant patients (Nordin and Roper 1955; Gruber et al 1984; Smith et al 1985). These patients may suffer fractures of the vertebrae and hips. There are no distinguishing features on bone biopsy or with any of the currently available serum markers of bone turnover. The cause and treatment are unknown (Nordin and Roper 1955; Gruber et al 1984; Smith et al 1985). Patients can be reassured that in the cases reported so far, osteoporosis has been limited to the pregnancy period, and that it does not necessarily recur in future pregnancies.

Hyperthyroidism and thyroid hormone therapy

Hyperthyroidism is associated with osteopenia, and in occasional patients with hypercalcemia (Mundy and Raisz 1979). This is due to the effects of thyroid hormone on bone cells to increase osteoclastic bone resorption (Mundy et al 1976). Hyperthyroidism is associated with a state of high bone turnover, presumably due to an increased frequency of activation of remodeling cycles and subsequent coupled bone formation (Eriksen 1986). Increased bone turnover is confirmed by an increase in serum alkaline phosphatase and markers of bone resorption such as urine hydroxyproline and urine deoxypyridinoline crosslinks (Harvey et al 1990). Although thyroid hormones have been shown to stimulate osteoclastic bone resorption in organ culture (Mundy et al 1976), thyroid hormones have not been thoroughly evaluated using currently available organ and cell culture systems to determine their effects on bone cells in more detail. Older studies suggested that 20% of patients with hyperthyroidism had increased total serum calcium and 50% had increased ionized calcium (Mundy and Raisz 1979), although those figures are much higher than most thyroidologists currently find in their clinics. Severe hypercalcemia is rare, and symptomatic osteoporosis (associated with fractures) is also rare in the majority of patients with Graves disease, who tend to be premenopausal females.

Possibly a more important clinical issue in the 1990s is the more subtle osteopenia seen in many middle-aged or elderly women treated with suppressive doses of thyroid hormone. A number of studies have now shown that when the plasma TSH is suppressed, bone mass is reduced (Diamond et al 1990; Baran and Braverman 1991; Greenspan et al 1991). This is necessary in treating patients with thyroid hormone for thyroid cancer, but is not necessary when replacement doses of thyroid hormone are needed in the treatment of hypothyroidism not associated with thyroid cancer. Under these circumstances, the plasma TSH should be kept in the normal range. There is some evidence that premenopausal women treated with thyroid hormone have reduced bone mineral density at the femoral neck, whereas postmenopausal women have reduced bone mineral density at the femoral neck, spine and radius (Diamond et al 1990). It is not surprising that postmenopausal women are especially vulnerable to overzealous thyroid hormone replacement therapy as an additional risk factor for osteoporosis. Since sensitive plasma TSH assays are now widely available, thyroid hormone replacement therapy that does not cause hyperthyroidism can be readily attained.

Osteoporosis in men

Osteoporosis in men has enough special features to make it different from osteoporosis in women that it deserves special consideration. Although not as common as in women, it is still a major clinical problem. The lifetime risk of osteoporotic fractures for white men in the US is about one-third that of women at all the major sites (Melton et al 1992). About one-third of all osteoporotic hip fractures world-wide occur in men, a total of more than 500 000 each year (Cooper and Melton 1992).

The vertebral fracture rate in men is about half that of women, not one-tenth as previously thought (Cooper and Melton 1992). Osteoporosis in men is clearly a major clinical problem.

The pathophysiologic factors responsible for osteoporotic fractures in men are slightly different than in women. Peak bone mass is greater in men. Loss of trabecular connectivity is not as prominent a feature in men as it is in women, possibly due to the absence of an abrupt menopause in men. Trabecular plate thinning may be the most prominent feature of the disturbance in bone microarchitecture that is present in men (Mosekilde 1990). Men are probably less susceptible to falls than women (Sattin et al 1990).

The major risk factors for osteoporosis in men are also slightly different from those in women. In a retrospective case control study of 105 male patients designed to detect particular risk factors that predispose men to vertebral osteoporosis, Seeman et al (1983) found that the outstanding factors prominent in the development of vertebral fractures in men were cigarette smoking, alcohol consumption and leanness. Lau et al (1988) found that alcohol, tobacco use and lower dietary calcium intake increased risk for hip fractures in men.

Secondary osteoporosis is relatively more common in men than it is in women. In men with osteoporotic vertebral fractures, 50% may have secondary causes (Scane and Francis 1993). The diseases associated with osteoporosis in men are hypogonadism due to pituitary tumors, hyperprolactinemia, Kleinfelter's syndrome, and hemochromatosis. Exogenous corticosteroids are also a relatively common cause of secondary osteoporosis in men (Seeman et al 1983; Jackson and Kleerekoper 1990).

There is a lack of published clinical trials of treatment in men. Short of such data, bisphosphonates or calcitonin can be used, and hypogonadal men should be treated with testosterone replacement unless contraindicated for other reasons.

Clinical features of osteoporosis

Pain

One of the most characteristic clinical features of osteoporosis is pain, particularly in the vertebrae. The source of the pain is unknown. Pain may or may not be associated with a detectable radiologic change. The radiologic changes observed usually involve one or more partial compression fractures of the vertebral bodies. However, severe pain occurs in some patients without any change in the X-ray appearance. It is likely that microfractures, which cannot be discerned by X-ray, have occurred in these patients. Pain is unusual in other skeletal sites in osteoporosis, even though many bones may be osteopenic. When pain does occur in the vertebral column, it may be extremely severe and last for a number of weeks. A component of the pain may be due to spasm of the large muscles of the back. This type of acute pain usually abates with rest. Other patients have more chronic and persistent back pain. The pain in patients with osteoporosis runs a variable course. In some patients, acute episodes of a few weeks' duration are separated by long periods of relative freedom from pain. Immobilization, which may be enforced because of pain, will itself cause further bone loss.

Fracture

There are three common sites of fracture in the osteoporotic (Melton and Riggs 1983; Kelsey 1984; Cummings et al 1985). The most common is in the vertebral bodies, which undergo compression or crush fractures. Fracture of the femoral neck is the most serious and life-threatening complication of this disease. Fractures of the distal forearm are less common, and usually occur after a fall on the outstretched hand. In the United States, there are approximately 600 000 vertebral fractures and 200 000 femoral neck fractures per year. The majority of these occur in osteoporotic individuals.

As already indicated, difficulties in detection and diagnosis of vertebral fracture have made assessment of the clinical features associated with this condition difficult to assess. It is probable that only one-third of patients with vertebral fractures seek medical attention as a consequence of the fracture. Different investigators have used different definitions of vertebral fracture based on either vertebral height, wedging or compression fracture. These results have been difficult to compare and it is not surprising that there have been considerable variations in recorded incidence and prevalence rates.

In recent years, considerable attention has been given to the effects of vertebral deformity and crush fracture on quality of life in the elderly. Not all compression fractures are associated with pain, and pain does not always correlate well with the radiological abnormalities. Patients may have multiple complaints that seriously interfere with their lives although they do not have pain. These complaints may include difficulty with bathing, performing household tasks such as bed-making or meal preparation, climbing stairs, gardening, and traveling to visit relatives and friends. These complaints, as well as the deformity itself, may lead to depression. Recently, the European Foundation for Osteoporosis (EFFO) has developed a questionnaire for patients with vertebral osteoporosis to assess objectively the effects of vertebral osteoporosis on the quality of life (Lips et al 1996).

Hip fracture is the most serious fear for the elderly osteoporotic, since it leads directly to death within one year for 15%, and about half of the survivors will require institutionalized care. Hip fracture is always associated with trauma, usually a fall, and prevention of factors predisposing to falls is vitally important in prevention. Recent data showing that improving calcium absorption through calcium and vitamin D intake, which also reduces the secondary hyperparathyroidism associated with old age, decreases hip fracture rates and is very encouraging (Chapuy et al 1992).

Deformity

Fractures of the vertebral column often follow a predictable sequence of events, and lead to characteristic deformity. The initial event is often a compression fracture in the midthoracic region. This may be followed by compression fractures of the lower dorsal or upper lumbar vertebrae, which together with compression fractures in the midthoracic region lead to a dorsal kyphosis or hunchback appearance (Figure 13.1). This is associated with loss of height. With further crush fractures, the abdomen becomes more prominent and as more lower lumbar vertebrae compress, the thoracic cage may occasionally come to rest on the pelvic rim to give a protruding abdomen or potbelly appearance.

Differential diagnosis of osteopenia

There are four major bone diseases that may present with the X-ray appearance of osteoporosis and low bone mineral density (Figure 13.3). It is extremely important to distinguish these diseases because they have different histologic features, pathogenesis, prognosis and therapy.

Osteomalacia

In this bone disease, there is an impairment in the mineralization of newly formed bone. The X-ray appearance is osteopenia, which may be indistinguishable from osteoporosis, unless pseudofractures are present at the sites where arteries cross bone surfaces at the scapula border, around the pelvic brim or on the medial aspect of the humeral head. Pseudofractures are rare. The histological picture shows a characteristic increase in nonmineralized osteoid tissue associated with decreased mineralization rates. Osteomalacia occurs in a setting where vitamin D or phosphate deficiency occurs and is usually characterized by abnormalities in the serum calcium, phosphate, and alkaline phosphatase concentrations. When phosphate depletion is the cause, the serum phosphorus is markedly depressed. In patients with vitamin D deficiency due to dietary lack or malabsorption, the serum calcium is low, the serum phosphorus is very low (due to decreased gut absorption and increased renal loss, caused by secondary hyperparathyroidism induced by the low serum calcium), and urine calcium excretion is also very low. Significant osteomalacia is occasionally seen without any detectable serum abnormality.

Osteitis fibrosa

In primary hyperparathyroidism, many patients develop osteopenia associated with increased bone turnover. The overall picture is not unlike that seen in occasional patients with thyrotoxicosis, but there are some important subtle differences. For example, in primary hyperparathyroidism subperiosteal osteoclastic bone resorption is characteristic and the increase in bone turnover is associated with marrow fibrosis. Although primary hyperparathyroidism occurs most commonly in postmenopausal women, it remains to be shown that untreated patients with mild disease are at increased risk of osteopenic fracture. Patients with primary hyperparathyroidism have hypercalcemia that should be detected if serum calcium is measured on several occasions.

Osteopenia associated with malignant disease

Osteopenia is common in myeloma, and occasionally occurs in other hematologic malignancies and sometimes with solid tumors. Osteopenia in myeloma may occur as discrete lytic lesions or as diffuse osteopenia. The changes are due to an increase in osteoclastic bone resorption produced by the bone resorbing factors produced by tumor cells. Hypercalcemia may be present (30% of patients with myeloma), but usually the serum calcium and phosphorus are normal.

Laboratory evaluation of the osteopenic patient

Abnormalities in serum calcium and phosphorus

There are no known abnormalities in calcium or phosphorus homeostasis in patients with primary osteoporosis. Serum calcium and phosphate are always normal. This is in contrast to most patients with osteomalacia and osteitis fibrosa cystica, where calcium and phosphate homeostasis are disturbed (discussed earlier). In some patients, particularly those with an increase in bone turnover, there may be an increase in urine calcium excretion.

Other noninvasive measurements have been used in an attempt to determine whether patients with osteoporosis have the high- low-turnover form of the disease. Unfortunately, investigators do not agree on their utility. Patients with high-turnover osteoporosis as a group have higher urine calcium excretion than patients with low-turnover osteoporosis. Nordin and colleagues have suggested that if patients have urinary calcium excretion greater than 150 mg/day, this is an indication of high-turnover osteoporosis (Nordin et al 1984). Bone Gla protein has also been used as a noninvasive measurement of the rate of bone turnover. The assays have been improved greatly in the last 2 years, with the development of IRMA assays using monoclonal antibodies directed against human bone Gla protein. Delmas et al (1983) and Epstein et al (1984) have each reported a gradual increase in the serum bone Gla protein from age 30 to 90 years, and this may be a predictor of increased risk of hip fracture. Serum bone Gla protein is increased in some patients with high-turnover osteoporosis, and is low in some patients with low-turnover osteoporosis. A recent study has shown that serum measurements of undercarboxylated bone Gla protein (also called osteocalcin) have a striking relationship to later development of hip fracture (Szulc et al 1993), a potentially important finding that requires confirmation. Assays for bone alkaline phosphatase have been improved by monoclonal antibodies that distinguish bone from liver isoenzymes. Newer markers of bone turnover such as urine pyridinoline crosslinks and serum pro-collagen peptides may turn out to be even more discriminating. After the menopause, there is a 50–100% increase of bone turnover as assessed by changes in bone markers such as pyridinoline crosslinks, bone alkaline phosphatase and bone Gla protein (Delmas 1993). However, it is not entirely clear that, with the therapeutic agents currently available, that such information is useful. It has been suggested that these markers may identify patients with high rates of bone turnover, which are associated with faster loss of bone and should possibly be treated aggressively with resorption inhibitors such as estrogen.

Bone biopsy

Quantitative histomorphometric evaluation of a core of bone taken from the iliac crest may provide useful pathophysiologic information, although this information only rarely alters clinical management. Probably the most important information is that it excludes the presence of osteomalacia if the specimen is undecalcified and that condition is suspected. Since in the United States osteomalacia is rare in the great majority of patients with osteopenia, it is hard to justify a bone biopsy unless osteomalacia seems a likely possibility for other reasons (such as malabsorption, chronic alcoholism, low serum 25-hydroxyvitamin D_3, anticonvulsant therapy, suggestive electrolyte abnormalities). In osteomalacia, there is an excess of nonmineralized bone (called osteoid tissue). In addition, there is a decrease in the mineralization rate of newly formed bone, which can be measured by labeling the active mineralization front with spaced courses of tetracycline. Tetracycline is fluorescent and the distance between the tetracycline lines in the biopsy represents the rate at which new bone is being mineralized. In osteomalacia, mineralization rates are markedly suppressed.

For the osteoporotic patient without osteomalacia, bone biopsy may indicate either high- or low-turnover osteoporosis. However, the biochemical markers also provide this information without an invasive procedure. Moreover, as noted above, it is arguable that this provides useful therapeutic information. It is possible that in the future, when more specific remedies become available, patients with high-turnover osteoporosis may be treated with agents that inhibit bone resorption and patients with low-turnover osteoporosis may be treated specifically with drugs that stimulate bone formation. The biopsy procedure is not only invasive, it is also not very sensitive for assessing cancellous bone volume. Moreover, bone in the iliac crest does not necessarily represent bone in the vertebral column, and even samples taken at adjacent sites in the iliac crest can show marked differences in cancellous bone volume. This should be taken into account when results using this insensitive technique are being evaluated. As a research technique, bone biopsy may give an indication of the structural basis of osteoporosis, including the disorder of cancellous bone architecture. It may also identify patients with unusual forms of osteoporosis, such as systemic mastocytosis, in which patients may have skeletal abnormalities such as osteopenia and crush fractures.

Bone mass measurements

Precise and accurate measurements of bone mass have markedly altered the management of patients with osteoporosis over the past decade. Progressive improvements in techniques have greatly influenced our understanding of patterns of bone loss associated with different types of osteoporosis, and have had major impact on clinical studies for monitoring changes in response to treatment. They have also greatly influenced clinical decision making such as when to treat and how aggressively. Bone mass measurements can be performed safely and quickly, are becoming progressively less expensive, and have been clearly shown to predict the relative risk of future fracture, more efficiently than can be estimated by an assessment of clinical risk factors. A decrease of one standard deviation below the mean for young normal individuals approximately doubles the risk of all fractures.

It is now possible to evaluate bone mineral density for the total skeleton and also in specific regions that provide estimates of the independent status of cortical and cancellous bone. Radiation exposure from dual energy X-ray absorptiometry is considerably less than for a chest X-ray or full dental X-ray. However, it should be appreciated that measurements of bone mass are not a measurement of bone mass for the total skeleton or in regional parts of the skeleton, and do not reflect the morphologic nature of the disease that is responsible for decreased bone mass. A wide range of techniques have been used, including radiogrammetry, single beam photon absorptiometry, dual beam photon absorptiometry (DPA), dual energy X-ray absorptiometry (DEXA) and quantitative computer tomography (QCT). Other techniques including ultrasound and magnetic resonance imaging are still in the investigational stage.

One major issue of interest with all of these techniques is the distinction of diagnostic threshold and therapeutic threshold. Although it is widely stated in the bone field that measurements of bone mineral density by any technique should be used primarily for diagnosis and not for decisions on therapeutic intervention, in practice this may be how these measurements are most often utilized.

DEXA

Although the usefulness and importance of these different techniques for bone mass measurement are evolving, DEXA is currently the most widely used and most useful. In this technique, a dual X-ray source is used to measure bone mass. It is reliable, rapid, relatively inexpensive, is associated with low radiation exposure, and has a low accuracy error in the order of 6%, depending on the site. The accuracy is greatest at the lumbar spine, but may be obscured by vascular calcifications, osteoarthritis or previous fracture. Although accuracy error is good for screening, low precision error is more useful for follow-up. The precision error with DEXA is of the order of 0.8–2%, depending on sites. Its usefulness in the prediction of fracture risk has been validated. It also has the advantage of being capable of measuring regional parts of the skeleton. New applications of dual energy X-ray absorptiometry, such as lateral spine scanning, which may provide better measurements of cancellous bone and body composition analysis are also possible. In recent years, the National Osteoporosis Foundation established a task force to provide guidelines for the clinical indications for bone mass measurements. This task force suggested that indications for bone mass measurements were as follows (Johnston et al 1989):

- In postmenopausal or estrogen-deficient women, measurements of bone mass can be used to help make decisions about hormone replacement therapy.

- In patients with X-rays of the spine that suggest osteopenia, bone mass measurements may be useful for more accurate determination of vertebral bone mass, relative risk of future fracture and provide useful information in order to make decisions regarding further diagnostic tests or therapy. Treatment interventions should not be based on bone mineral density alone, but should also be considered in light of other risk factors such as family history, previous fractures, length of time since menopause. In prediction of fracture risk, hip fracture is best predicted by bone mineral density measurements of the hip. The risks of other osteoporotic fractures can be made by measurements at any of the common sites (for example, wrist or spine).

- In patients being treated with long-term glucocorticoid therapy in order to guide glucocorticoid dose and the use of preventative measures.

- In patients with asymptomatic primary hyperparathyroidism in whom a decision has to be made whether or not to intervene surgically.

- Monitoring bone mass to assess the efficacy of therapy. This remains primarily an investigational tool, which is used in conjunction with other parameters of successful therapy such as reduced fracture rate. If serial measurements of bone mass are to be performed, they must be performed at some distance apart in time, determined by the precision of the instrument and the anticipated annual rate of bone loss. It is probably not useful with currently available instruments to measure more frequently than yearly. If serial measurements are to be performed, then the same instrument should be used. Moreover, bone mass has to be compared in relation to the appropriate reference population.

DEXA measurements are usually expressed either as a Z score (standard deviation from the age-adjusted normal mean) or as a T score (standard deviation from the peak bone mass). The T score is now used in the WHO criteria for the diagnostic assessment of osteoporosis (see earlier). By these WHO criteria, approximately one-third of postmenopausal Caucasian women have osteoporosis.

In individual patients with osteoporotic fracture, there is overlap with bone mineral density measurements with those of normals, which critics of this measurement frequently point to. The counterargument is that bone mineral density measurement is not a diagnostic technique for fracture, but rather an assessment of fracture risk. In fact, it is now widely documented that the fracture risk increases by 50–100% for every one standard deviation below the mean in the T score. Most data for this assessment have been accumulated with measurements of the radius, but it is also true for whatever bone mineral density is measured. It should be noted that DEXA does not assess the trabecular microarchitecture, and since this is an important parameter of increased fracture risk, improvements in this technique and others that include assessment of microarchitecture should improve fracture risk prediction.

A practical issue with DEXA measurements is whether it is necessary to measure more than one site. There is good correlation in most individual patients between sites and one site is enough for diagnosis. However, in about 10% of patients, one site may be normal and another low.

Computerized tomography

CT scans have been used for many years to determine bone mineral content in cancellous bone in the vertebral spine (Cann and Genant 1980; Genant et al 1982; Laval-Jeantet et al 1984; Rosenthal et al 1985). The major drawback to this technique has been that results can be obscured by the presence of subcutaneous tissue as well as by intramedullary fat, which is common in the elderly population. To ensure long-term reproducibility, measurements are standardized with the use of a phantom detector (usually an aluminum bar). Measurements can be made by most hospital scanners with the use of commercially available phantoms, but the accuracy is questionable (Riggs and Melton 1986). The radiation exposure is considerably higher and patient acceptance is less because of patient discomfort during the procedure. More precise and reproducible measurements are made when the machine can be dedicated to this use, although even in the best of hands precision is probably not as good as with DEXA.

CT techniques are evolving and improving dramatically. The future lies in their capacity to assess accurately trabecular microarchitecture. If this becomes possible, and it can be shown that this improves the prediction of fracture risk, then computerized tomography may challenge DEXA as the gold standard.

Ultrasound

Ultrasound is now being widely used for the assessment of bone mineral density. It has a number of advantages over other techniques, including portability, the assessment of bone microarchitecture, and the fact that it is relatively cheap. It is mostly performed at the heel, but may also be performed on the patella, tibia or phalanges. An additional advantage is that there is no radiation exposure. It is probably comparable to DEXA for diagnostic assessment, although as yet there is not adequate documentation of its value in monitoring therapy. The technique is evolving and future developments and validation are being watched with considerable interest.

Bone mineral density and fracture risk

There is now considerable evidence that bone mineral density is related to fracture risk. A number of convincing studies have suggested a strong relationship between fracture risk and bone mineral density. The site of measurement is probably not important. The relationship between bone mineral density and fracture risk has been assessed by a number of prospective studies that include fracture rate at the site of measurement as well as at other sites (Cooper and Melton 1992; Cummings et al 1990, 1993; Riggs and Melton 1995). The largest of these studies involved a cohort of 8134 women studied for almost 2 years, and this showed that for each decrease in bone mineral density of one standard deviation below the normal mean, there was a 2.6-fold increase in the age-adjusted risk of hip fractures. This was a short-term study, but is consistent with what has been found in other studies in smaller numbers of women followed for up to 10 years, where for a similar decrease in BMD at the normal mean, there was a 2.4-fold increase in the age-adjusted hip fracture risk rate (Melton et al 1993). Of course, these measurements are useful in population or epidemiology-based studies, but care should be taken in extrapolations made to the individual patient.

Bone markers

Simple markers of rates of bone turnover such as measurement of urinary hydroxyproline (for collagen breakdown products), or serum alkaline phosphatase and osteocalcin (for rates of bone formation), have been used for many years as assessments of bone turnover. This field has been advanced considerably in the past 5 years with the introduction of more sophisticated and specific markers of both bone resorption and bone formation. Bone formation can now be assessed by measuring not only serum alkaline phosphatase but the bone-specific isoenzyme by either ELISA or IRMA assay. Measurements of serum osteocalcin have been improved with better antibodies directed against both the intact human molecule and the large N-mid-fragment. A third measure of bone formation is serum Type I collagen carboxyterminal extension peptide, although this does not appear to be as sensitive as the other measurements. For bone resorption, use of one of the myriad assays for pyridinoline or deoxypyridinoline crosslinks of collagen has become the gold standard. Until recently, these various assays utilized HPLC methods on urine products, but have now been replaced by radioimmunoassay. Deoxypyridinoline crosslinks are specific for collagen. These crosslinks are present in the urine in free form (40%), the rest are associated with peptides. Some of the commercially available assays measure only free crosslinks, and others the peptide-bound crosslinks associated with either N or C terminal peptides.

The introduction of these better techniques for measuring rates of bone resorption and bone formation has raised the important issue of what place the measurement of these markers should occupy in the management of patients with osteoporosis. Specific questions ask whether their place is (1) relative to measurements of bone mineral density; (2) in the prediction of fracture risk; (3) in monitoring the efficacy of therapy; (4) in distinguishing states of high turnover and low turnover; or (5) in distinguishing fast losers from slow losers. It is becoming increasingly clear that the higher rates of bone turnover are more frequent in the elderly, and are more likely to be associated with later fragility fractures. These tests in general have considerably less accuracy and precision than bone mineral density, and are not surrogates for measuring bone mineral density. They should not be used in the diagnosis of osteoporosis. However, the precision is much better than the expected rate of change, and so they are excellent for measuring response to therapy, at least in larger numbers of patients in investigative studies. Their place in the assessment of individual patients is still uncertain. Despite this, they offer information not obtainable from bone mineral density such as the effects of specific antiresorptive therapies within the first few months after introduction of therapy, and evidence of compliance with therapy. They will clearly become increasingly important adjuncts to measurements of bone mineral density.

Risk factors and osteoporosis

Since osteoporosis is presently a disease that is easier to prevent than to treat, over the years considerable attention has been given to identification of those people who are at increased risk of developing the disease, and particularly those at risk of fracture. The list of risk factors has changed a little with increased knowledge made possible by precise measurements of bone mass. However, the literature has become somewhat confused because the risk factors for osteoporotic fracture are not necessarily the same as those for decreased bone mineral density. In other words, not all risk factors predispose to osteoporotic fracture because of their direct effects on bone mineral density (Cummings et al 1993). The major risk factors for development of an osteoporotic hip fracture (the most serious consequence of osteoporosis) are decreased bone mineral density coupled with increased propensity to fall. The risk of falling may be enhanced by the use of barbiturates or psychotropic drugs in the elderly (Kelsey and Hoffman 1987; Ray et al 1987). Many of the other factors linked to decreased bone mass and osteoporotic fracture involve relatively loose associations. It is impossible at present to define precisely the degree of risk associated with any one factor to the later development of osteoporotic fracture. It is possible that many of the so-called risk factors are interrelated or overlap, with one being responsible for or causing another.

The major risk factors for osteoporosis are listed below.

Female sex

Osteoporosis is clearly more common in females than in males. A number of factors may be important. Women have less bone mass at maturity and more rapid rates of loss than men due to the abrupt cessation of ovarian function that occurs at the menopause. Bone loss occurs at the rate of 3–5% per year during the first 3 years after estrogen withdrawal and although it then slows a little, it is still greater than in men 10 years after menopause.

Race/ethnicity

Peak bone mass is in part a genetic trait. Osteoporosis is rare in African-Americans and Mexican-Americans, but common in Caucasians and Asians. African-Americans have a higher bone mass at maturity than Caucasians, and it is likely that this is also true for Mexican-Americans. Hip fracture rates in African-American women are about 50% of those of Anglo-Americans, and Mexican-American women are intermediate between the two. Peak bone mass in these groups shows the same trend.

Diet

It is widely held that osteoporosis is more common in patients whose dietary calcium intake is low (Consensus Conference 1984; Riggs et al 1986). Osteoporosis is more common in patients who have increased phosphate and protein content in the diet. Increased dietary phosphate is associated with negative calcium balance (due to calcium binding in the gut lumen) and subjects who ingest large amounts of protein have increased calcium loss in the urine (Heaney and Recker 1982), presumably because acid radicals decrease renal tubular reabsorption of calcium. A fuller description of the potential role of calcium deficiency in osteoporosis was discussed earlier.

Smoking

There is evidence that smokers are more prone to osteoporosis as well as to hip fractures (Daniell 1976; Seeman et al 1983; Aloia et al 1985). Smokers are leaner and are less likely to be obese, which is also a protective factor against osteoporosis. Smoking is associated with earlier menopause in women (Jick et al 1977). However, smoking is also a risk factor for osteoporosis in men (Seeman et al 1983), so other mechanisms are presumably involved.

Alcohol

Alcoholics have less bone than controls and some alcoholics have severe osteoporosis without other apparent cause (Saville 1965). Alcoholics are also more likely to fall. The association between alcohol intake, alcoholism and osteoporosis was reviewed earlier.

Inactivity

Physical exercise is associated with relative increase in bone mass, although intense physical activity may be associated with amenorrhea and causes decreased bone mass (discussed earlier). Athletes in general have greater bone mineral density than their age-matched controls (Nilsson and Westlin 1971). However, although absolute immobilization causes osteopenia, it is not entirely clear that low levels of physical activity are a significant risk factor (Johnell and Nilsson 1984). In prospective studies, postmenopausal women enrolled in a regular exercise program have gained bone rather than lost it, as controls do (Aloia et al 1978; Krolner et al 1983). Pocock et al (1986) have recently evaluated the relationship between physical fitness, as measured by capacity to pedal at a fixed speed on an exercise bicycle against a work load, and bone mineral density. They found a positive correlation between physical fitness and bone mineral density in the femoral neck and lumbar spine as measured by dual beam photon absorptiometry.

Leanness

Osteoporosis is more common in the thin than it is in the obese (Daniell 1976; Seeman et al 1983).

Coffee ingestion

Osteoporosis has been linked to excessive caffeine ingestion, which has a calciuric effect (Heaney and Recker 1982). Daniell (1976) found that a high caffeine intake was associated with decreased cortical thickness and higher fracture rates in postmenopausal women.

Diseases associated with secondary osteoporosis

There are some diseases that make the patients more likely to develop osteoporosis. These include Cushing's syndrome, thyroid hormone suppressive therapy, previous gastric surgery, which impairs both vitamin D absorption and metabolism and dietary calcium absorption, and hypogonadism in males.

Methods of determining efficacy of therapy in osteoporosis

Fracture rate

The ultimate assessment of the efficacy of any form of treatment for osteoporosis is determination of the rate of new fractures while patients are being treated with that form of therapy. However, the rates of occurrence of new clinically apparent fractures are low enough in untreated patients that this form of assessment takes thousands of patients and years of study to provide useful information (Liberman et al 1995). As a shortcut, investigators have changed the definition of a new "fracture" so that it is based on a radiologic change assessed by changes in shape of vertebral bodies on lateral X-rays. However, as noted earlier, there is no uniform agreement on criteria. Moreover, it is unclear that these radiologic abnormalities will progress. Such an approach increases by 25 times the number of so-called fractures. The FDA currently requires fracture assessment as a criterion of therapeutic efficacy. Radiologic abnormalities and bone mass measurements are not always concordant, as demonstrated by the recent fluoride and etidronate studies (Riggs et al 1990; Storm et al 1990).

Serial measurements of bone mineral density or bone mass

One method for evaluating any form of therapy is to use a serial measurement of bone mineral density. However, the expected rate of change is similar to the precision of the instrument, and it is likely to take 1–2 years to see an effect. Moreover, such an approach requires observation of individual patients for a number of years since it will take this period to produce a new steady state because of the effects on remodeling space (Parfitt 1980). Thus, prolonged observation in large numbers of patients is required for valid evaluation of therapy, at least for 2–3 years. Studies showing beneficial effects of antiresorptive agents such as calcitonin or bisphosphonates should be interpreted as inconclusive unless they have been assessed after this period of treatment.

Serial measurements of bone markers

Serial measurements of bone markers (serum alkaline phosphatase or osteocalcin, urine deoxypyridinoline or pyridinoline crosslinks of collagen) should give an indication of response to therapy within 6–12 weeks of commencement. The precision of these tests is better than the anticipated rate of change, and they should become increasingly useful in the short term in assessing treatment efficacy.

Pain

Assessing efficacy of any treatment by relief from pain is unreliable. Pain in the back is due not only to vertebral fracture but may be associated with muscle spasm (frequent in patients with vertebral body compression fractures), or other unrelated causes, such as disc disease or degenerative arthritis. Moreover, in addition to the placebo effects, some agents used as therapies in osteoporosis have an analgesic effect. Calcitonin is the classic example (Pecile et al 1975).

Treatment

Therapy can be considered in terms of preventative treatment and treatment for established disease. Preventative treatment of osteoporosis should ideally begin during adolescence and involve those activities that ensure attainment of optimal peak bone mass, namely an adequate dietary calcium intake and avoidance of sedentary activities. In later life, other lifestyle factors that may be avoided or modified include sedentary habits, prolonged immobilization, malnutrition and vitamin D deficiency. Other lifestyle activities after the menopause that are helpful include reasonable physical activity, avoidance of excess alcohol and tobacco, and avoidance or limitation of harmful medications such as corticosteroids. Recent evidence indicates that prophylactic therapy with adequate dietary calcium and vitamin D prevents against later development of hip fractures in institutionalized individuals (Chapuy et al 1992). To reduce the rate of bone loss after the menopause, estrogen is the most effective useful agent available, particularly in the first few years postmenopausally when the loss of bone due to estrogen deficiency appears to be exponential.

Although many studies have suggested that moderate exercise is beneficial to bone mass, definitive proof is still lacking. Excessive exercise leading to amenorrhea in women is harmful (discussed earlier). Patients should be encouraged to walk several miles per day. It is usually stated that exercise should be weight-bearing, and that walking and jogging are better than, for example, swimming. This has been reinforced by the evidence that astronauts lose bone during space flight and that immobilization and denervation cause osteopenia. However, nonweight-bearing exercise may also help. It is clear that there is a strong correlation between lean body muscle mass and bone mineral density, and any exercise that maintains or increases lean body muscle mass should be beneficial to the skeleton. One beneficial aspect of exercise in the elderly may be to decrease the likelihood of falls because of its effects on muscle strength and coordination.

Planned physical activity should improve bone mass, reduce the likelihood of falls and subsequent fracture, and benefit patients with vertebral fracture. Although weight-bearing exercise clearly increases bone mass, Pocock et al (1986) also found that bone mass in the femoral neck and lumbar spine is also positively correlated with fitness. Patients with severe osteoporosis may benefit from a rehabilitation program that involves psychiatrists, physical therapists, occupational therapists and rehabilitation nurses and social workers. Bracing of the thoracolumbar spine for vertebral fractures, pain relief, measures to prevent constipation and risk of falls, the use of low-heeled and soft-soled shoes with assistive devices such as canes and walkers, the assessment of environmental hazards such as poor vision, polypharmacy, shoewear, throw rugs, electrical cords, long dresses and nightgowns, poorly lit stairways and icy streets, adding bilateral handrails on stairs and handrails on bathrooms may all be beneficial. A successful exercise program that is weight-bearing, diverse, associated with a slow progression to accommodate the fitness level, and compatible with the state of cardiovascular fitness may increase bone mass, increase lean body muscle mass, improve flexibility, decrease pain and markedly reduce risk of falling.

Since prevention of fracture and maintenance of bone mass and the structural integrity of bone in patients with osteoporosis depend to a large degree on patient motivation and understanding the problem so that appropriate lifestyle changes can be made, patient education is very important. In this regard, foundations such as the National Osteoporosis Foundation (NOF) in the United States, the National Osteoporosis Society in the United Kingdom and EFFO (European Federation for Osteoporosis) in Europe are very important. These foundations provide state-of-the-art educational information for both patients and physicians. Through the use of patient brochures and newsletters, as well as information on web sites on the Internet on such issues as diet, physical activity, living with bone pain and avoiding fractures, they serve an increasingly more important service as patients (either current or future) become increasingly more aware of this condition. Moreover, these groups have held enormously successful educational physician conferences at international, national and regional levels, have provided grants for research for studies through their own grant programs and have assisted by lobbying for funds in this field through traditional government granting agencies.

For patients with established disease, the same approach to lifestyle factors is important. Avoidance of excessive intake of tobacco and lack of physical activity are probably the most important, as well as ensuring an adequate calcium and vitamin D intake. The appropriate available pharmacological therapies are estrogen, bisphosphonates and calcitonin. Estrogen is preferred in postmenopausal women because it can be taken orally and is much cheaper. Moreover, it has other beneficial effects on cardiovascular mortality. However, for those women who will not or should not take estrogen, or for men, then bisphosphonates or calcitonin are appropriate alternatives. There are multiple preparations of estrogen, bisphosphonates and calcitonin, as well as several different modes of administration for each. This is covered in more detail in Chapter 5. Antiestrogens and newer bisphosphonates are still under trial, and there are still so many questions about fluoride therapy that its use routinely outside investigative units is not recommended.

Available drug therapies (estrogen, calcitonin, fluoride, bisphosphonates) have been considered in more detail in Chapter 5. Potential future approaches are reviewed in Chapter 14.

The clinical problem of osteoporosis is so great and the numbers of patients so enormous that care cannot be administered entirely by subspecialists such as endocrinologists or rheumatologists. For example, there are approximately 6000 endocrinologists and rheumatologists in the United States, but there are literally tens of millions with this disease. Many of these patients will receive care from other physicians including primary care physicians and orthopedists. Many countries recognize this problem and are now writing clinical practice guidelines for physicians who see these patients based on the strongest evidence available. These guidelines will consider not just issues such as the therapeutic value of a given intervention, but also the costs relative to the potential gain, an increasingly important consideration in the current medical climate of spiraling health care costs. A special complicating issue is that some interventions, particularly those relative to primary prevention, will not show benefit for many years hence. In the United States, the National Osteoporosis Foundation (NOF) has been primarily responsible for the development of clinical osteoporosis guidelines, which will be launched publicly in 1998.

References

Adams ND, Mundy GR (1983) Therapy of hyper- and hypoparathyroidism. In: Conn HF, ed, *Current therapy* (WB Saunders: Philadelphia) 480–4.

Aloia JF, Cohn SH, Ostuni JA et al (1978) Prevention of involutional bone loss by exercise, *Ann Intern Med* **89**: 356–8.

Aloia JF, Vaswani A, Ellis K et al (1985) A model for involutional bone loss, *J Lab Clin Med* **106**: 630–7.

Armbrecht HJ, Zenser TV, Davis BB (1980) Effect of age on the conversion of 25-hydroxyvitamin D_3 to 1,25-dihydroxyvitamin D_3 by kidney of rat, *J Clin Invest* **66**: 1118–23.

Atkinson M, Nordin BEC, Sherlock S (1956) Malabsorption and bone disease in prolonged obstructive jaundice, *Q J Med* **25**: 299–312.

Avery DH, Overall JE, Calil HM et al (1983) Plasma calcium and phosphate during alcohol intoxication. Alcoholics versus nonalcoholics, *J Stud Alcohol* **44**: 205–14.

Baran DT, Braverman LE (1991) Thyroid hormones and bone mass, *J Clin Endocrinol Metab* **72**: 1182–3.

Baran DT, Teitelbaum SL, Bergfeld MA et al (1980) Effect of alcohol ingestion on bone and mineral metabolism in rats, *Am J Physiol* **238**: E507–E510.

Bassett CAL (1968) Biologic significance of piezoelectricity, *Calcif Tissue Res* **1**: 252–72.

Bauer RL (1986) Ethnic differences in hip fracture incidence in Bexar County, *Clin Res* **34**: 358A.

Baylink DJ (1983) Glucocorticoid-induced osteoporosis, *N Engl J Med* **309**: 306–8.

Bikle DD, Genant HK, Cann C et al (1985) Bone disease in alcohol abuse, *Ann Intern Med* **103**: 42–8.

Birge SJ Jr, Whedon GD (1968) Bone. In: McCally M, ed, *Hypodynamics and hypogravics* (Academic Press: New York) 213–35.

Body JJ, Heath H III (1983) Estimates of circulating monomeric calcitonin: physiological studies in normal and thyroidectomized man, *J Clin Endocrinol Metab* **57**: 897–903.

Bordier PJ, Miravet L, Hioco D (1973) Young adult osteoporosis, *Clin Endocrinol Metab* **2**: 277–92.

Bressot C, Meunier PJ, Chapuy MC et al (1979) Histomorphometric profile, pathophysiology and reversibility of corticosteroid-induced osteoporosis, *Metab Bone Relat Res* **1**: 303–11.

Canalis EM, Dietrich JW, Maina DM et al (1977) Hormonal control of bone collagen synthesis in vitro: effects of insulin and glucagon, *Endocrinology* **100**: 668–74.

Cann CE, Genant HK (1980) Precise measurement of vertebral mineral content using computed tomography, *J Comput Assist Tomogr* **4**: 493–500.

Cann CE, Martin MC, Genant HK et al (1984) Decreased spinal mineral content in amenorrheic women, *JAMA* **251**: 626–9.

Chamus JP, Prier A, Lievre JA et al (1979) L'ostéoporose mastocytaraire, *Revue du Rhumatisme et les Maladies Osteo-articulaires* **46**: 29–35.

Chapuy MC, Arlot ME, Duboeuf F et al (1992) Vitamin D_3 and calcium to prevent hip fractures in the elderly women, *N Engl J Med* **327**: 1637–42.

Cobb CF, Van Thiel DH, Ennis MF (1979) Is acetaldehyde an adrenal stimulant? *Curr Surg* **36**: 431–7.

Cohn SH, Abesamis C, Yasumura S et al (1977) Comparative skeletal mass and radial bone mineral content in black and white women, *Metabolism* **26**: 171–8.

Consensus Conference (1984) Osteoporosis, *JAMA* **252**: 799–802.

Cooper C, Melton LJ (1992) Epidemiology of osteoporosis, *Trends Endocrinol Metab* **3**: 224–9.

Cummings SR, Nevitt MC (1994) Falls, *N Engl J Med* **331**: 872–3.

Cummings SR, Kelsey JL, Nevitt MC et al (1985) Epidemiology of osteoporosis and osteoporotic fractures, *Epidemiol Rev* **7**: 178–208.

Cummings SR, Black DM, Nevitt MC et al (1990) Appendicular bone density and age predict hip fracture in women, *JAMA* **263**: 665–8.

Cummings SR, Black DM, Nevitt MC et al (1993) Bone density at various sites for prediction of hip fractures, *Lancet* **341**: 72–5.

Daniell HW (1976) Osteoporosis of the slender smoker: vertebral compression fractures and loss of metacarpal cortex in relation to postmenopausal cigarette smoking and lack of obesity, *Arch Intern Med* **136**: 298–304.

Darby AJ, Meunier PJ (1981) Mean wall thickness and formation periods of trabecular bone packets in idiopathic osteoporosis, *Calcif Tissue Int* **33**: 199–204.

Deftos IJ, Weisman MH, Williams GW (1980) Influence of age and sex on plasma calcitonin in human beings, *N Engl J Med* **302**: 1351–3.

Delmas PD (1993) Biochemical markers of bone turnover in osteoporosis. In: Christiansen C, ed, *Proceedings of the 4th International Symposium on Osteoporosis and Consensus Development Conference*, Hong Kong, 1993, no 48.

Delmas PD, Stenner D, Wahner HW et al (1983) Increase in serum bone gamma carboxyglutamic acid protein with aging in women: implications for the mechanism of age-related bone loss, *J Clin Invest* **71**: 1316–21.

Dempster DW, Shane E, Horbert W et al (1986) A simple method for correlative light and scanning electron microscopy of human iliac crest bone biopsies: qualitative observations in normal and osteoporotic subjects, *J Bone Miner Res* **1**: 15–21.

de Vernejoul MC, Bielakoff J, Herve M (1983) Evidence for defective osteoblastic function: a role for alcohol and tobacco consumption in osteoporosis in middle-aged men, *Clin Orthop* **179**: 107–15.

Diamond T, Nery L, Hales I (1990) A therapeutic dilemma: suppressive doses of thyroxine significantly reduce bone mineral measurements in both pre-menopausal and postmenopausal women with thyroid carcinoma, *J Clin Endocrinol Metab* **72**: 1184–8.

Drinkwater BL, Nilson K, Chesnut CH III et al (1984) Bone mineral content of amenorrheic and eumenorrheic athletes, *N Engl J Med* **311**: 277–81.

Eastell R, Cedel SL, Wahner HW et al (1991) Classification of vertebral fractures, *J Bone Miner Res* **6**: 207–15.

Eisenhardt L, Thompson KW (1939) Brief consideration of present status of so-called basophilism with a tabulation of verified cases, *J Biol Med* **11**: 507–22.

Eisman JA (1995) Vitamin D receptor gene alleles and osteoporosis: an affirmative view, *J Bone Miner Res* **10**: 1289–93.

Epstein S, Poser J, McClintock R (1984) Differences in serum bone Gla protein with age and sex, *Lancet* **i**: 307–10.

Eriksen EF (1986) Normal and pathological remodeling of human trabecular bone: three dimensional reconstruction of the remodeling sequence in normals and in metabolic bone disease, *Endocrinol Rev* **7**: 379–408.

Fallon MD, Whyte MP, Craig RB et al (1980) Mast cell proliferation in postmenopausal osteoporosis, *Clin Res* **28**: 738A.

Faulkner KG, Cummings SR, Black D et al (1993) Simple measurements of femoral geometry predicts hip fracture, *J Bone Miner Res* **8**: 1211–17.

Frame B, Nixon RK (1968) Bone marrow mass cells in osteoporosis of aging, *N Engl J Med* **279**: 626–30.

Fricht CB, Johnson TS, Martin BJ et al (1978) Secondary amenorrhoea in athletes, *Lancet* **ii**: 1145–6.

Gallagher JC, Riggs BL, Eisman J et al (1979) Intestinal calcium absorption and serum vitamin D metabolites in normal subjects and osteoporotic patients: effect of age and dietary calcium, *J Clin Invest* **64**: 729–36.

Gallagher JC, Riggs BL, Jerpbak CM et al (1980) The effect of age on serum immunoreactive parathyroid hormone in normal and osteoporotic women, *J Lab Clin Med* **95**: 373–85.

Garnero P, Borel O, Sornay-Rendu E et al (1995) Vitamin D receptor gene polymorphisms do not predict bone turnover and bone mass in healthy premenopausal women, *J Bone Miner Res* **10**: 1283–8.

Garnero P, Sornayrendu E, Chapuy MC et al (1996) Increased bone turnover in late postmenopausal women is a major determinant of osteoporosis, *J Bone Miner Res* **11**: 337–49.

Genant HK, Cann CE, Ettinger B et al (1982) Quantitative computed tomography of vertebral spongiosa: a sensitive method for detecting early bone loss after oophorectomy, *Ann Intern Med* **97**: 699–705.

Gennari C (1993) Intestinal calcium transport and aging. In: Christiansen C, ed, *Proceedings of the 4th International Symposium on Osteoporosis and Consensus Development Conference*, Hong Kong, 1993, no 59.

Goldhaber P (1965) Heparin enhancement of factor-stimulating bone resorption in tissue culture, *Science* **147**: 407–8.

Greenspan SL, Greenspan FS, Resnick NM et al (1991) Skeletal integrity in premenopausal and postmenopausal women receiving long-term L-thyroxine on bone density, *Am J Med* **91**: 5–14.

Greenspan SL, Maitland LA, Myers ER et al (1994) Femoral bone loss progresses with age: a longitudinal study in women over age 65, *J Bone Miner Res* **9**: 1959–65.

Griffith GC, Nichols G Jr, Asher JD et al (1965) Heparin osteoporosis, *JAMA* **193**: 91–4.

Gruber HE, Gutteridge DH, Baylink DJ (1984) Osteoporosis associated with pregnancy and lactation: bone biopsy and skeletal features in three patients, *Metab Bone Dis Relat Res* **5**: 159–65.

Hahn TJ, Halstead LR, Baran DT (1982) Effects of short-term corticosteroid administration on the intestinal calcium absorption and circulating vitamin D metabolite concentrations in man, *J Clin Endocrinol Metab* **52**: 111–15.

Hahn TJ, Halstead LR, Teitelbaum SL et al (1979) Altered mineral metabolism in glucocorticoid-induced osteopenia: effects of 25-hydroxyvitamin D_3 administration, *J Clin Invest* **64**: 655–65.

Harms HM, Kaptaina U, Kulpmann WR et al (1989) Pulse amplitude and frequency modulation of parathyroid hormone in plasma, *J Clin Endocrinol Metab* **69**: 843–51.

Harvey RD, McHardy KC, Reid IW et al (1990) Measurement of bone collagen degradation in hyperthyroidism and during thyroxine replacement therapy using pyridinium crosslinks as specific urinary markers, *J Clin Endocrinol Metab* **72**: 1189–94.

Heaney RP (1993) Why does bone mass decrease with age and menopause? In: Christiansen C, ed, *Proceedings of the 4th International Symposium on Osteoporosis and Consensus Development Conference*, Hong Kong, 1993, no 41.

Heaney RP, Recker RR (1982) Effects of nitrogen, phosphorus, and caffeine on calcium balance in women, *J Lab Clin Med* **99**: 46–55.

Heaney RP, Recker RR, Saville PD (1978) Menopausal changes in bone remodeling, *J Lab Clin Med* **92**: 964–70.

Heaney RP, Gallagher JC, Johnston CC et al (1982) Calcium nutrition and bone health in the elderly, *Am J Clin Nutr* **36**: 986–1013.

Heath H III, Sizemore GW (1977) Plasma calcitonin in normal man: differences between men and women, *J Clin Invest* **60**: 1135–40.

Hustmyer FG, Peacock M, Hui S et al (1994) Bone mineral density in relation to polymorphism at the vitamin D receptor gene locus, *J Clin Invest* **94**: 2130–4.

Jackson WU (1958) Osteoporosis of unknown cause in young people, *J Bone Joint Surg Br* **40**: 420–41.

Jackson JA, Kleerekoper M (1990) Osteoporosis in men—diagnosis, pathophysiology and prevention, *Medicine* **69**: 137–52.

Jaffe MD, Willis PW (1965) Multiple fractures associated with long-term sodium heparin therapy, *JAMA* **193**: 158–60.

Jick H, Porter J, Morrison AS (1977) Relation between smoking and age of natural menopause, *Lancet* **i**: 1354–5.

Johnell O (1993) Fracture outcomes. Consequences of osteoporosis for individuals and community. In: Christiansen C, ed, *Proceedings of the 4th International Symposium on Osteoporosis and Consensus Development Conference*, Hong Kong, 1993, no 12.

Johnell O, Nilsson BE (1984) Life-style and bone mineral mass in perimenopausal women, *Calcif Tissue Int* **36**: 354–6.

Johnston CC, Melton LJ, Lindsay R et al (1989) Clinical indication for bone mass measurement, *J Bone Miner Res* **4** (Suppl 2): 1989.

Johnston CC, Miller JZ, Slemenda CW et al (1992) Calcium supplementation and increases in bone mineral density in children, *N Engl J Med* **327**: 82–7.

Jorgensen HL, Scholler J, Sand JC (1996) Relationship of common allelic variation at the vitamin D receptor locus to bone mineral density and bone turnover, *Br J Obstet Gynaecol* **103**: 28–30.

Kalbfleisch JM, Lindeman RD, Ginn HE et al (1963) Effects of thanol administration on urinary excretion of magnesium and other electrolytes in alcoholic and normal subjects, *J Clin Invest* **42**: 1471–5.

Kanis JA (1993) What is vertebral fracture. In: Christiansen C, ed, *Proceedings of the 4th International Symposium on Osteoporosis and Consensus Development Conference*, Hong Kong, 1993, no 2.

Kelly PJ, Hopper JL, Macaskill GT et al (1991) Genetic factors in bone turnover, *J Clin Endocrinol Metab* **72**: 808–13.

Kelsey JF (1984) Osteoporosis: prevalence and incidence. In: Christiansen C, ed, *Proceedings of the NIH Consensus Development Conference*, April, 25–28, 1984.

Kelsey JL, Hoffman S (1987) Risk factors for hip fracture, *N Engl J Med* **316**: 404–6.

Kitamura N, Shigeno C, Shiomi K et al (1990) Episodic fluctuation in serum intact parathyroid hormone concentration in men, *Clin Endocrinol Metab* **70**: 252–63.

Krolner B, Taft B, Nielsen PS et al (1983) Physical exercise as prophylaxis against involutional vertebral bone loss: a controlled trial, *Clin Sci* **64**: 541–6.

Lau E, Donnan S, Barker DJ et al (1988) Physical activity and calcium intake in fracture of the proximal femur in Hong Kong, *Br Med J* **297**: 1441–3.

Laval-Jeantet AM, Cann CE, Dallant P (1984) A postprocessing dual energy technique for vertebral CT densitometry, *J Comput Assist Tomogr* **8**: 1164–7.

Liberman UA, Weiss ST, Broll M et al (1995) Effect of oral alendronate on bone mineral density and the incidence of fractures in postmenopausal osteoporosis, *N Engl J Med* **333**: 1437–43.

Lindsay R, Hart DM, Aitken JM et al (1976) Long-term prevention of postmenopausal osteoporosis by oestrogen: evidence for an increased bone mass after delayed onset of oestrogen treatment, *Lancet* **i**: 1038–41.

Lindsay R, Hart DM, Forrest C et al (1980) Prevention of spinal osteoporosis in oophorectomised women, *Lancet* **ii**: 1151–3.

Lips P, Agnusdel D, Caulilin F et al (1996) The development of a European questionnaire for quality of life in patients with vertebral osteoporosis, *Scand J Rheumatol* **25**: 84–5.

Lutter JM, Cushman S (1982) Menstrual patterns in female runners, *Phys Sportsmed* **10**: 60–72.

Mack PB, LaChance PA (1967) Effect of recumbency and space flight on bone density, *Am J Clin Nutr* **20**: 1194–205.

Marcus R, Cann C, Madvig P et al (1985) Menstrual function and bone mass in elite women distance runners, *Ann Intern Med* **102**: 158–63.

Matkovic V, Kostial K, Simonovic I et al (1979) Bone status and fracture rates in two regions of Yugoslavia, *Am J Clin Nutr* **32**: 540–9.

Melton LJ, Riggs BL (1983) Epidemiology of age-related fractures. In: Avioli LV, ed, *The osteoporotic syndrome* (Grune and Stratton: New York) 45–72.

Melton LJ, Kan SH, Frye MA et al (1989) Epidemiology of vertebral fractures in women, *Am J Epidemiol* **129**: 1000–11.

Melton LJ, Chrischilles EA, Cooper C et al (1992) Perspective: how many women have osteoporosis? *J Bone Miner Res* **7**: 1005–10.

Melton LJ III, Atkinson EJ, O'Fallon WM et al (1993) Long-term fracture prediction by bone mineral assessed at different skeletal sites, *J Bone Miner Res* **8**: 1227–33.

Meunier PJ (1993) Is steroid-induced osteoporosis preventable? *N Engl J Med* **328**: 1781–2.

Minaire P, Meunier P, Edouard C et al (1974) Quantitative histological data on disuse osteoporosis. Comparison with biological data, *Calcif Tissue Res* **17**: 57–73.

Morrison NA, Yeoman R, Kelly PJ et al (1992) Contribution of transacting factor alleles to normal physiological variability: vitamin D receptor polymorphism and circulating osteocalcin, *Proc Natl Acad Sci USA* **89**: 6665–9.

Morrison NA, Qi JC, Tokita A et al (1994) Prediction of bone density from vitamin D receptor alleles, *Nature* **367**: 284–7.

Mosekilde L (1990) Consequences of the remodeling process for vertebral trabecular bone structure—a scanning electron microscopy study (uncoupling of unloaded structures), *Bone Miner* **10**: 13–35.

Mundy GR (1994) Boning up on genes, *Nature* **367**: 216–17.

Mundy GR (1995) The genetics of osteoporosis, *Endocrinologist* **5**: 176–9.

Mundy GR, Raisz LG (1974) Drugs for disorders of bones: pharmacological and clinical considerations, *Drugs* **8**: 250–89.

Mundy GR, Raisz LG (1979) Thyrotoxicosis and calcium metabolism, *Miner Electrolyte Metab* **2**: 285–92.

Mundy GR, Shapiro JL, Bandelin JG et al (1976) Direct stimulation of bone resorption by thyroid hormones, *J Clin Invest* **58**: 529–34.

Newcomer AD, Hodgson SF, McGill DB et al (1978) Lactase deficiency. Prevalence in osteoporosis, *Ann Intern Med* **89**: 218–20.

Nilsson BE, Westlin NE (1971) Bone density in athletes, *Clin Orthop* **77**: 179–82.

Nordin BEC, Roper A (1955) Post-pregnancy osteoporosis—a syndrome? *Lancet* **i**: 431.

Nordin BEC, Crilly G, Smith DA (1984) Osteoporosis. In: Nordin BEC, ed, *Metabolic bone and stone disease*, 2nd edn (Churchill Livingston: Edinburgh) 1–70.

Nordin BEC, Horsman A, Marshall DH et al (1979) Calcium requirement and calcium therapy, *Clin Orthop* **140**: 216–39.

Pacifici R, Susman N, Carr PL et al (1986) Single versus dual energy computer tomography of vertebral bone in osteoporotic women, *Clin Res* **34**: 432A.

Panin N, Gorday WJ, Paul BJ (1971) Osteoporosis in hemiplegia, *Stroke* **2**: 41–7.

Parfitt AM (1980) Morphologic basis of bone mineral measurements: transient and steady state effects of treatment in osteoporosis, *Miner Electrolyte Metab* **4**: 273–87.

Parfitt AM (1981) Bone remodeling in the pathogenesis of osteoporosis, *Medical Times* **109**: 80–92.

Parfitt AM (1984) Age-related structural changes in trabecular and cortical bone: cellular mechanism and biomechanical consequences. a) Difference between rapid and slow bone loss. b) Localized bone gain, *Calcif Tissue Int* **36**: S123–S128.

Parfitt AM (1987) Trabecular bone architecture in the pathogenesis and prevention of fracture, *Am J Med* **82** (Suppl 1B): 68–72.

Parfitt AM, Matthews CHE, Villaneuva AR et al (1983) Relationship between surface, volume, and thickness of iliac trabecular bone on aging and in osteoporosis: implications for the microanatomic and cellular mechanism of bone loss, *J Clin Invest* **72**: 1396–409.

Paterson CR, McAllion S, Stellman JL (1984) Osteogenesis imperfecta after the menopause, *N Engl J Med* **310**: 1694–6.

Peacock M (1995) Vitamin D receptor gene alleles and osteoporosis: a contrasting view, *J Bone Miner Res* **10**: 1294–7.

Pecile A, Ferri S, Braga PC et al (1975) Effects of intracerebroventricular calcitonin in the conscious rabbit, *Experientia* **31**: 332–3.

Peng TC, Gitelman HJ (1974) Ethanol-induced hypocalcemia, hypermagnesemia and inhibition of the serum calcium-raising effect of parathyroid hormone in rats, *Endocrinology* **94**: 608–11.

Peng TC, Cooper CW, Munson PL (1972) The hypocalcemic effect of ethyl alcohol in rats and dogs, *Endocrinology* **91**: 586–93.

Plum F, Dunning MF (1958) The effect of therapeutic mobilization on hypocalciuria following acute pyelomyelitis, *Arch Intern Med* **101**: 528–36.

Pocock NA, Eisman JA, Yeates MG et al (1986) Limitations of forearm bone densitometry as an index of vertebral or femoral neck osteopenia, *J Bone Miner Res* **1**: 369–75.

Preger L, Steinbach HL, Moskowitz P et al (1968) Roentgenographic abnormalities in phenotypic females with gonadal dysgenesis, *Am J Roentgenol* **104**: 899–910.

Ray WA, Griffin MR, Schaffner W et al (1987) Psychotropic drug use and the risk of hip fracture, *N Engl J Med* **316**: 363–9.

Reid IR, King AR, Alexander CJ (1988) Prevention of steroid-induced osteoporosis with (3-amino-1-hydroxypropylidene)-1,1-bisphosphonate (APD), *Lancet* **i**: 143–6.

Reid IR, Evans MC, Stapleton J (1992) Lateral spine densitometry is a more sensitive indicator of glucocorticoid-induced bone loss, *J Bone Miner Res* **7**: 1221–5.

Reifenstein EC (1956) The rationale for use of anabolic steroids in controlling the adverse effects of corticoid hormones upon protein and osseous tissues, *South Med J* **49**: 933–60.

Riggs BL, Melton LJ (1986) Involutional osteoporosis, *N Engl J Med* **314**: 1676–86.

Riggs BL, Melton LJ (1995) The worldwide problem of osteoporosis: insights afforded by epidemiology, *Bone* **17**: S505–S511.

Riggs BL, Wahner HW, Dunn WL (1981) Differential changes in bone mineral density of the appendicular and axial skeleton with aging, *J Clin Invest* **67**: 328–35.

Riggs BL, Jowsey J, Kelly PJ et al (1973) Studies on pathogenesis and treatment in postmenopausal and senile osteoporosis, *Clin Endocrinol Metab* **2**: 317–22.

Riggs BL, Wahner HW, Seeman E et al (1982) Changes in bone mineral density of the proximal femur and spine with aging: differences between the postmenopausal and senile syndromes, *J Clin Invest* **70**: 716–23.

Riggs BL, Wahner HW, Melton LJ III et al (1986) In women dietary calcium intake and rates of bone loss from midradius and lumbar spine are not related, *J Bone Miner Res* **1** (Suppl): 96 (abst).

Riggs BL, Hodgson SF, O'Fallon WM et al (1990) Effect of fluoride treatment on the fracture rate in postmenopausal women with osteoporosis, *N Engl J Med* **322**: 802–9.

Rigotti NA, Nussbaum SR, Herzog DB et al (1984) Osteoporosis in women with anorexia nervosa, *N Engl J Med* **311**: 1601–6.

Riis BJ, Hansen MA, Jensen AM et al (1996) Low bone mass and fast rate of bone loss at menopause: equal risk factors for future fracture. A 15-year follow-up study, *Bone* **19**: 9–12.

Rivier C, Bruhn T, Vale W (1984) Effect of ethanol on the hypothalamic–pituitary–adrenal axis in the rat: role of corticotropin-releasing factor (CRF), *J Pharm Exp Ther* **229**: 127–31.

Rose GA (1966) Immobilization osteoporosis, *Br J Surg* **53**: 769–74.

Rosenthal DI, Ganott MA, Wyshak G et al (1985) Quantitative computed tomography for spinal density measurement: factors affecting precision, *Invest Radiol* **20**: 306–10.

Sambrook P, Birmingham J, Kelly P (1993) Prevention of corticosteroid osteoporosis. A comparison of calcium, calcitriol, and calcitonin, *N Engl J Med* **328**: 1747–52.

Samuels MH, Veldhuis J, Cawley C (1993) Pulsatile secretion of parathyroid hormone in normal young subjects: assessment by deconvolution analysis, *J Clin Endocrinol Metab* **77**: 399–403.

Sattin RW, Lambert Huber DA, DeVito CA et al (1990) The incidence of fall injury events among the elderly in a defined population, *Am J Epidemiol* **131**: 1028–37.

Saville PD (1965) Changes in bone mass with age and alcoholism, *J Bone Joint Surg* **47**: 492–9.

Scane AC, Francis RM (1993) Risk factors for osteoporosis in men, *Clin Endocrinol* **38**: 15–16.

Seeman E, Melton LJ, O'Fallon WM et al (1983) Risk factors for spinal osteoporosis in men, *Am J Med* **75**: 977–83.

Shapiro JR, Rowe DW (1983) Collagen genes and brittle bones, *Ann Intern Med* **99**: 700–4.

Shapiro JR, Rowe D (1984) Imperfect osteogenesis and osteoporosis, *N Engl J Med* **310**: 1738–40.

Sitran M, Meredith S, Rosenberg IH (1978) Vitamin D deficiency and bone disease in gastrointestinal disorders, *Arch Intern Med* **138**: 886–8.

Slovik DM, Adams JS, Neer RM et al (1981) Deficient production of 1,25-dihydroxyvitamin D_3 in elderly osteoporotic patients, *N Engl J Med* **305**: 372–4.

Smith DM, Nance WE, Kang KW et al (1973) Genetic factors in determining bone mass, *J Clin Invest* **52**: 2800–8.

Smith EL, Reddan W, Smith PE (1981) Physical activity and calcium modalities for bone mineral increase in aged women, *Med Sci Sports Exerc* **13**: 60–4.

Smith R (1980) Idiopathic osteoporosis in the young, *J Bone Joint Surg Br* **62**: 417–27.

Smith R, Stevenson JC, Winearls GC (1985) Osteoporosis of pregnancy, *Lancet* **i**: 1178–80.

Sowers M (1996) Pregnancy and lactation as risk factors for subsequent bone loss and osteoporosis, *J Bone Miner Res* **11**: 1052–60.

Spector TD, Keen RW, Arden NK et al (1994) Vitamin D receptor gene (VDR) alleles and bone density in postmenopausal women: a UK twin study, *J Bone Miner Res* **9**: no 91.

Spotila LD, Constantinou CD, Sereda L et al (1991) Mutation in a gene for type-I procollagen (COL1A2) in a woman with postmenopausal osteoporosis—evidence for phenotypic and genotypic overlap with milk osteogenesis imperfecta, *Proc Natl Acad Sci U S A* **88**: 5423–7.

Storm T, Thamsborg G, Steiniche T (1990) Effect of intermittent cyclical etidronate therapy on bone mass and fracture rate in women with postmenopausal osteoporosis, *N Engl J Med* **322**: 1265–71.

Szulc P, Chapuy MC, Meunier PJ et al (1993) Serum undercarboxylated osteocalcin is a marker of the risk of hip fracture in elderly women, *J Clin Invest* **91**: 1769–74.

Thompson K, Goltfredsen A, Christiansen C (1986) Is postmenopausal bone loss an age-related phenomenon? *Calcif Tissue Int* **39**: 123–7.

Tinetti ME, Baker DI, McAvay G (1994) A multifactorial intervention to reduce the risk of falling among elderly people living in the community, *N Engl J Med* **331**: 821–7.

Trotter MI, Broman GE, Peterson RR (1960) Densities of bones of white and negro skeletons, *J Bone Joint Surg Am* **42**: 50–8.

Tsai K-S, Heath H III, Kumar R et al (1984) Impaired vitamin D metaboism with aging in women: possible role in pathogenesis of senile osteoporosis, *J Clin Invest* **73**: 1668–72.

Valimake MJ, Harkonen M, Eriksson CJP et al (1984) Sex hormones and adrenocortical steroids in men acutely intoxicated with ethanol, *Alcohol* **1**: 89–93.

Whedon GD, Shorr E (1957) Metabolic studies in paralytic-acute anterior pyelomyelitis: II. Alterations in calcium and phosphorus metabolism, *J Clin Invest* **36**: 966–81.

Yamagata Z, Miyamura T, Iijima S et al (1994) Vitamin D receptor gene polymorphism and bone mineral density in healthy Japanese women, *Lancet* **344**: 1027.

Zarrabeitia MT, Riancho JA, Amado JA (1991) Cytokine production by peripheral blood cells in postmenopausal osteoporosis, *Bone Miner* **14**: 161–7.

CHAPTER 14

Potential future treatments for osteoporosis

The most demanding need in bone research is better therapies for established osteoporosis. Currently, no available treatment is either totally satisfactory or universally acceptable. This is the reason that the pharmaceutical industry is now spending billions of dollars in the search for better modalities of treatment than those currently available. The task is daunting. There remain a number of fundamental questions that haunt investigators searching for better treatments, the answers to which are necessary to determine that current approaches are worthwhile. These questions include:

- Is bone loss in patients with osteoporosis irreversible?
- Can aging bone cells respond to drug therapy?
- Is bone architecture irreversibly destroyed in patients with osteoporosis?
- Are there suitable in vivo animal models for evaluating new drugs?

One of the major issues that interfere with advances in this area is incomplete understanding of the complexities of the normal bone remodeling sequence, which in turn prevents full understanding of the pathophysiology of bone loss responsible for osteoporosis. Moreover, there remains a lack of reliable in vitro systems for screening new potential drug therapies, and the animal models currently available are less than optimal for studying new treatment regimens. At the present time, the major need is clearly in the area of development of new agents for stimulating bone formation. The only widely used agent known to stimulate bone formation is fluoride, and a dark cloud still remains over this agent. In contrast, there are a number of available agents that effectively inhibit bone resorption (estrogens, calcitonin, bisphosphonates).

Ideal therapy for patients with established osteoporosis would be an agent that inhibits osteoclastic bone resorption and stimulates new bone formation. (Ultimately, selection of therapy should depend on a particular patient's situation. For example, the teenager or the perimenopausal woman with a strong family history require measures directed to maintain current bone mass (Figure 14.1).) There is no currently available therapeutic agent that convincingly achieves both resorption inhibition and significantly increased formation. The currently available resorption inhibitors (estrogen, bisphosphonates, calcitonin) have negligible to very modest effects on bone formation over prolonged periods. As a consequence, they may prevent further bone loss and stabilize bone mass, but do not substantially increase bone mass. There is currently no acceptable formation stimulator that is widely available.

Bone resorption inhibitors

Three classes of bone resorption inhibitors are currently used extensively for the treatment or

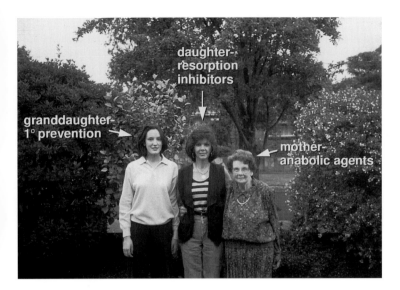

Figure 14.1

This figure shows three generations of women. The elderly lady on the right has severe osteoporosis, characterized by loss of height, kyphosis, recurrent fractures and back pain. The issues for her daughter and granddaughter are primary and secondary prevention respectively to avoid developing severe established osteoporosis, whereas the patient requires ideally a drug that will stimulate bone formation and prevent further bone loss.

prevention of osteoporosis. These are estrogen, calcitonin and the bisphosphonates. Of these, estrogen is the agent that has been used the longest. Although it has been used for over 50 years, evidence for its efficacy dates back only about 15 years. Estrogen reverses the accelerated phase of bone loss associated with the postmenopausal period, and is useful even if used for the first time 20 or more years after the menopause. Unfortunately, not all women will accept estrogen therapy, and in many it is contraindicated. In the next few years, the contraindications for estrogen therapy will continue to be clarified and hopefully reduced, and the use of estrogen preparations should become more widespread. In particular, modes of administration such as transdermal patches, which limit unwanted side effects, should become more widespread (Stevenson 1993). However, these considerations notwithstanding, it seems unlikely that more than 30–40% of the patients who should otherwise be taking estrogen therapy will in fact take it. Moreover, at this point in time the exact mode of action of estrogen to inhibit bone resorption remains unclear. Recent advances have been made in this area, including determination of the effects of estrogen to regulate cytokine production such as interleukin-6 and interleukin-1 (Pacifici et al 1987, 1991; Girasole et al 1992; Jilka et al 1992), and the demonstration that there are functional estrogen receptors in osteoclasts (Oursler et al 1991). Which of these mechanisms of estrogen action on bone cells is pre-eminent is unclear at this time.

Over the last 5 years, a lot of attention has been focused on an interesting series of compounds known as antiestrogens, and many companies are now actively involved in the development of compounds in this category. These compounds are now more widely known as Selective Estrogen Response Modifiers (SERMs). The companies with active SERMs programs include SmithKline Beecham, Zeneca, Pfizer, Nova Nordisk, and Eli Lilly. Theoretically, the ideal antiestrogen would be a compound that had all the beneficial effects of estrogen on bone and on the cardiovascular system, including appropriate lowering of blood lipids, without the deleterious effects of estrogen on the uterus and the breast. Although some of these compounds clearly fit this category, with others it remains unclear. The potential market is enormous, and is potentially even greater than the current estrogen market in postmenopausal women. The forerunner of this group of drugs is raloxifene, and it is likely to be the eventual gold standard against which the other antiestrogens will be compared, since it is the first to be evaluated for this use (Black et al 1994). The actual molecular mechanism by which these compounds can exert estrogen-like effects in some tissues and antiestrogen-like effects in others is not clear (Pennisi 1996). Interactions between the estrogen receptor, which is a transcription factor for estrogen-target proteins, and its ligands as well as the eventual gene promoters are still being unraveled (McDonnell et al 1992; Tzukerman et al 1994). There are a number of levels for potential specificity. One of these is at the receptor itself, which has different domains that may be differentially activated in different tissues. In part, this may be associated with co-activator and suppressor proteins that are involved in estrogen receptor action, and have been recently identified by O'Malley et al (1995). However, there is also now evidence for more than one estrogen receptor, and the involvement of different estrogen receptors in the antiestrogen effects is unknown. It is also clear that these compounds cannot be considered as one single class, but probably represent novel compounds, with possibly different actions. Raloxifene has been clearly shown to prevent bone loss, and to lower serum cholesterol in ovariectomized rats without any uterotrophic activity (Black et al 1994). The effects on bone and lipids are comparable to those of estrogen. Estrogen and related compounds enhance transforming growth factor β (TGFβ) production in bone cells. Yang et al (1996) believe that raloxifene (and possibly other related compounds) may have a preferential effect on TGFβ III in bone. Another interesting compound in this group is centochroman, which appears to be a very effective inhibitor of bone resorption (Hall et al 1995).

The potential for these compounds is enormous, and the first of these (Raloxifene) has been approved by the FDA. It appears likely that they will have similar effects on bone as the bisphosphonates, but also may have the added advantage of beneficial effects on the cardiovascular system.

Calcitonin is probably not as effective as estrogen or the bisphosphonates as an inhibitor of osteoclastic bone resorption, although it has not been as widely used in the United States. However, it has very large markets in Japan, where estrogens are not popular, and in Italy. The use of intranasal preparations should improve patient acceptability, although expense will remain a problem. Moreover, its effects on inhibition of bone resorption may be transient and its effects to increase bone mass are modest at best.

The bisphosphonates are now established as useful agents for use in osteoporosis, as well as for other causes of increased bone resorption. Etidronate in short-term studies was initially thought to improve fracture risk (Storm et al 1990), although its effects on bone mass are very modest, like those of other resorption inhibitors. Follow-up studies on fracture risk have been less encouraging. Newer bisphosphonates (most notably alendronate) are more potent and less toxic, and their usefulness in situations where estrogen cannot be used is now well established (see Chapter 5).

New approaches to resorption inhibition

During the next few years, continued efforts will be made to improve the efficacy of current bone resorption inhibitors. In the case of calcitonin, this will mean improvements in the mode of administration by, for example, intranasal aerosols or rectal suppositories. Transdermal estrogen patches avoid the first pass effect of the liver and reduce estrogenic side effects, since estradiol concentration can be maintained in the systemic circulation using very low dosage (Balfour and McTavish 1992). Current experience suggests that transdermal estrogens may be a preferable alternative to oral estrogen, with all the benefits for bone, but with avoidance of some undesirable metabolic effects due to circumvention of the hepatic first pass effect. This is also discussed in Chapter 5.

There has been great interest recently in estrogen-like compounds for their potential to be used as surrogates for estrogen for the treatment of osteoporosis (see above). Small synthetic estrogen agonists/antagonists (depending on the target tissue) have been studied for many years and have been investigated extensively for their potential role in breast cancer, in particular tamoxifen. The ideal compound for bone would be one that had protective estrogen-like effects on bone and the cardiovascular system, but lacked estrogen's effect on the uterus. Tamoxifen has some of these properties but has estrogen-like agonist effects on the uterus. The benzothiophene derivative raloxifene appears to have a very promising spectrum of activity with estrogen-like effects on bone and lipids, but no apparent effects on the uterus (Black et al 1994). Recent studies have shown that raloxifene, like estrogen, protects against the bone loss associated with ovariectomy in the distal femur and proximal tibiae of rats. In the same animals, raloxifene did not have estrogenic effects on uterine tissue. It is unknown why these compounds should have different effects from estrogen in different tissues, and whether there are additional receptors for such compounds other than the estrogen receptor. It appears likely in the coming years that with the promise provided so far with raloxifene there will be a flood of these compounds pursued by a number of companies and, unless troublesome side effects occur, they may be widely used as alternatives to estrogen.

The bisphosphonates are considered in detail in Chapter 5. The new generation bisphosphonates such as pamidronate, risedronate, alendronate, ibandronate, and tiludronate are very effective inhibitors of osteoclastic bone resorption. Although all these compounds have poor oral absorption and their long-term effects on the skeleton are still not adequately explored, it appears very likely that they are such effective inhibitors of bone resorption and, to date, appear so relatively nontoxic that they will be widely used over the next decade.

The flavanoids, and in particular ipriflavone, have received considerable attention recently as inhibitors of bone resorption, particularly in Italy and in Japan. These orally active compounds have been tested experimentally in Paget's disease of bone, primary hyperparathyroidism and in osteoporosis. They inhibit bone resorption by mechanisms that are not entirely clear and their effects on bone resorption from both clinical and experimental studies appear to be relatively modest (either as resorption inhibitors or formation stimulators) (Miyauchi et al 1996). Ipriflavone has been used in patients in Europe with promising effects on markers of bone turnover, although no data on effects on fracture rate are available as yet (Brandi 1993).

Although current resorption inhibitors are effective, it is possible in the future that more satisfactory agents will be developed and become available. The currently available agents (with the exception of calcitonin) have modes of action that are unknown and their beneficial effects on bone resorption were discovered by serendipity rather than by rational drug development. However, as information on the cellular and molecular mechanisms involved in bone resorption is accumulating, it may be possible to develop more rational therapeutic approaches to inhibiting osteoclast function (Baron 1993; Mundy 1993). For example, it is now realized that a number of tyrosine kinases are essential for both normal osteoclast formation and osteoclast action. The colony stimulating factor-1 (CSF-1) receptor, also known as the c-fms oncogene, is a receptor tyrosine kinase (Felix et al 1990a,b; Yoshida et al 1990; Kodama et al 1991a,b). The src proto-oncogene, which is required for normal osteoclast ruffled border formation, is a nonreceptor tyrosine kinase that may be inhibited by a number of small molecular weight compounds such as the antibiotic herbimycin A (Soriano et al 1991; Yoneda et al 1993). Recently, several pharmaceutical and biotechnology companies have developed large programs to identify small molecular weight inhibitors of the src tyrosine kinase for their potential in osteoporosis. Recent studies have shown that a number of adhesion proteins are important for normal osteoclastic bone resorption. These proteins are dependent on availability of RGD (arginine–glycine–asparagine) sequences in attachment proteins (Horton and Davies 1989). Peptide antagonists for RGD sequences may be effective inhibitors of osteoclastic bone resorption. Similarly, other cytoskeletal inhibitors may be useful as therapeutic agents for the treatment of enhanced osteoclast activity. Recently, there has been clarification of the molecular mechanisms by which protons are generated within osteoclasts and then pumped across the ruffled border. These mechanisms involve carbonic anhydrase isoenzyme Type II as well as a complex vacuolar ATPase representing the osteoclast proton pump. Inhibitors of both the proton pump mechanism as well as carbonic anhydrase have been identified, and these agents inhibit osteoclastic bone resorption in vitro. Finally, proteolytic enzymes that are responsible for bone matrix degradation during osteoclastic bone resorption, including an array of lysosomal enzymes as well as collagenase, may be inhibited by different agents (Vaes et al 1968; Eilon and Raisz 1978). Thus, the future looks bright for the development of better and more rational therapeutic approaches to the inhibition of osteoclastic bone resorption.

Stimulators of bone formation

In aging patients with osteoporosis there is a decrease in osteoblast function characterized by a decrease in the capacity of osteoblasts to fill in completely the defects left by osteoclastic resorption with new bone. This is referred to by bone histomorphometrists as decreased mean wall thickness (Darby and Meunier 1981). What is needed in this situation is an agent that stimulates osteoblasts to increase their bone forming activities. This is the only mechanism by which bone mass can be increased. The agents that are known to have a stimulatory effect on new bone formation are fluoride, low-dose intermittent parathyroid hormone and the peptide growth factors.

Fluoride

Fluoride has been widely used in the treatment of postmenopausal osteoporosis for many years. It has always been a controversial drug because many physicians have doubted its efficacy and have been concerned by the frequency of side effects, and particularly the risk of increased bone fragility. This issue remains unresolved. New preparations of fluoride such as monofluorophosphate and slow release sodium fluoride may reduce some of these side effects, although not all of these studies are positive, and some investigators remain unconvinced that fluoride therapy reduces vertebral fracture rates in non-toxic doses.

Mechanism of action

Fluoride therapy increases bone formation. These effects are seen in spinal trabecular bone, not cortical bone. The mechanism by which fluoride stimulates bone formation is not clear. One group has suggested that fluoride acts directly on bone cells to inhibit the activity of an osteoblast acid phosphatase which is responsible for the dephosphorylation of tyrosine kinases (Farley et al 1983; Lau et al 1989). Such an effect would lead to enhanced tyrosine kinase activity, and potentially enhance the effects of growth factor to cause proliferation of bone cells. An alternative theory proposed by Burgener et al (1995) is that fluoride increases tyrosine kinase activity in osteoblasts, and this effect is potentiated by small amounts of aluminum (Caverzasio et al 1996). Although there is a dramatic increase in bone formation in response to fluoride therapy, the new bone may be structurally abnormal when higher doses are used. Fluoride is incorporated into the mineral phase of bone and newly formed bone frequently shows evidence of mineralization defects. The bone tends to be spongy and irregular and mineralizes poorly. If supplemental oral calcium and vitamin D are given with fluoride, this mineralization defect does not occur.

Mode of administration

Three different types of preparation of fluoride are used: sodium fluoride, sodium monoflourophosphate, and now slow release sodium fluoride. The latter two are associated with fewer gastrointestinal side effects and are much safer compounds than plain sodium chloride. This is very important because the therapeutic window for fluoride is very narrow. Following therapy with sodium fluoride, serum concentrations of 10 $\mu M/l$ may lead to maximal beneficial effects, but 15 $\mu M/l$ may be toxic. The importance of the bioavailability of the preparation has recently been emphasized in view of the narrow therapeutic window (Pak et al 1989; Nagant et al 1990). The use of concomitant oral calcium and vitamin D is necessary to prevent osteomalacia.

Efficacy

Fluoride therapy increases bone mass in the vertebrae in approximately 70% of osteoporotic patients. Bone mass is increased by 10% per year as measured by bone mineral density. The increase is progressive without a plateau, and is dramatic. Similar effects are not produced with any other current form of therapy. The responses may be even greater when assessed by quantitative computerized tomography. Many uncontrolled studies have reported the benefits of fluoride therapy. However, recent randomized controlled studies show there may be an increased risk of fractures in the appendicular skeleton (Riggs et al 1990). Fracture rates are unchanged in the vertebrae.

The problem with fluoride therapy was apparent with several NIH-sponsored studies in the US during the 1980s (Riggs et al 1990; Kleerekoper et al 1991). Although there was an impressive increase in bone mineral density in the vertebral spine, there was not a concomitant improvement found in vertebral fracture rates. This led to considerable scepticism regarding the benefits of fluoride. Some investigators felt that these negative results were due to the dose of fluoride being too high in these studies and considered lower doses or alternative forms of therapy, including slow release sodium fluoride and sodium monofluorophosphate. These have been shown to be effective in some studies (Pak et al 1996), but not in others, as reported by Meunier for the FAVOS study in patients at the World Osteoporosis Congress in May, 1996.

Adverse reactions

There is an increased risk of fracture in patients treated with fluoride which is presumably related to structurally abnormal bone and the mineralization defect which is caused by excessive fluoride administration. In uncontrolled studies, increases in spinal fracture rates have not been observed (Farley et al 1990). In addition, there are other less serious side effects which occur in 30–40% of patients treated with this form of therapy. These include synovitis, anemia, gastric irritation (discomfort, nausea, vomiting), and a periarticular pain syndrome in the lower extremities associated with stress microfractures. These dose-related side effects may be so irritating that approximately 30% of patients will not continue to take this therapy. The non-skeletal side effects can be reduced by discontinuation of therapy for one month and then resumption at a lower dose. They can also be limited by using slow-release or enteric-coated preparations. The critical factor, however, may be careful selection of dose with measurement of serum fluoride levels.

Indications

At the current time, fluoride should probably not be used except in investigational studies until clearer information is available on doses which decrease bone fragility. The theoretical indication is for the patient with a low turnover form of osteoporosis, where stimulation of bone formation is required. The most effective dose is probably in the range of 60–75 mg of NaF daily, although side effects are more likely in this range. Beneficial effects may be seen with as little as 30 mg of NaF per day.

One of the major problems with fluoride therapy is that about 30% of patients do not respond, and so far it has not been possible to predict those who would not respond prior to initiating therapy.

Low-dose parathyroid hormone

Parathyroid hormone when administered intermittently and in low dose has long been known to have an anabolic or bone forming effect in rodents, dogs and humans (Parsons and Potts 1972). This anabolic effect is likely to be mediated by the production of peptide bone growth factors such as insulin-like growth factor I (IGF-I) and TGFβ by bone cells in response to PTH (Canalis et al 1989). In contrast, when parathyroid hormone is administered in high doses and continuously, the major effect is an increase in bone turnover with a prominent increase in osteoclastic bone resorption. The effect seems to occur predominantly on cancellous bone in the axial skeleton. Studies have been in progress for some years to determine if this anabolic effect of parathyroid hormone can be useful therapeutically in patients with osteoporosis (Slovik et al 1986; Reeve et al 1980, 1989). A number of pharmaceutical companies have programs on PTH, PTH-rP, or synthetic analogs as potential anabolic agents. The anabolic effect of PTH is enhanced by a concomitant administration of 1,25-dihydroxyvitamin D_3. Current data suggest that beneficial effects in patients may plateau after several years, and then decline, particularly in cortical bone. There are a number of unanswered issues with this therapy, including the long-term effects on cortical bone, the optimal timing and dosage schedule, the need for concomitant administration of 1,25-dihydroxyvitamin D_3, whether the effects are mediated through the same receptor responsible for osteoclastic bone resorption, and whether the anabolic effects can be mimicked by oral agents. A thorough review of the status of PTH as a potential therapeutic agent has recently been written (Reeve 1996) and the potential for PTH-rP or analogs (Vickery et al 1996) has been summarized by Stewart (1996).

Peptide growth factors

In recent years, increased understanding of the peptide growth regulatory factors responsible for the control of the cellular events involved in bone formation (reviewed in Chapter 4) has led to the real possibility that these factors may be potential drugs for stimulating the growth of bone in patients with bone loss. Although this area of study is still very young, sufficient progress has been made in recent years to believe that the introduction of such agents in the relatively near future is not so very far-fetched.

Nevertheless, there are many potential problems associated with the use of peptide growth factors in the therapy of osteoporosis. The obvious major problem is that of delivery. Since all the peptide growth factors are potent peptides that have short half-lives, they must be administered parenterally, a serious limitation to their use in patients with chronic diseases such as osteoporosis. Moreover, most of the peptide growth factors that have been identified so far affect the functions of many cells outside bone. As a consequence, systemic administration could well lead to deleterious side effects such as hypoglycemia (for IGF-I) or fibrosis due to mesenchymal cell proliferation (TGFβ). This suggests that their usefulness may be limited to either local administration, unless mechanisms can be developed for targeting them to bone (for example, by linking them to bone-seeking bisphosphonates) or by developing small molecular weight compounds, which could be administered orally but could modulate their local production in the bone cell microenvironment. This latter idea is not so far-fetched. For example, retinoic acid has been shown to enhance expression of both TGFβ and the bone morphogenetic proteins in bone cells (Harris et al 1992).

Transforming growth factor β (TGFβ)

Transforming growth factor β has dramatic effects on bone in vivo (Noda and Camilliere 1989; Mackie and Trechsel 1990; Marcelli et al 1990) (Figures 14.2 and 14.3). Numerous studies

Figure 14.2

Effects of TGFβ (5 μg/day for 5 days) on calvarial bone, showing an increase in width of the bone as well as in the periosteum following local injections of TGFβ over the calvarium of normal mice. (See also Chapter 4.)

Figure 14.3

Effects of TGFβ in increasing new bone formation over the calvaria of normal mice (from the same experiments as those described in Figure 14.2).

have now shown that it causes an impressive increase in bone formation and stimulates all the events involved in bone formation including chemotaxis of osteoblast precursors (Pfeilschifter et al 1990), mitogenesis of osteoblast precursors, and differentiated function in committed osteoblasts (Bonewald and Mundy 1990). Although TGFβ can mediate all these effects, it is likely that other growth regulatory factors work in concert with TGFβ on bone in vivo.

TGFβ represents a number of factors in a family of TGFβ superfamily members, including the bone morphogenetic proteins. TGFβ I and TGFβ II seem to have identical effects on bone cells in vitro and in vivo. However, these effects are different from those of the BMPs, at least as far as is known in vitro.

Despite these dramatic effects of TGFβ on bone formation, there remain a number of unanswered questions. These include the relationship of TGFβ with binding proteins that render it biologically inert, those effects that are due to TGFβ alone and those that are secondary effects, the mechanism of activation in the bone microenvironment, and its interactions with other growth regulatory factors in the bone formation process.

TGFβ has a complex relationship with several binding proteins, which mask its activity and form latent TGFβ complexes. In one latent form produced in bone, TGFβ is released as the precursor molecule, which is then cleaved extracellularly to form active TGFβ. In another type of latent complex, TGFβ and its precursor are bound to a binding protein called latency-associated peptide similar to the peptide present in platelets. Although little is known of the precise molecular mechanisms by which active TGFβ is released from these latent complexes, it appears that this can be accomplished by changing local pH to an acidic microenvironment, and by certain proteolytic enzymes such as plasmin (Bonewald and Mundy 1990). Both these mechanisms represent possible ways in which TGFβ could be activated in the bone cell microenvironment. For example, the area under the ruffled border of the osteoclast is acidic, and latent TGFβ complexes could be expected to be present there. Moreover, it has been shown that cells with the osteoblast phenotype express plasminogen activator when incubated with osteotropic hormones such as parathyroid hormone (Hamilton et al 1985). It is possible that several mechanisms are responsible for the activation of TGFβ in the bone cell microenvironment, and that these mechanisms may be essential for understanding the effects of these powerful bone growth stimulators and the regulation of its activity.

Bone morphogenetic proteins (BMPs)

Bone morphogenetic proteins belong to the TGFβ superfamily. They are a group of six or more fairly homologous growth regulatory factors probably derived from a common ancestral precursor (Wang et al 1988; Wozney et al 1988). These peptides share about 35% homology with TGFβ. Although their effects on normal bone have not been studied extensively, it has been shown that, unlike TGFβ, they can induce ectopic bone when injected into rodent subcutaneous tissue in vivo. They may also be important in fracture repair and in the repair of bone defects. Whether all the bone morphogenetic proteins have the same biological effects is unknown.

BMPs have not yet been examined extensively for specificity for bone cell targets, nor has a receptor mechanism been identified. Thus, it is not clear whether their effects are ubiquitous or specific to bone cells and related cells. Since this is unknown and it is similarly unknown whether systemic administration is possible without toxicity, whether they will have any role in the treatment of osteoporosis remains impossible to know. It may be that they will have an important therapeutic place in the repair of fractures, particularly open fractures, or repair of bone defects either surgical or congenital.

We have studied the effects of these members of the TGFβ superfamily on bone formation in vitro using freshly isolated fetal rat calvarial cells. In this system, over a period of several weeks, the cells initially proliferate and then differentiate to form mineralized bone nodules. In this model, TGFβ stimulates cell proliferation and initial events, including expression of proto-oncogenes that have been related to cell proliferation, but inhibits differentiated function (Harris et al 1992). In contrast, the BMPs, and particularly BMP-2, hasten and enhance differentiated function of these cells, which includes expression of proteins such as osteocalcin and alkaline phosphatase, both of which have been related to bone mineralization, as well as the formation of mineralized nodules. Thus, it is likely that there is a cascade of growth factor expression during bone cell differentiation, with TGFβ stimulating proliferation of bone cells and ultimately BMP expression, and then BMP in turn ultimately being responsible for expression of proteins involved in the differentiated function of the osteoblasts, which includes the formation of normal mineralized bone.

Other growth factors

A number of other growth factors have been found in bone matrix where they are apparently stored (Hauschka et al 1986), and then presumably released during bone resorption (Pfeilschifter and Mundy 1987). These growth factors include IGF-I and II, platelet-derived growth factor (PDGF), heparin-binding growth factors (acidic and basic fibroblast growth factors), as well as TGFβ and the bone morphogenetic proteins. IGF-I has achieved the most attention. It has powerful effects on bone formation in vitro. It also stimulates the formation of new bone in vivo (Spencer et al 1991), although it has never been compared directly with TGFβ. It has been implicated in the anabolic response of parathyroid hormone. Canalis and co-workers (1989) have shown that when cultures of embryonic fetal rat calvariae are cultured with PTH and then the PTH is withdrawn, there is an increase in the IGF-I content in the conditioned media. Similar effects are seen in isolated fetal rat calvarial cells. IGF-II has also been implicated as a coupling factor in bone formation. However, unlike IGF-I, its production in bone cells does not seem to be hormone-regulated. Both IGF-I and IGF-II have a complicated set of binding proteins that can determine their biological activities. The importance of interactions between the IGF-I and IGF-II and these binding proteins in bone has not yet been fully resolved, although some believe that the combination of IGF-I with specific binding proteins that enhance their effects has therapeutic potential. Recently, IGF-I and PDGF have been shown to be effective in the repair of bone defects in models of periodontal disease (Lynch et al 1989). This is presumably due to an increase in bone formation.

IGF-I and IGF-II can each cause hypoglycemia because of insulin-like effects on glucose uptake in peripheral tissues. This is a major limitation with their use as therapeutic agents to stimulate bone formation, particularly if delivered systemically, and clearly limits their potential as systemic therapies.

There have been recent disturbing reports that IGF-I may have a bone resorption stimulating effect depending on its mode of administration. When delivered in an intermittent manner, it has been shown to stimulate bone resorption in vivo (Ibbotson et al 1992). However, its effects when delivered by continuous infusion seem to be predominantly anabolic or bone stimulatory.

Recently, the heparin binding fibroblast growth factors, which are present in stored form in the bone matrix, have been shown to stimulate bone formation in vivo when injected locally or systemically in mice (Figure 14.4). They have profound effects on bone, similar in magnitude to those of TGFβ, but possibly even greater (Dunstan et al 1992). Moreover, unlike TGFβ, they appear not to

Figure 14.4

Effects of acidic fibroblast growth factors on calvarial bone of the mouse showing marked increase in new bone formation (Dunstan et al 1993).

have deleterious effects of stimulating bone resorption. Both acidic and basic fibroblast growth factors produce these effects. The therapeutic potential is still under investigation.

It seems very likely that there are bone forming proteins and bone growth factors that have yet to be discovered. These are also likely to be present in the bone matrix.

Other agents that in preliminary studies have been shown to stimulate bone formation include zeolite A and strontium. Zeolite A is a silicon-containing compound that causes mitogenesis in osteoblastic cells and increases new bone formation in beagle dogs (Drezner et al 1993). Strontium, and in particular the divalent-salt S12911, is also a potential bone stimulating agent, which may increase trabecular bone mass in ovariectomized rats without impairing mineralization in vivo. Other agents that may cause marginal stimulatory effects on bone formation in vivo are anabolic steroids and vitamin D metabolites, although their effects, if real, are so modest that their role for this indication is limited.

Other compounds and approaches

Over the years, considerable attention has been given to the concept of so-called coherence therapy or activate–depress–free–repeat (ADFR) to stimulate bone formation in patients with osteoporosis (Frost 1979, 1981, 1983). The theoretical background to this therapeutic regimen involves the concept that if bone resorption can be stimulated transiently, and then inhibited, the coupling phenomenon will ensure that subsequent cellular events involved in bone formation will proceed and lead to a net increase in bone mass (Figure 14.5). Bone remodeling units are stimulated (for example, by oral phosphate that enhances PTH secretion), and then osteoclastic resorption is inhibited by bisphosphonates or calcitonin. Since these manipulations theoretically favor bone formation, the consequence should be a net increase in bone mass. However, there is still no experimental evidence to support this attractive concept and its validation will require extensive additional experimentation.

Pharmaceutical companies attempting to develop new drugs in the bone field have to face some unpleasant realities. These include the enormous costs of bringing a new drug to the market, which are particularly severe in the osteoporosis field because of the FDA requirements to show beneficial effects on fracture rates, at least for drugs to be used in the United States. These issues are compounded somewhat by the current financial problems of the pharmaceutical industry and the decline in research and development

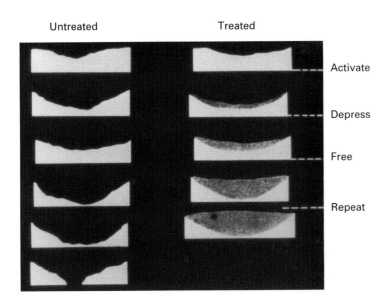

Figure 14.5

The ADFR concept as a method for increasing net bone mass. (See text for explanation.)

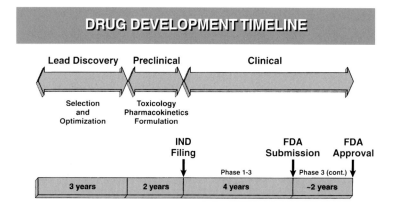

Figure 14.6

The typical time lines for drug development in the United States. For osteoporosis, these times are probably underestimates. Clinical studies in osteoporosis require a fracture assessment in large numbers of patients, which prolongs the approval time considerably.

budgets associated with the threat of reduced profits due to managed care. Establishing practice guidelines for osteoporosis may limit use of drugs, particularly those that are either expensive, or require treatment in many patients to see benefits in one. In the European community, price controls on drugs already exist. An additional important point for industry is the size of the available therapeutic market, and the potential that any drug can expect to have. For example, it seems likely that the bisphosphonate market will eventually be shared by a number of similar compounds, and the same appears likely for the estrogen/antiestrogen market. The great need in the field is for stimulators of bone formation, which will correct deficits in bone mass rather than simply stabilize it. Since the lag time from discovering a new lead for the bone field to the introduction of a drug in the clinic may be 10 or more years (Figure 14.6), it seems likely that resorption inhibitors will be the mainstay for treatment for the next 10 years. Hopefully, following that time, there will be acceptable drugs that will effectively and substantially stimulate bone formation.

References

Balfour JA, McTavish D (1992) Transdermal estradiol—a review of its pharmacological profile, and therapeutic potential in the prevention of postmenopausal osteoporosis, *Drugs and Aging* **2**: 487–507.

Baron R (1993) Biology of the osteoclast. In: Mundy GR, Martin TJ, eds, *Physiology and pharmacology of bone. Handbook of experimental pharmacology* (Springer-Verlag: Berlin) 111–47.

Black LJ, Sato M, Rowley ER (1994) Raloxifene (LY139481 HCl) prevents bone loss and reduces serum cholesterol without causing uterine hypertrophy in ovariectomized rats, *J Clin Invest* **93**: 63–9.

Bonewald LF, Mundy GR (1990) Role of transforming growth factor β in bone remodeling, *Clin Orthop Rel Res* **250**: 261–76.

Brandi ML (1993) New treatment strategies: ipriflavone, strontium, vitamin D metabolites. In: Christiansen C, ed, *Proceedings of the 4th International Symposium on Osteoporosis and Consensus Development Conference*, Hong Kong, 1993, 443–5.

Burgener D, Bonjour JP, Caverzasio J (1995) Fluoride increases tyrosine kinase activity in osteoblast-like cells: Regulatory role for the stimulation of cell proliferation and Pi transport across the plasma membrane, *J Bone Miner Res* **10**: 164–71.

Canalis E, Centrella M, Burch W et al (1989) Insulin-like growth factor I mediates selective anabolic effects of parathyroid hormone in bone cultures, *J Clin Invest* **8**: 60–5.

Caverzasio J, Imai T, Ammann P et al (1996) Aluminium potentiates the effect of fluoride on tyrosine phosphorylation and osteoblast replication in vitro and bone mass in vivo, *J Bone Miner Res* **11**: 46–55.

Darby AJ, Meunier PJ (1981) Mean wall thickness and formation periods of trabecular bone packets in idiopathic osteoporosis, *Calcif Tissue Int* **33**: 199–204.

Drezner M, Nesbitt T, Quarles LD (1993) Zeolite A: a

potential successful therapy for osteoporosis. In: Christiansen C, ed, *Proceedings of the 4th International Symposium on Osteoporosis and Consensus Development Conference*, Hong Kong, 1993, no 31.

Dunstan CR, Evans RA, Somers NM (1992) Bone death in transient regional osteoporosis, *Bone* **13**: 161–5.

Dunstan CR, Boyce BF, Izbicka E et al (1993) Acidic and basic fibroblast growth factors promote bone growth in vivo comparable to that of TGFβ, *J Bone Miner Res* **8** (Suppl 1): no 250.

Eilon G, Raisz LG (1978) Comparison of the effects of stimulators and inhibitors of resorption on the release of lysosomal enzymes and radioactive calcium from fetal bone in organ culture, *Endocrinology* **103**: 1969–75.

Farley JR, Wergedal JE, Baylink DJ (1983) Fluoride directly stimulates proliferation and alkaline phosphatase activity of bone-forming cells, *Science* **222**: 330–2.

Farley SM, Wergedal JE, Farley JR et al (1990) Fluoride decreases spinal fracture rate: A study of over 500 patients. In: Christiansen C, Overgaard K, eds, *Osteoporosis 1990, Volume 3. Third Intl Symposium on Osteoporosis*, Copenhagen, 1330–4.

Felix R, Cecchini MG, Fleisch H (1990a) Macrophage colony stimulating factor restores in vivo bone resorption in the op/op osteopetrotic mouse, *Endocrinology* **127**: 2592–4.

Felix R, Cecchini MG, Hofstetter W et al (1990b) Impairment of macrophage colony-stimulating factor production and lack of resident bone marrow macrophages in the osteopetrotic op/op mouse, *J Bone Miner Res* **5**: 781–9.

Frost HM (1979) Treatment of osteoporoses by manipulation of coherent bone cell populations, *Clin Orthop* **143**: 227–44.

Frost HM (1981) Coherence treatment of osteoporoses, *Orthop Clin North Am* **12**: 649–69.

Frost HM (1983) The ADFR concept revisited, *Calcif Tissue Int* **36**: 349–53.

Girasole G, Jilka RL, Passeri G et al (1992) 17β Estradiol inhibits interleukin-6 production by bone marrow-derived stromal cells in osteoblasts in vitro: a potential mechanism for the anti-osteotropic effect of estrogens, *J Clin Invest* **89**: 883–91.

Hall TJ, Nyugen H, Schaueblin M et al (1995) The bone-specific estrogen centhroman inhibits osteoclastic bone resorption in vitro, *BBRC* **216**: 662–8.

Hamilton JA, Lingelbach S, Partridge NC et al (1985) Regulation of plasminogen activator production by bone-resorbing hormones in normal and malignant osteoblasts, *Endocrinology* **116**: 2186–91.

Harris SE, Harris MA, Feng JQ et al (1992) Expression of bone morphogenetic proteins (BMPs) during differentiation of fetal rat calvarial osteoblasts in vitro, *J Bone Miner Res* **7** (Suppl 1): no 112.

Hauschka PV, Mavrakos AE, Iafrati MD et al (1986) Growth factors in bone matrix, *J Biol Chem* **261**: 12 665–74.

Horton MA, Davies J (1989) Perspectives—adhesion receptors in bone, *J Bone Miner Res* **4**: 803–8.

Ibbotson KJ, Orcutt CM, D'Souza SM et al (1992) Contrasting effects of parathyroid hormone and insulin-like growth factor-I in an aged ovariectomized rat model of postmenopausal osteoporosis, *J Bone Miner Res* **7**: 425–32.

Jilka RL, Hangoc G, Girasole G et al (1992) Increased osteoclast development after estrogen loss—mediation by interleukin-6, *Science* **257**: 88–91.

Kleerekoper M, Peterson EL, Nelson DA et al (1991) A randomized trial of sodium fluoride as a treatment for postmenopausal osteoporosis, *Osteoporosis Int* **1**: 155–61.

Kodama H, Nose M, Niida S et al (1991a) Essential role of macrophage colony-stimulating factor in the osteoclast differentiation supported by stromal cells, *J Exp Med* **173**: 1291–4.

Kodama H, Yamasaki A, Nose M et al (1991b) Congenital osteoclast deficiency in osteopetrotic op/op mice is cured by injections of macrophage colony stimulating factor, *J Exp Med* **173**: 269–72.

Lau KH, Farley JR, Freeman TK et al (1989) A proposed mechanism of the mitogenic action of fluoride on bone cells: inhibition of the activity of an osteoblastic acid phosphatase, *Metabolism* **38**: 858–68.

Lynch SE, Williams RC, Polson AM et al (1989) A combination of platelet-derived and insulin-like growth factors enhances periodontal regeneration, *J Clin Periodontol* **16**: 545–8.

Mackie EJ, Trechsel U (1990) Stimulation of bone formation in vivo by transforming growth factor β-remodeling of woven bone and lack of inhibition by indomethacin, *Bone* **11**: 295–300.

Marcelli C, Yates AJP, Mundy GR (1990) In vivo effects of human recombinant transforming growth factor β on bone turnover in normal mice, *J Bone Miner Res* **5**: 1087–96.

McDonnell DP, Vegeto E, O'Malley BW (1992) Identification of a negative regulatory function for steroid receptors, *Proc Natl Acad Sci U S A* **89**: 10 563–7.

Miyauchi A, Notoya K, Taketomi S (1996) Novel ipriflavone receptors coupled to calcium influx regulate osteoclast differentiation and function, *Endocrinology* **137**: 3544–50.

Mundy GR (1993) Cytokines of bone. In: Mundy GR, Martin TJ, eds, *Physiology and pharmacology of bone. Handbook of experimental pharmacology* (Springer-Verlag: Berlin) 185–214.

Nagant C, De-Vogelaer JP, Stein F (1990) Fluoride treatment for osteoporosis, *Lancet* **336**: 48–9.

Noda M, Camilliere JJ (1989) In vivo stimulation of bone formation by transforming growth factor-β, *Endocrinology* **124**: 2991–4.

O'Malley BW, Onate SA, Tsai SY et al (1995) Sequence and characterization of a coactivator for the steroid hormone receptor superfamily, *Science* **270**: 1354–7.

Oursler MJ, Osdoby P, Pyfferoen J et al (1991) Avian osteoclasts as estrogen target cells, *Proc Natl Acad Sci U S A* **88**: 6613–17.

Pacifici R, Rifas L, Teitelbaum S et al (1987) Spontaneous release of interleukin-1 from human blood monocytes reflects bone formation in idiopathic osteoporosis, *Proc Natl Acad Sci U S A* **84**: 4616–20.

Pacifici R, Rifas L, McCracken R et al (1991) Ovarian steroid treatment blocks a postmenopausal increase in blood monocyte interleukin-1 release, *Proc Natl Acad Sci U S A* **86**: 2398–402.

Pak C, Sakhaee K, Zerwekh JE et al (1989) Safe and effective treatment of osteoporosis with intermittent slow release sodium fluoride: augmentation of vertebral bone mass and inhibition of fractures, *J Clin Endo Metab* **68**: 150–9.

Pak C, Sakhaee K, Bell NH et al (1996) Comparison of nonrandomized trials with slow-release sodium fluoride with a randomized placebo-controlled trial in postmenopausal osteoporosis, *J Bone Miner Res* **11**: 160–8,

Pak C, Zerwekh JE, Antich PP et al (1996) Slow-release sodium fluoride in osteoporosis, *J Bone Miner Res* **11**: 561–4.

Parsons JA, Potts JT Jr (1972) Physiology and chemistry of parathyroid hormone, *Clin Endocrinol Metab* **1**: 33–78.

Pennisi E (1996) Drug's link to genes reveals estrogen's many sides, *Science* **273**: 1171.

Pfeilschifter J, Mundy GR (1987) Modulation of transforming growth factor β activity in bone cultures by osteotropic hormones, *Proc Natl Acad Sci U S A* **84**: 2024–8.

Pfeilschifter J, Bonewald L, Mundy GR (1990) Characterization of the latent transforming growth factor β complex in bone, *J Bone Miner Res* **5**: 49–58.

Reeve J (1996) PTH: a future role in the management of osteoporosis? *J Bone Miner Res* **11**: 440–5.

Reeve J, Meunier PJ, Parsons JA et al (1980) Anabolic effect of human parathyroid hormone fragment on trabecular bone in involutional osteoporosis: a multicentre trail, *Br Med J* **280**: 1340–4.

Reeve J, Davie U, Arlot M et al (1989) Parathyroid peptide (hPTH-1–34) in the treatment of osteoporosis. In: Kleerekoper M, Krane SM, eds, *Clinical disorders of bone and mineral metabolism* (Mary Ann Liebert: New York) 621–7.

Riggs BL, Hodgson SF, O'Fallon WM et al (1990) Effect of fluoride treatment on the fracture rate in postmenopausal women with osteoporosis, *N Engl J Med* **322**: 802–9.

Slovik DM, Rosenthal DI, Doppelt SH et al (1986) Restoration of spinal bone in osteoporotic men by treatment with human parathyroid hormone (1-34) and 1,25-dihydroxyvitamin D$_3$, *J Bone Miner Res* **1**: 377–81.

Soriano P, Montgomery C, Geske R et al (1991) Targeted disruption of the c-src proto-oncogene leads to osteopetrosis in mice, *Cell* **64**: 693–702.

Spencer EM, Liu CC, Si ECC et al (1991) In vivo actions of insulin-like growth factor-I (IGF-I) on bone formation and resorption in rats, *Bone* **12**: 21–6.

Stevenson JC (1993) ERT—new generation transdermal patches. In: Christiansen C, ed, *Proceedings of the 4th International Symposium on Osteoporosis and Consensus Development Conference*, Hong Kong, 1993, no 763.

Stewart AF (1996) PTHrP(1-36) as a skeletal anabolic agent for the treatment of osteoporosis, *Bone* **19**: 303–6.

Storm T, Thamsborg G, Steiniche T et al (1990) Effect of intermittent cyclical etidronate therapy on bone mass and fracture rate in women with postmenopausal osteoporosis, *N Engl J Med* **322**: 1265–71.

Tzukerman MT, Esty A, Santiso-Mere D et al (1994) Human estrogen receptor transcriptional capacity is determined by both cellular and promoter context and mediated by two functionally distinct intramolecular regions, *Mol Endocrinol* **8**: 21–30.

Vaes E (1968) The action of parathyroid hormone on the excretion and synthesis of lysosomal enzymes and on the extracellular release of acid by bone cells, *J Cell Biol* **39**: 676–97.

Vickery BH, Avnur Z, Cheng Y et al (1996) RS-66271, a C-terminally substituted analog of human parathyroid hormone-related protein (1-34), increases trabecular and cortical bone in ovariectomized, osteopenic rats, *J Bone Miner Res* **11**: 1943–53.

Wang EA, Rosen V, Cordes P et al (1988) Purification and characterization of other distinct bone-inducing factors, *Proc Natl Acad Sci U S A* **85**: 9484–8.

Wozney JM, Rosen V, Celeste AJ et al (1988) Novel regulators of bone formation: molecular clones and activities, *Science* **242**: 1528–34.

Yang NN, Venugopalan M, Hardikar S et al (1996) Identification of an estrogen response element activated by metabolites of 17β-estradiol raloxifene, *Science* **273**: 1222–5.

Yoneda T, Lowe C, Lee CH et al (1993) Herbimycin A, a pp60[c-src] tyrosine kinase inhibitor, inhibits osteoclastic bone resorption in vitro and hypercalcemia in vivo, *J Clin Invest* **91**: 2791–5.

Yoshida H, Hayashi SI, Kunisada T et al (1990) The murine mutation osteopetrosis is in the coding region of the macrophage colony stimulating factor gene, *Nature* **345**: 442–4.

INDEX

Page numbers in *italics* refer to figures and tables, where they occur on pages without accompanying text. The alphabetical order of the index is letter-by-letter.

A375 human melanoma cells 63, 117, 130
c-abl 22
achondroplasia 69
acid phosphatase
 fluoride actions 96, 244
 as osteoclast marker 17
 in Pagetic osteoclasts 181
activate–depress–free–repeat (ADFR) treatment, in osteoporosis 249
acute phase response, bisphosphonates 89
adenylate cyclase 50
adhesion molecules
 bone matrix 36–7
 in myeloma bone disease 154
 osteoblasts 31
 osteoclasts 23
 in tumor metastasis 129–32
adolescence, osteoporosis prevention 233
age, bone mass changes with 1–3, 210
alcoholism
 osteoporosis 215, 221, 224, 231
 vitamin D deficiency 202
alendronate 86, *87*, 88
 adverse effects 89–90
 in osteoporosis 242
 in Paget's disease 190
alfacalcidol 97, *203*
alkaline phosphatase 31, 41
 serum
  in chronic renal failure 204
  in hypophosphatemic rickets 205
  in myeloma 148, 149, 155
  in osteoporosis 226
  in Paget's disease 187
α-2 HS glycoprotein 36, 37

α2 macroglobulin 67
aluminium intoxication 41, 203–4
alveolar bone, osteoclast formation 15
amenorrhea 222–3
amniotic cells, PTH-rP expression 115
anabolic steroids 249
anorexia nervosa 222, 223
anovulation, in premenopausal women 222–3
anticoagulants, tumor metastasis and 133
antiestrogens 241–3
apical ectodermal ridge (AER) 69
apoptosis, osteoclast 4, *6*, *19*, 20
 bisphosphonate actions 87
 estrogen actions 84
appositional bone formation 30, 39
arachidonic acid metabolites 56–9
arteriography, parathyroid gland localization 177
Asians, vitamin D deficiency 201
athletes
 amenorrheic 222–3
 osteoporosis risk 231
attachment molecules, *see* adhesion molecules

back pain, in osteoporosis 224, 232
band keratopathy 173
basement membrane, degradation 132, 133
Batson's vertebral plexus 126–7
Bcl-X$_L$ gene 16
biglycan 36
biliary cirrhosis, primary 203, 221
biopsy, bone, *see* bone biopsy
bisphosphonates 86–91
 adverse reactions 88–90
 in corticosteroid-treated patients 219
 efficacy 88
 in hypercalcemia of malignancy 88, *89*, *90*, 119
 indications 90–1
 mechanism of action 87
 mode of administration 87–8

 in myeloma 155–6, 157, 158
 newer generation 86, 88, 243
 in osteolytic bone metastases 88, *90*, 138–9
 in osteoporosis 88, *90*, 234, 242
 in Paget's disease 88, *90*, 189–90
 in primary hyperparathyroidism 88, 90–1, 176
blindness, in osteopetrosis 197
BMPs, *see* bone morphogenetic proteins
bone
 architecture, in Paget's disease 182
 microarchitecture, in osteoporosis 212–13
 organ culture systems 15, 33–4
 structural composition 34–7
bone acidic glycoprotein (BAG) 36, 37
bone biopsy
 in osteomalacia 200–1
 in osteoporosis 226–7
 in Paget's disease 188
bone fluid 32
 calcium fluxes 112
bone formation 4–6, 30
 appositional 30, 39
 cellular events 7–8
 coupling to resorption, *see* coupling phenomenon
 endochondral 30, 37–9
 factors regulating 45–71
 intramembranous 30, 37
 methods of studying 32–4
 in Paget's disease 182
 parathyroid hyperplasia and 167
 therapeutic stimulation 240, 244–9
 types 37–42
 see also mineralization; osteoblasts
bone Gla protein (osteocalcin) 35–6
 chemo-attractant effects 7, 133
 1,25-dihydroxyvitamin D$_3$ and 56
 knockout mice 35, 40
 in mineralization 40

bone Gla protein (osteocalcin) (cont.)
  serum 35–6
    in myeloma 157
    in osteoporosis 226, 230
bone lining cells 30, 32
  osteoclast interactions 23–5, 31
bone loss, age-related 1
  factors affecting 211, 214–17
  pathophysiology 210–13
bone markers
  in myeloma 157
  in osteoporosis 226, 229–30
  in Paget's disease 187
  in primary hyperparathyroidism 175
  serial measurements 232
bone marrow
  failure, in osteopetrosis 197
  in Paget's disease 182–3, 184
  transplantation, in osteopetrosis 198
bone marrow cells
  isolation of osteoclasts 14
  long-term cultures 15–16
  osteoclast precursors 17–18
bone mass
  age-related changes 1–3, 210
  measurement 227–9
  peak 2, 210–11
  serial measurements 228, 232
  see also bone mineral density
bone matrix
  growth regulatory factors, see growth factors, bone matrix-derived
  mineralization, see mineralization
  nonmineralized 39
  proteins 31, 34–7
bone "membrane" 32
  calcium fluxes 112
bone mineral density (BMD)
  defining osteoporosis 208
  fracture risk and 229
  measurement 227–9
  in primary hyperparathyroidism 175
  serial measurements 228, 232
  see also bone mass
bone morphogenetic proteins (BMPs) 37, 70–1
  in coupling phenomenon 8–9
  in endochondral bone formation 38
  osteoblastic bone metastases and 140, 141
  receptors 70–1
  therapeutic potential 247–8
bone pain
  in metastatic bone disease 127
  in myeloma 147, 158
  in Paget's disease 186
  in rickets/osteomalacia 201–2
bone remodeling 1–9, 39

cellular events 3–7
cortical and cancellous bone 3
disorders 1
unit 4
bone resorption 12–25
  cellular events 4–6
  coupling to formation, see coupling phenomenon
  factors regulating 45–71
  induction 46
  in metastatic bone disease 6, 133, 134–8
  molecular mechanisms 20–1
  in primary hyperparathyroidism 170–1, 172
  role of osteoblasts 12, 23, 31
  therapeutic inhibition 240–3
  see also osteoclasts
bone scans (scintigraphy)
  in metastatic bone disease 124, 125
  in myeloma 149
  in Paget's disease 188, 189
  role of bisphosphonates 88
bone sialoprotein II 23
bone sialoproteins (BSP) 36–7, 40
bone structural unit (BSU) 4
bone turnover
  in elderly 212
  in osteoporosis 226, 229–30
  in primary hyperparathyroidism 172, 175
breast, PTH-rP function 51
breast cancer 132
  bone metastases 124, 125
    frequency 123, 125
    mechanisms of osteolysis 134, 135–6, 137–8
    mouse model 135–6, 137–8, 139
    pathophysiology 130, 131, 133, 137
  estrogen therapy and 85
  hypercalcemia 113, 127, 128
  PTH-rP production 114
brown tumors 171

C433 stromal cells 33
C57BL/KaLwRij mice, aging 152
cadherin-6 (cadherin-K) 31
cadherins, osteoblast 31
calcifediol, see 25-hydroxyvitamin D_3
calcification
  heterotopic 88, 91
  phosphate therapy-associated 100, 101
calcitonin 45, 52–3
  in calcium homeostasis 52, 91, 108–9
  effects on bone/bone cells 17, 52–3, 91, 92

pharmacologic use 53, 91–2
  adverse effects 92
  in corticosteroid-treated patients 219
  efficacy 92
  indications 91
  mechanism of action 91–2
  in myeloma 156–7
  in osteoporosis 92, 234, 242
  in Paget's disease 53, 92, 189
  preparations/mode of administration 91
  in primary hyperparathyroidism 176
receptors 52, 91
  as osteoclast marker 17
serum, in osteoporosis 217
calcitriol, see 1,25-dihydroxyvitamin D_3
calcium
  absorption
    age-related decline 214
    in chronic renal failure 203
    vitamin D actions 98
  dietary intake 95, 214–15, 231
  extracellular fluid
    error correction 110
    set-point 109–10, 166–7
  homeostasis 45, 108–12
    bone membrane fluxes 32, 112
    bone remodeling and 112
    calcitonin and 52, 91, 108–9
    1,25-dihydroxyvitamin D_3 and 55, 56, 108
    IL-1 actions 60–1, 116
    PTH and 48–9, 108, 110–11
    role of kidney vs. bone 111–12
  intracellular 49
  in mineralization 39, 40
  oral therapy 94–5
    adverse reactions 95
    in corticosteroid-treated patients 219
    efficacy 95
    in elderly 215
    indications 95
    mechanism of action 94–5
    mode of administration 95
    preparations 94, 95
  serum
    in osteomalacia/rickets 202
    in osteoporosis 226
    in Paget's disease 187
    in primary hyperparathyroidism 166–7, 173–4, 175–6
    see also hypercalcemia; hypocalcemia
  tumor metastasis and 136–7
  urinary excretion 48, 50, 108
    in hypercalcemia of malignancy 111–12, 128
    methods of promoting 119, 157

calcium (cont.)
    in osteomalacia/rickets 202
    in osteoporosis 226
calcium phosphate, amorphous 39
calvaria, rodent
    isolation of bone cells 14–15, 32, 33
    tumor metastasis 138
cancellous (trabecular) bone 34
    age-related changes 2–3
    in osteoporosis 212–13, 224
    in primary hyperparathyroidism 171
    remodeling 3
canine distemper virus 184–5
carbonic anhydrase type II 20, 196, 243
    inherited deficiency 21–2, 194, 195, 197
cardiac failure, in Paget's disease 186–7
cartilage
    bone formation on 37–9
    differentiation, role of PTH-rP 38, 51, 52
cathepsin K 21
    deficiency 198
Cbfa-1 transcription factor 37
celiac disease 203
cell adhesion molecules (CAMs)
    in myeloma bone disease 154
    in tumor metastasis 129–32, 133
centochroman 242
CFU-GM, see colony forming units for granulocyte–macrophages
"chalk bone disease" 193
chick osteoclasts, isolation methods 13–14
children, corticosteroid therapy 219
chloride, serum, in primary hyperparathyroidism 174
cholecalciferol (vitamin D_3) 54, 97
chondroblasts 41
chondrocytes
    differentiation 38, 51
    in endochondral bone formation 38
    transformation into osteoblasts 38–9
chondroitin sulfate 36
chromosome 11 deletions 165, 167
cisplatinum, in myeloma 157
cleidocranial dysplasia 37
clodronate 86, 87
    efficacy 90
    method of administration 88
    in myeloma 156, 158
coffee ingestion, osteoporosis and 215, 231–2
coherence therapy, osteoporosis 249
collagen
    deoxypyridinoline crosslinks 157, 187, 230
    in mineralization 39, 40, 41
    pyridinoline crosslinks 226, 230
    synthesis 34–5
        factors influencing 55, 57
    type I 31, 34–5
        carboxyterminal extension peptide 230
        chemo-attractant effects 7, 133
        genes 34
        heritable disorders 34–5, 222
        "hole zones" 34, 39
        osteoclast interactions 23
        post-translational modification 34, 40
    type X 38
collagenase
    bone collagen degradation 21, 23
    type IV, in tumor metastasis 133
colony forming units for granulocyte–macrophages (CFU-GM) 19, 60
    in Paget's disease 182, 184
colony-stimulating factor 1 (CSF-1, M-CSF)
    deficiency 22, 194
    in osteoclast differentiation 19, 65, 196
    receptor (c-fms) 65, 243
colony-stimulating factors (CSFs) 9, 19, 65
compact bone, see cortical bone
computed tomography (CT)
    in osteoporosis 229
    quantitative (QCT), parathyroid gland localization 176
cortactin 22, 70
cortical bone 34
    age-related changes 2–3
    in primary hyperparathyroidism 171
    remodeling 3
corticosteroids (glucocorticoids)
    and calcitonin therapy 53, 92, 93, 94
    in myeloma 156–7
    in primary hyperparathyroidism 176
    -induced osteoporosis 218–19, 221, 224, 228
    in myeloma 155, 156
    in osteopetrosis 198
    PTH-rP expression and 51
coupling phenomenon 5, 6–7
    osteoblastotropic factors mediating 8–9, 71
    in osteoporosis 217
cranial nerve compression, in osteopetrosis 197
craniosynostosis 69
Crohn's disease 203
Crouzon syndrome 69
CSF, see colony-stimulating factor

Cushing's syndrome 218–19, 221
cyclic AMP
    activation by PTH 49
    urinary excretion 48, 128
cyclins, PTH actions 48
cytotoxic drugs
    in myeloma 155, 157
    see also gallium nitrate; plicamycin

deafness
    in osteopetrosis 197
    in Paget's disease 186
decorin 36
deflazocort 219
deformity
    in osteopetrosis 197
    in osteoporosis 225
    in Paget's disease 186
    in rickets 202
deoxypyridinoline crosslinks of collagen 157, 187, 230
desferrioxamine 204
DEXA (dual energy X-ray absorptiometry) 227, 228–9
diabetes mellitus 221
diacylglycerol 49
diaphyseal dysplasia, progressive 198
diaphysis 38
diarrhea, phosphate therapy-associated 100–1
Dictostelium discoideum 87
diet, osteoporosis and 214–15, 231
dihydrotachysterol 54, 97, 203
1,25-dihydroxyvitamin D_3 (calcitriol) 45, 53–6
    actions on osteoclasts 17, 20, 55
    in calcium homeostasis 55, 56, 108
    in hypercalcemia of malignancy 118
    metabolism 54
    in myeloma 150
    PTH interactions 46, 48, 55, 56
    receptors, see vitamin D, receptors
    serum
        in hypophosphatemic rickets 205
        in osteoporosis 216
        in vitamin D-dependent osteomalacia 204–5
    therapy 56, 97–8, 203
        adverse effects 98
        in chronic renal failure 204
        in corticosteroid-treated patients 219
        efficacy 98
        indications 98
        and low-dose PTH 245
        mode of administration 97–8
        in oncogenic osteomalacia 206

1,25-dihydroxyvitamin D_3 (calcitriol) (*cont.*)
   in osteopetrosis 55, 198
   in vitamin D-dependent osteomalacia 205
24,25-dihydroxyvitamin D_3 56
drug development, new 249–50
dual energy X-ray absorptiometry (DEXA) 227, 228–9

E-cadherin 31
   in osteoclast formation 18–19
   in tumor metastasis 129, 130, 131–2
echistatin 14, 23
elderly
   bone cell senescence 214
   osteoporosis 209, 218
     prevention 233
   primary hyperparathyroidism 162
   vitamin D
     deficiency 202, 214–15
     metabolism 216
     therapy 98, 214, 215
endochondral bone formation 30, 37–9
endometrial cancer 85
endothelin-1 142
Engelmann's disease 198
environmental factors, osteoporosis 215
epidermal growth factor (EGF)
   prostaglandin production and 57
   PTH interaction 46
   PTH-rP expression and 51
epiphyseal (growth) plates 38
   in rickets 202–3
ergocalciferol (vitamin D_2) 54, *97*, 203
esophageal ulceration, bisphosphonate-induced 89–90
estrogen 83–6
   adverse reactions 85–6
   contraindications 241
   in corticosteroid-treated patients 219
   deficiency, bone loss and 211
   efficacy 85
   indications 83–4
   mechanism of action 50–1, 64, 84–5, 241
   mode of administration 85, 241
   in osteoporosis 83–4, 85, 233, 234, 241
   preparations 85
   in primary hyperparathyroidism 84, 176
   receptors 84, 242
   transdermal 85, 242
ethnic differences
   bone mass 2, 210
   osteoporosis 215, 231

etidronate 86, *87*
   adverse effects 88–9, 204
   efficacy *89*, *90*
   in myeloma 156
   in osteoporosis 242
   in Paget's disease 189–90
European Federation for Osteoporosis 233
exercise
   -induced amenorrhea 222–3
   in osteoporosis prevention 231, 233

falls 213, 230, 233
femoral head, cortical bone content 2
femoral neck
   cortical bone content 2
   fractures, *see* hip fractures
   geometry 213
FGFs, *see* fibroblast growth factors
fibroblast growth factor receptors (FGFR) 68, 70
   disease-causing mutations 69
   low affinity proteoglycan 70
fibroblast growth factors (FGFs) 68–70
   bone formation in vivo and 68–9
   in coupling process 9
   in inherited skeletal disorders 69
   limb development and 69
   osteoblastic bone metastases and 141
   signal transduction 70
   therapeutic potential 248–9
   in vitro effects on bone cells 68
fibronectin 36, 133
5T murine model of myeloma (Radl) 148, 152
flavanoids 243
fluoride 240
   intoxication 41, 198
   therapy 6, 95–7
     adverse reactions 97
     in corticosteroid-treated patients 219
     efficacy 96, 244–5
     indications 97, 245
     mechanism of action 96, 244
     mode of administration 96, 244
     in myeloma 158
     in osteoporosis 95–7, 234, 244–5
fluorosis, endemic 198
c-fms (M-CSF receptor) 65, 243
c-fos 70
   knockout mice 22–3, 194
   in osteoclast formation 22–3, 196
fractures
   fluoride-associated 97, 245
   in metastatic bone disease 127
   in osteopetrosis 197
   osteoporotic 224–5

   assessing efficacy of therapy 232
   estrogen therapy and 85
   in men 223–4
   pathophysiology 212–13
   prediction of risk 228, 229
   prevalence 209
   prevention 233
   risk factors 230
   in Paget's disease 186
furosemide, in myeloma 157

gallium nitrate 101–2
   in myeloma 102, 157
   in Paget's disease 102, 190
gastrointestinal disorders
   osteomalacia in 203
   in primary hyperparathyroidism 172–3
gender differences, *see* sex differences
genes, immediate-early 70
genetic factors
   osteoporosis 210–11, 215
   Paget's disease 180–1, 185–6
giant cell tumors 14, 64
glucocorticoids, *see* corticosteroids
gluten enteropathy 203
β-glycan 70
glycipan 70
glycosaminoglycans 36
gonadotropin releasing hormone antagonists 222
GP-130 protein 7, 63, 64
granulocyte colony-stimulating factor (G-CSF) 65
granulocyte–macrophage colony-stimulating factor (GM-CSF)
   in osteoclast differentiation 19, 65
   tumors producing 63, 117
granulocyte–macrophage committed progenitor cells (CFU-GM), *see* colony forming units for granulocyte–macrophages
granulomas, in Paget's disease 182
growth factors
   bone matrix-derived 37, 66–71
     osteolytic bone metastases and 136–8
   controlling bone cell function 45
   osteoblast 8, 9, 31
   parathyroid gland 166, 167
   therapeutic potential 246–9
   see also specific growth factors
growth hormone 71

Harrison's groove 202
hemochromatosis 224
heparan sulfate proteoglycans 36, 70
heparin therapy 220

hepatic disease
  osteomalacia 203
  osteoporosis 220
hepatitis C 198
Her-2/Neu oncogene 132
herbimycin A 243
heterotopic ossification and calcification 88, 91
hip fractures 224, 225
  estrogen therapy and 85
  in men 223
  pathophysiology 213
  prediction of risk 228, 229
  prevalence 209
  risk factors 230
HL-60 cells 15, 16, 55
HLA antigens, in Paget's disease 180
Hodgkin's disease 124
"hole zones", collagen 34, 39
hormones
  calcium-regulating 108–9
  controlling bone cell function 41–56
  controlling mineralization 41
  in osteoporosis 216–17
  see also calcitonin; 1,25-dihydroxyvitamin D_3; estrogen; parathyroid hormone; parathyroid hormone-related peptide
Howship's lacuna 13
HTLV type I 150
humoral hypercalcemia of malignancy (HHM)
  historical background 49–50
  pathophysiology 114–15, 127–8
"hungry bone" syndrome 177
hydrogen ions, in bone matrix degradation 20–1
hydroxyapatite 39, 41
1α-hydroxylase
  deficiency 204–5
  PTH-rP actions 50
hydroxyproline, serum, in Paget's disease 187
25-hydroxyvitamin D_3 (calcifediol) 97, 203
  serum 202, 216
hypercalcemia 107–19
  causes 107
  in chronic renal failure 204
  defenses against 109
  familial hypocalciuric (FHH) 165, 167
  humoral factors 113–18
  IL-1-induced 60–1, 116
  lactational 51–2
  in metastatic bone disease 127–8
  in myeloma, see myeloma, hypercalcemia
  in Paget's disease 187
  pathophysiology 109–18

  in primary hyperparathyroidism 162, 168, 173–4, 175
  treatment 118–19
hypercalcemia of malignancy 127–8
  causes 107
  humoral, see humoral hypercalcemia of malignancy
  IL-1 and 61, 115–16
  IL-6 and 64, 117–18
  pathophysiology 109, 111–12, 113–18, 127–8
  TNF/lymphotoxin and 62–3, 117
  treatment 118–19
    bisphosphonates 88, 89, 90, 119
    calcitonin 92, 93, 94
    gallium nitrate 101–2
    oral phosphate 100, 101
    plicamycin 98–9, 100
hyperostosis corticalis generalisata 197
hyperparathyroidism
  primary 1, 46, 162–77
    asymptomatic 168, 169, 175
    bisphosphonate therapy 88, 90–1, 176
    bone disease 6, 170–2
    bone mass measurement 228
    clinical presentation 168–73
    diagnosis 173–5
    estrogen therapy 84, 176
    etiology 165–8
    history 162
    indications for surgery 175
    management 175–6
    medical therapy 176
    oral phosphate therapy 100, 176
    pathology 163–5
    pathophysiology of hypercalcemia 109, 113–18
    in postmenopausal women 84
    surgical management 177
    vs. osteoporosis 225–6
  secondary 202
    in chronic renal failure 47–8, 166, 203
    in osteoporosis 214
  "tertiary" 166
hyperprolactinemia 222, 223, 224
hypertension, in primary hyperparathyroidism 173
hyperthyroidism (thyrotoxicosis) 6, 217, 223
Hyp mutant mice 205
hypocalcemia
  defenses against 109
  in rickets/osteomalacia 202
hypochondroplasia 69
hypogonadism 224
hypophosphatasia 41

hypophosphatemia
  oral phosphate therapy 100
  in primary hyperparathyroidism 174
hypophosphatemic osteomalacia/rickets 98, 201, 205

ia osteopetrotic rat 17–18, 194
ibandronate 88, 158
IGF, see insulin-like growth factor I
IL-1; IL-6, see interleukin-1; interleukin-6
immediate-early genes 70
immobilization osteoporosis 216, 220
Indian hedgehog 38, 50, 52
indomethacin 57, 118
inflammatory diseases, chronic 63
inositol 1,4,5-triphosphate 49
insulin deficiency 221
insulin-like growth factor I (IGF I) 8, 71
  in coupling process 9, 71
  PTH interactions 47, 71, 248
  therapeutic potential 248
insulin-like growth factor II (IGF II) 8, 71
  therapeutic potential 248
insulin-like growth factor binding proteins 71, 248
insulin-like growth factor receptor I 71
INT-2 oncogene 167
integrins 36
  $\alpha 4_\beta 1$ 154
  $\alpha v_\beta 3$ 23, 36, 130
  in osteoclast function 4, 23, 25
  in tumor metastasis 130
γ-interferon 64–5
  in osteopetrosis 198
interleukin-1 (IL-1) 59–61
  bone resorption and 4–6, 60–1
  1,25-dihydroxyvitamin D_3-induced release 55
  in hypercalcemia of malignancy 115–16
  hypercalcemic effects 60–1, 116
  in myeloma 61, 116, 151–2
  osteolytic bone metastases and 138
  in osteoporosis 61, 84, 218
  in postmenopausal bone loss 84
  prostaglandin-mediated effects 57, 61
  PTH interaction 46
interleukin-1 receptor antagonist (IL-1 RA) 61–2, 84
interleukin-2 (IL-2) 55
interleukin-4 (IL-4) 64
interleukin-6 (IL-6) 62, 63–4
  in hypercalcemia of malignancy 64, 117–18

interleukin-6 (IL-6) (cont.)
   in myeloma 64, 152, 153–4
   neutralizing antibodies 64, 118, 152
   in osteoporosis 64, 84
   in Paget's disease 64, 183
   PTH interaction 46
   PTH-rP interaction 64, 118
intramembranous bone formation 30, 37
ipriflavone 243
irradiation, neck 166

Jackson–Weiss syndrome 69
JAK/STAT pathway 63
Jansen's metaphyseal chondrodysplasia 51, 115
joint disease
   in Paget's disease 186
   in primary hyperparathyroidism 173
c-jun 70
juvenile osteoporosis 218

kidney
   calcium excretion, see calcium, urinary excretion
   in calcium homeostasis 108, 111–12
   see also entries beginning with renal
Klinefelter's syndrome 224

lactase deficiency 215
lactation
   osteoporosis and 215–16, 223
   role of PTH-rP 51–2, 115
lactational hypercalcemia 51–2
laminin
   receptors 132, 133
   synthetic antagonists 131, 133, 139
   in tumor metastasis 129, 130–1, 133
latency associated peptide 67, 247
latent TGFβ binding protein 141
   135–190 kDa 67
   1 (LTBP-1) 67
leanness, osteoporosis and 224, 231
leukotrienes 58–9
limb development 69
linkage analysis
   multiple endocrine neoplasia 2 (FMEN-2) 167–8
   Paget's disease 180–1
lipids, bone 40
5-lipoxygenase 58
liver disease, see hepatic disease
Looser's zones (pseudofractures) 202, 203, 206
loss of heterozygosity
   in multiple endocrine neoplasia 167
   in parathyroid adenoma 165
lung cancer
   frequency of bone metastases 123, 125
   hypercalcemia 113
lymphocytes, 1,25-dihydroxyvitamin D_3 actions 55
lymphoma
   bone lesions 124
   osteoclast activating factors 150
   pathophysiology of hypercalcemia 113, 114, 115–16, 118
lymphotoxin (tumor necrosis factor β) 62–3
   hypercalcemia of malignancy and 62–3, 117
   in myeloma 62, 151

macrophage colony-stimulating factor (M-CSF), see colony-stimulating factor 1
macrophages
   bone resorption 12
   peritoneal 15
   vs. osteoclasts 17
Madin–Darby canine kidney (MDCK) cells 131
MAD signal transduction molecules 67, 71
magnetic resonance imaging (MRI), parathyroid gland localization 176
malabsorption 221
MAP kinase pathway 63, 70
marble bone disease, see osteopetrosis
mastocytosis 220
Mat Ly/Lu variant of rat Dunning prostate cancer 141
matrix, bone, see bone matrix
matrix Gla protein 36
matrix metalloproteinase, breast carcinoma 133
matrix metalloproteinase-1 (collagenase) 21, 23
matrix vesicles 31, 41–2
MC3T3-E1 osteoblast-like cells 32
MCF-7 breast carcinoma cells 131–2
MDA-(MB-)231 breast carcinoma cells 131–2, 135–6, 138, 139
Meador's syndrome 218–19
mean wall thickness, decreased 214, 244
measles virus, in Paget's disease etiology 183–5
medroxyprogesterone 84
melanoma 125, 132
MEN, see multiple endocrine neoplasia
metalloproteinase, breast carcinoma 133

metaphyseal chondrodysplasia, Jansen's 51, 115
metastasis, tumor 128–33
   cell adhesion molecules 129–32
   cell motility and 132, 133
   multistep process 128–9
   protective mechanisms 133
   proteolytic enzymes 132, 133
metastatic bone disease 123–42
   classification 123, 124
   clinical effects 127–8
   favored sites 125–7
   frequency 123–4, 125
   method of studying 130–1
   osteoblastic, see osteoblastic bone metastases
   osteolytic (destructive), see osteolytic bone metastases
   pathophysiology 128–33
   treatment 138–9
MH-85 tumor 63, 117
mineralization 39–42
   bisphosphonate-induced defects 88–9
   cellular components involved 41
   fluoride-induced defects 96, 97
   hormonal control 41
   lag time 201
   potentially important factors 39–41
   proposed scheme 41–2
   role of osteoblasts 31
   in vitamin D deficiency 53
mi osteopetrotic mouse 194, 195
mithramycin, see plicamycin
mitochondria, in mineralization process 41
monocyte–macrophage colony-stimulating factor (M-CSF), see colony-stimulating factor 1
monocyte–macrophage lineage, osteoclast origin 17, 19–20
monocytes
   bone resorption 12
   prostaglandin release 56
monocytic cell lines, human 15
mouth ulceration, bisphosphonate-induced 89–90
Mov 13 mouse 35
mucosal ulceration, bisphosphonate-induced 89–90
multiple endocrine neoplasia
   type 1 (MEN-1, FMEN-1) 164, 165
      etiology 166
      gastrointestinal symptoms 173
      pathophysiology 167
   type 2 (MEN-2, FMEN-2) 164, 165, 167–8
muscle mass, osteoporosis and 216
myeloma 124, 147–58
   bone lesions 147–8
      animal models 148, 152–3
      pathogenetic factors 150–2

myeloma (cont.)
  pathophysiology 6, 148–52
  cells, bone/bone cell products affecting 153–4
  hypercalcemia 124, 127, 148
    pathogenesis 113, 154–5
    treatment 155–7
  IL-1 production 61, 116, 151–2
  IL-6 and 64, 152, 153–4
  lymphotoxin production 62, 151
  osteopenia 148, 217, 226
  osteosclerotic 124, 148, 149–50
  renal calcium excretion 128
  treatment 155–8
    bone lesions without hypercalcemia 158
    bone markers in 157
    gallium nitrate 102, 157
    indications 155
    inhibition of bone resorption 155–7
    practical guide 157

National Osteoporosis Foundation 228, 233
National Osteoporosis Society 233
nephrocalcinosis, in primary hyperparathyroidism 169
nerve compression/entrapment
  in metastatic bone disease 127
  in osteopetrosis 197
  in Paget's disease 186
neuromuscular symptoms, primary hyperparathyroidism 173
neuropsychiatric symptoms, primary hyperparathyroidism 173
NFκB-deficient mice 194
nitric oxide 23
NM23 oncogene 132
NPS-R-568 176

OB-cadherin 31
obesity, osteoporosis and 216
OIM mouse 35
op/op osteopetrotic mice 19, 22, 65, 194
organ culture systems, bone 15, 33–4
ossification, heterotopic 88, 91
osteitis fibrosa cystica 46, 162, 168, 170–2
  vs. osteoporosis 225–6
osteoblastic bone metastases 6, 123, 124, 139–42
  differential diagnosis 187–8, 197
  pathophysiology 140–2
osteoblasts 30–1
  in bone formation 4, 5, 7–8
  cessation of activity 8
  derivation from chondrocytes 38–9
  factors regulating 8–9, 45–71

functions 31
growth factors 8, 9, 31
lineage cells 30–2
matrix proteins synthesized by 31, 35
methods of studying 32–4
in myeloma 148
as osteoclast helper cells 12, 23, 31
in osteopetrosis 196
precursors 30
  chemotactic factors 7–8
  differentiation 8
  proliferation 8
senescence 214
surfaces, in osteomalacia 200
see also bone formation
osteocalcin, see bone Gla protein
osteoclast activating factors (OAFs) 17, 24, 25
  in myeloma 150–2
osteoclastpoietic factor (OPF) 65–6
osteoclasts 12–25
  activation 4, 5
  apoptosis, see apoptosis, osteoclast
  in bone resorption 4, 5, 20–3
  factors regulating 45–71
  identification criteria 16–17
  immortalization 16
  inhibiting agents 17, 25
  isolation methods 13–15
  "killer" 84, 213
  in long-term marrow cultures 15–16
  mature multinucleated 20
  methods for studying 13–16
  morphology 12–13
  motility 21
  in myeloma bone disease 148, 149, 150–2, 153–4
  nuclei 12–13
  origin/cell lineage 17–20
  osteoblasts as helper cells 12, 23, 31
  in osteopetrosis 193–6
  Pagetic 181, 182
    abnormal marrow environment 182–3, 184
    intranuclear inclusion bodies 185, 185
    virus infection 184–5
  precursors 17–18, 19–20
  regulation of activity 23–5
  ruffled border 13
  tumor cell-mediated stimulation 134–8
  see also bone resorption
osteocytes 30, 31–2
  functions 35
  isolation methods 32
osteocytic osteolysis 12, 32, 48
osteogenesis imperfecta 221–2

animal models 35
molecular basis 34–5
osteogenin (BMP-3) 70
osteoid tissue 39
  relative surfaces 200
  seam thickness 200
  volume 200
osteolysis
  familial expansile 181
  in myeloma, see myeloma, bone lesions
  osteocytic 12, 32, 48
  in primary hyperparathyroidism 170–1, 172
osteolytic bone metastases 123, 124
  cancellous bone 3
  hypercalcemia and 127–8
  pathophysiology 6, 133, 134–8
  role of PTH-rP 114, 115, 135–6
  treatment 138–9
    bisphosphonates 88, 90, 138–9
    gallium nitrate 102
  see also metastatic bone disease
osteomalacia 53, 200–6
  bisphosphonate-induced 89
  causes 201
  in chronic renal failure 203–4
  definition 200
  in gastrointestinal/hepatic disorders 203
  hypophosphatemic 201, 205
  nutritional 201–3
  oncogenic (tumor-induced) 205–6
  pathology 200–1
  vitamin D-dependent 201, 204–5
  vitamin D therapy 98, 203
  vs. osteoporosis 209, 225
  see also rickets
osteonectin 36
osteopenia 209
  definition 208
  differential diagnosis 225–6
  laboratory evaluation 226–30
  in malignant disease 226
  in myeloma 148, 217, 226
  in osteomalacia 202
  pathophysiology 210–12
  in primary hyperparathyroidism 170, 175
  see also osteoporosis
osteopetrosis 16, 193–8
  absence of hypercalcemia 116
  animal models 22–3, 193–5, 196
  clinical features 196–7
  differential diagnosis 197–8
  hemopoietic cell transplantation 17–18
  lessons in osteoclast biology from 21–2, 194, 196
  pathophysiology 193–6

osteopetrosis (cont.)
  treatment 55, 198
osteopontin 36
  osteoclast interactions 23, 25
osteoporosis 208–34
  animal models 35
  "circumscripta" 187
  classification 217
  clinical features 224–5
  definition 208
  differential diagnosis 225–6
  factors influencing 214–17
  fractures, see fractures, osteoporotic
  idiopathic 216, 218
  IL-1 and 61, 84, 218
  IL-6 and 64, 84
  juvenile 218
  laboratory evaluation 226–30
  in men 223–4, 234
  pathophysiology 6, 210–13
  postmenopausal 217–18
  prevalence/public health burden 209
  primary 217–18
  risk factors 230–2
  secondary 217, 218–23, 224, 232
  senile 216, 217–18
  terminology 209
  treatment 233–4
    activate–depress–free–repeat (ADFR) 249
    assessing efficacy 232
    bisphosphonates 88, 90, 234, 242
    bone formation stimulators 244–9
    bone resorption inhibitors 240–3
    calcitonin 92, 234, 242
    estrogen 83–4, 85, 233, 234, 241
    fluoride 95–7, 234, 244–5
    future prospects 240–50
    new drug development 249–50
    oral calcium 94, 95
    vitamin D 98
  type I (accelerated) 217, 218
  type II 216, 217, 218
osteoprotegerin (OPG) 63
osteosarcoma
  cell lines 32
  in Paget's disease 187
osteosclerosis
  in myeloma 124, 148, 149–50
  in primary hyperparathyroidism 171–2
  vs. osteopetrosis 197
ovarian cancer, cell adhesion molecules 130
22-oxa-1,25-dihydroxyvitamin D_3 (OCT) 56
oxygen-derived free radicals 23

p53 gene deletions 165
PA6 cells 32–3
Paget's disease of bone 1, 180–90
  bone marrow cell cultures 16, 184
  clinical features 186
  complications 186–7
  epidemiology 180–1
  etiology 183–6
  laboratory evaluation 187–8
  pathophysiology 6, 64, 181–3
  treatment 188–90
    bisphosphonates 88, 90, 189–90
    calcitonin 53, 92, 189
    gallium nitrate 102, 190
    plicamycin 99, 190
PA-III rat prostate adenocarcinoma model 140, 141
pain
  bone, see bone pain
  in osteoporosis 224, 232
pamidronate 86, 87
  adverse effects 89–90, 156
  efficacy 90
  in myeloma 155–6, 157, 158
  in osteolytic bone metastases 138–9
  in Paget's disease 190
pancreatitis
  acute 173
  chronic 203, 220
paramyxoviruses, in Paget's disease etiology 183–5
paraneoplastic syndromes 63, 64, 117
parathyroid gland
  adenoma 163–4
    etiology 165–6
    localization 176–7
    surgical management 175
  carcinoma 163, 164
    etiology 165
  growth factors 166, 167
  hyperplasia 163, 164
    etiology 165, 166, 167
  irradiation 166
  localization 176–7
parathyroid hormone (PTH) 45–52
  anabolic effect 9, 45, 47–8, 111
  bone formation and 47–8
  bone resorption and 45–7
  in calcium homeostasis 48–9, 108, 110–11
  1,25-dihydroxyvitamin D_3 interactions 46, 48, 55, 56
  estrogen interactions 84
  hypercalcemic responses 113–14, 115
  IGF-I mediated action 47, 71, 248
  low-dose therapy, in osteoporosis 245–6
  nonparathyroid tumors producing 115

  in osteoporosis 216
  in primary hyperparathyroidism 166
  PTH-rP homology 50
  pulsatile secretion 48, 110–11, 216
  receptors 47, 49, 50
    knockout mice 51, 115
  serum 174–5, 204
  signal transduction 49
parathyroid hormone-related peptide (PTH-rP) 46, 49–52
  anabolic effect 48
  1,25-dihydroxyvitamin D_3 analogs and 56
  discovery 49–50
  in HTLV-I infection 150
  in humoral hypercalcemia of malignancy (HHM) 114–15, 128
  hypercalcemic responses 113–15
  IL-6 interaction 64, 118
  knockout mice 38, 50, 51, 115
  in myeloma 152
  neutralizing antibodies 114, 135–6, 139
  osteoblastic bone metastases and 141, 142
  osteolytic response 114, 115, 135–6
  physiologic role 38, 50–2, 115
  post-translational processing 51
  receptor, see parathyroid hormone (PTH), receptors
  regulation of expression 50–1
  secretion pattern 111
  therapeutic use 245, 246
  transfected tumor cells 114–15
  transgenic mice 51, 52
parenteral nutrition, chronic 204
PC3 human prostatic carcinoma cells 140, 141
PDGF, see platelet-derived growth factor
peptic ulcer disease, in primary hyperparathyroidism 172–3
Pfeiffer syndrome 69
pharmaceutical industry, new drug development 249–50
phosphate
  dietary intake 231
  in mineralization 39
  oral therapy 100–1
    adverse effects 100–1
    in hypophosphatemic rickets 205
    mechanism of action 100
    mode of administration 100
    in oncogenic osteomalacia 206
    in primary hyperparathyroidism 100, 176

phosphate (*cont.*)
  serum
    in hypophosphatemic rickets 205
    in myeloma 155
    in osteomalacia/rickets 202
    in osteoporosis 226
    in Paget's disease 187
    see also hypophosphatemia
  urinary excretion, PTH-rP actions 50
phosphatidyl inositol 3 kinase (PI3 kinase) 22
phospholipase C-γ (PLC-γ) 70
phosphoproteins, bone matrix 40
"phosphotonin" 206
physical activity, osteoporosis and 231, 233
plasmacytoma, solitary 147–8
plasminogen activator, in tumor metastasis 141
platelet-derived growth factor (PDGF) 71
  effects on osteoblasts 7–8
  therapeutic potential 248
plicamycin (mithramycin) 98–100
  adverse effects 100
  efficacy 99
  indications 100
  mechanism of action 99
  mode of administration 99
  in myeloma 156
  in Paget's disease 99, 190
  in primary hyperparathyroidism 176
POEMS syndrome 149, 150
postmenopausal women
  bone loss 2, 211–12
    cancellous/cortical bone 3
    estrogen therapy 83, 84, 85
    pathogenesis 63, 84–5
  corticosteroid therapy 219
  dietary calcium intake 95
  osteoporosis 216, 217–18
    prevention 231, 233
  primary hyperparathyroidism 84
PRAD1 oncogene rearrangements 165–6
pregnancy, osteoporosis and 215–16, 223
premarin 84, 85
pre-osteoclasts
  early 19–20
  late 20
procollagen, type I 34
progestins 85, 176
prostaglandins (E series) 56–8
  hypercalcemia of malignancy and 118
  IL-1 action and 57, 61, 118
prostate cancer, bone metastases *124*, 126–7
  animal models 138, 140–1

frequency 123, *125*
  osteoblastic 140, 141–2
prostate specific antigen (PSA) 141–2
protein
  high dietary intake 215, 231
  malnutrition 215
protein kinase C 49
proteins, bone matrix 31, 34–7
protein tyrosine phosphatase (PTP) epsilon 87
proteoglycans 36, 40, 70
proteolipids, bone 40
proteolytic enzymes
  bone matrix degradation 20, 21
  inhibitors 243
  in tumor metastasis 132, 133
proton pump, osteoclast 21, 243
protons, in bone matrix degradation 20–1
pruritus, in primary hyperparathyroidism 173
pseudofractures (Looser's zones) 202, 203, 206
psychiatric symptoms, primary hyperparathyroidism 173
PTH, *see* parathyroid hormone
PTH-rP, *see* parathyroid hormone-related peptide
PU.1 hematopoietic transcription factor 194
pyknodysostosis 198
pyridinoline crosslinks, collagen 226, 230
pyrophosphate, inorganic 40, 41

quail-chick chimeras 17, 18
quality of life, in vertebral osteoporosis 225

racial differences, *see* ethnic differences
radiation therapy, neck 166
radius, cortical bone content 2
raloxifene 241–3
rat Leydig cell tumor 63, 117
renal cancer 123, *125*
renal failure
  bisphosphonate-induced 90
  chronic
    osteomalacia 202, 203–4
    secondary hyperparathyroidism 47–8, 166, 203
    vitamin D therapy 98
  in myeloma 154–5, 156, 157
  in primary hyperparathyroidism 169
renal stones (calculi)
  bisphosphonate therapy 88, 91
  in Paget's disease 187
  in primary hyperparathyroidism 162, 168, 169

renal tubular acidosis, in primary hyperparathyroidism 169–70
resorption pit 13
respiratory syncytial virus 184
retinoblastoma (rb) gene deletions 165
retinoic acid 246
  receptor (RXR) 56
RET proto-oncogene 168
RGD amino acid sequences
  in matrix proteins 4, 23, 36
  peptide antagonists 23, 243
rickets 38, 53, 200–6, 209
  hypophosphatemic 205
  nutritional 201–3
  oncogenic (tumor-induced) 205–6
  vitamin D-resistant 205
  vitamin D therapy 98, 203
  see also osteomalacia
risedronate *87*, 88
"rugger jersey" spine 47–8

saline-induced diuresis 119, 157
"salt and pepper" skull 171
sarcomas, in Paget's disease 187
selective estrogen response modifiers (SERMs) 241–2
sestamibi scanning, parathyroid gland localization 176–7
severe combined immunodeficiency (SCID) mice, model of myeloma 148, 152–3
sex differences
  age-related bone loss 211
  bone mass 2, 210
  osteoporosis 230–1
  in primary hyperparathyroidism *168*
Shc 70
skeleton, natural history 1–3
skull
  in Paget's disease 186, 187, *188*
  "salt and pepper" 171
smad genes 67
smoking, osteoporosis and 215, 224, 231
sodium fluoride (NaF) 96, 97, 244, 245
  slow-release 96, 244
sodium monofluorophosphate 96, 244
space flight 220, 233
spleen, osteoclast precursors 17–18
squamous cell carcinoma, PTH-rP secretion 50, 114
c-src
  inhibitors 243
  knockout mice 22, 194, *195*, *196*
  modulation by PTH 49
  in osteoclast action 22, 36, 196
  PDGF interaction 71
ST2 cells 32–3
stromal cell lines 32–3

strontium 249
subtilisins 51
Sudek's osteodystrophy 88, 91
sunlight, inadequate exposure 215
SV40 large T antigen 16, 33
syndecans 70

tamoxifen 242
technetium bone scans 88
teeth, in primary
    hyperparathyroidism 171
tetracycline labeling 200, 201, 227
TGF, see transforming growth factor
thiazide diuretics 157, 219, 220
thrombospondin 36
thyroid carcinoma
    bone metastases 123, 125
    familial medullary (FMTC) 167–8
thyroid hormone therapy 223
thyrotoxicosis (hyperthyroidism) 6, 217, 223
tiludronate 86, 87
tissue inhibitor of matrix
    metalloproteinase-2 (TIMP-2) 139
T-lymphocytes, 1,25-
    dihydroxyvitamin D_3 actions 55
TNF, see tumor necrosis factor
tobacco use, osteoporosis and 215, 224, 231
trabecular bone, see cancellous
    (trabecular) bone
TRAMP (transgenic
    adenocarcinoma mouse
    prostate) model 141
transforming growth factor α
    (TGFα)
    hypercalcemic effects 116
    prostaglandin production and 57
    PTH interaction 46
transforming growth factor β
    (TGFβ) 7, 31, 66–7
    in coupling phenomenon 9
    effects on osteoblasts 7, 8, 66
    effects on osteoclasts 66–7
    estrogen actions and 84, 85, 242
    latent binding proteins 67, 247
    latent complex 67
    osteoblastic bone metastases
        and 141
    in osteocytes 32
    osteolytic bone metastases
        and 136
    PTH interaction 46, 47

PTH-rP expression and 51
receptors 67
superfamily 8–9, 37, 70
    see also bone morphogenetic
        proteins
therapeutic potential 246–7
transgenic mice 67
tumor metastasis and 133
TRAP promoter 16
T score 228
tumor cells
    bone destruction 12, 134–8
    metastasis, see metastasis, tumor
    motility 132, 133
tumor necrosis factor (TNF) 46, 61–3
    hypercalcemia of malignancy
        and 62–3, 117
    in postmenopausal bone loss 63
    see also lymphotoxin
tumors
    colony-stimulating factors
        (CSFs) 65, 117
    IL-1 production 61, 115–16
    osteoclastpoietic factor
        (OPF) 65–6
    osteomalacia/rickets induced
        by 205–6
    PTH-rP secretion 50, 114–15
    TGFα production 116
    see also breast cancer; metastatic
        bone disease; myeloma;
        prostate cancer
tumor suppressor genes 165, 167
Turner's syndrome 220
tyrosine kinase receptors 243

ultrasound
    in osteoporosis 229
    parathyroid gland
        localization 176
urokinase (uPA), in bone
    metastases 141
uvomorulin, see E-cadherin

Van Buchem's disease 197
VCAM-1 154
venous sampling, parathyroid gland
    localization 177
vertebrae
    cancellous bone content 2
    metastatic disease 127
    "rugger jersey" appearance 47–8
vertebral fractures 224–5

calcitonin therapy and 92
diagnostic criteria 209
in men 224
pathophysiology 212, 213
prediction of risk 228
prevalence 209
vertebral plexus, Batson's 126–7
viral hypothesis, Paget's
    disease 183–5
vitamin D
    in bone mineralization 41
    deficiency 41, 53, 98, 201–3
        osteoporosis and 214–15
    -dependent osteomalacia 201, 204–5
    excess 53
    metabolism 54
        in elderly 216
        in liver disease 220
    receptors 55, 56
        mutations 205
        polymorphisms 210–11, 215
    therapy 97–8
        in corticosteroid-treated
            patients 219
        in elderly 98, 214, 215
        in "hungry bone"
            syndrome 177
        in hypophosphatemic
            rickets 205
        in osteopetrosis 55, 198
        preparations 97, 203
        in vitamin D deficiency 98, 203
    see also 1,25-dihydroxyvitamin D_3
vitamin D_2 (ergocalciferol) 54, 97, 203
vitamin D_3 (cholecalciferol) 54, 97
vitamin K 35
vitronectin receptor
    antibodies (23C6) 14, 17
    in tumor metastasis 130

World Health Organization (WHO),
    definition of osteoporosis 208, 228
wrist fractures 213, 224

X-rays
    in Paget's disease 187–8
    in rickets 202–3

Zeolite A 249
zolendronate 87
Zollinger–Ellinson syndrome 173
Z score 228